This volume, and its companion volume on the oocyte, provide an authoritative and wide-ranging account of the gametes and their reproductive role and function in humans. Acknowledged authorities from around the world provide a detailed and timely account of the spermatozoon. The volume starts with an evolutionary perspective before focusing on the molecular and cellular biology of the sperm cell and its structure and function. The development and maturation of sperm are described as is their movement and transport in the male and female genital tract. Practical issues such as sperm storage and assisted conception are fully covered. The causes of male infertility are also an important theme. The volume concludes with a thought-provoking chapter on ethical considerations.

The volume will be an essential source of information for all clinicians and scientists with an interest in human reproduction.

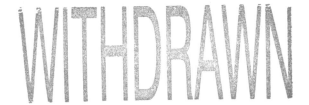

Gametes – the spermatozoon

Cambridge Reviews in Human Reproduction

SERIES EDITORS

*Professor J. G. Grudzinskas, Dr J. L. Yovich, Professor J. L. Simpson,
Professor T. Chard*

This major new series on human reproduction provides a comprehensive and integrated review of the reproductive process. The first six volumes concentrate on the essential reproductive events leading up to birth. The series provides a synthesis of the scientific, clinical and physiological elements of the reproductive process. Each volume focuses on a well-defined aspect of reproduction and provides a multidisciplinary though self-contained review.

Each volume has been prepared by an international and authoritative team of writers involving many of the world's leading experts. The series is edited to the highest standard to insure an integrated and uniformly high level of presentation. An important feature of the series is the inclusion of high-quality line illustrations.

The series provides an essential source of information for all trainees in obstetrics, gynacecology, andrology and reproductive medicine and will also be of interest to reproductive biologists and geneticists, physiologists and endocrinologists.

Titles in the series:

THE UTERUS

GAMETES – THE OOCYTE

GAMETES – THE SPERMATOZOON

Contents

Contributors

J. AITKEN

MRC Unit of Reproductive Biology, 37 Chalmers Street, Edinburgh EH3 9EW, UK

C. R. AUSTIN

47 Dixon Road, Buderim, Queensland 4556, Australia

C. L. R. BARRATT

Department of Obstetrics and Gynaecology, Jessop Hospital for Women, Leavygreave Road, Sheffield S3 7RE, UK

L. J. BURKMAN

Division of Reproductive Endocrinology, Department of Gynecology and Obstetrics, State University of New York, 140 Hodge Avenue, Buffalo, New York 14222, USA

R. A. CARDULLO

Department of Biology, The University of California, Riverside, CA 92521, USA

J. M. CUMMINS

School of Veterinary Studies, Murdoch University, Murdoch WA 6150, Australia

M. R. CURRY

Department of Veterinary Basic Sciences, Royal Veterinary College, Royal College Street, London NW1 0TU, UK

R. JANSEN

187 Macquarie Street, Sydney 2000, Australia

A. M. JEQUIER

Perth Andrology, Suite 18, The Perth Surgicentre, 38 Ranelagh Crescent, South Perth, Western Australia 6151, Australia

R. H. MARTIN

Division of Medical Genetics, Department of Paediatrics, Faculty of Medicine, University of Calgary, Alberta, Canada TXT 5C7

P. L. MATSON

Regional IVF Unit, St Mary's Hospital, Whitworth Park, Manchester M13 0JH, UK

H. D. M. MOORE

Department of Obstetrics and Gynaecology, Jessop Hospital for Women, Leavygreave Road, Sheffield S3 7RE, UK

D. MORTIMER
SIVF, Sydney IVF Pty Ltd, 4 O'Connell Street, Sydney 2000, Australia

C. D. THALER
Department of Biology, University of California, Riverside, CA 92521, USA

P. F. WATSON
Department of Veterinary Basic Sciences, Royal Veterinary College, Royal College Street, London NW1 0TU, UK

D P. WOLF
Division of Reproductive Biology and Behavior, Oregon Regional Primate Research Center, 505 NW 185th Avenue, Beaverton, Oregon 97006, USA

J. L. YOVICH
PIVET Medical Centre, 166–168 Cambridge Street, Leederville, Perth WA 6007, Australia

Editors' preface

The aim of this book is to provide a complete and up-to-date account of the physiology, endocrinology and biochemistry of spermatozoa, with particular emphasis on the human and on the relationship of clinical abnormalities to sperm function. The book begins with a detailed account of the evolution of the spermatozoon, an extraordinary perspective of events leading to our present state of knowledge of human spermatozoa by Colin Austin. The molecular and cellular aspects of the mammalian sperm surface are detailed by Thaler and Cardullo, whilst Watson and Curry deal with sperm structure and function and Jim Cummins with tests of sperm function. The genetic aspects of sperm function are considered by Renée Martin. The mobility of spermatozoa (Lani Burkman) and then transportation from the male (Harry Moore) and female genital tract (David Mortimer) are extensively described.

Clinical disorders affecting semen quality are addressed by Anne Jequier, followed by authoritative reviews on sperm storage (David Wolf) and cell biology of sperm (John Aitken). Phillip Matson addresses the formation and significance of sperm antibodies, and Chris Barratt gives a comprehensive account of spermatogenesis. A current review of sperm preparation procedures for various assisted conception techniques is provided by John Yovich. Finally, Rob Jansen reflects on the bioethical issues and challenges resulting from progress in research on human spermatozoa and its current clinical implications.

J. G. Grudzinskas
and J. L. Yovich
March 1995

1

Evolution of human gametes – spermatozoa

C. R. AUSTIN

Introduction

The proper background to a discussion on the evolution of human gametes would seem naturally to be a survey of facts relating to the evolution of living forms and, more particularly, that of the human species; such a survey is set out at the beginning of the companion paper to the present one, which appears in the publication *Gametes: The Oocyte*. The evidence reviewed there supports the theory that living cells first appeared on Earth between 3900 and 3400 Myr (million years ago), metazoan species developed during the Cambrian period (1600–600 Myr), mammal-like reptiles appeared between 300 and 400 Myr, 'modern' animals emerged around 100 Myr, the Primate stock first became discernible as a separate entity about 65 Myr, and more distinct human ancestors materialized during the Miocene period between 26 Myr and 7 Myr, with relics that could be classed as those of Hominidae between 15 and 5 Myr. Then the first evidence of the erect posture and bipedal progression appeared at about 4 Myr and finally the forerunner of modern man *Homo erectus* between 3 Myr and 1.5 Myr.

When it comes to thoughts on the evolution of gametes, specifically spermatozoa, nothing has as yet been found in the fossil record to help us. Fossil relics of single cells have indeed been identified, as implied above, but as yet no gametes, so inferences relating to their evolution have to be based on the close study of their current morphology in relation to the taxonomic order of the species.

Morphology of sperms

Size and form

Variations in the structure of animal spermatozoa far exceed those of eggs in their range and prominence (see for instance Bishop & Walton, 1960; Dunbar

& O'Rand, 1991, for mammalian sperms and Baccetti & Afzelius, 1976, for non-mammalian). These sources provide data on selected features of a wide variety of sperms, and there seems to be a broad correlation between sperm characters and taxonomic order.

In Table 1, a variety of sperm characteristics is set out against groups of organisms, which are listed in the systematic order given, for instance, by Holmes (1979), but the arrangement of sperm characteristics is somewhat arbitrary. Nevertheless, some seemingly valid trends or relationships do emerge. 'Pauciciliated' sperms, namely those depending on very few (one, two or sometimes three) cilia for locomotion, are found particularly in the algae and sporozoa (Fig. 1), though they do occur (less regularly) in quite a wide array of other organisms, including advanced invertebrates such as the Crustacea and Annelida, and fish among the vertebrates (Table 1). In the algae and sporozoa, such sperms closely resemble ciliated spores (zoospores), involved with asexual reproduction. A much more clear-cut association exists between 'multiciliated' sperms (spermatozoids) and mosses and liverworths (Bryophyta), ferns, horsetails and clubmosses (Pteridophyta), and cycads (Cycadales) (Fig. 1). (The term 'cilium' as used in this paper identifies the slim filament based on the familiar $9+2$ microtubule pattern, while 'flagellum' is used to describe the more robust structure containing a ring of coarse fibres around the microtubule array.)

'Amoeboid' and 'spiral' sperms also have a wide distribution, the former possessed by members of the algae, Mesozoa, Nematoda and Crustacea, and the latter by Protozoa along with three vertebrate groups, Reptilia, Aves and Prototheria.

'Threadlike', 'fusiform', 'barrel-shaped', 'spherical', and 'disc-shaped' sperms seem to have had rather limited exploitation. Similarly, the morphology that includes an 'undulating membrane' has evidently not proved particularly advantageous, for it seems to be displayed only by turbellarian flatworms (Hendelberg, 1969) and Amphibia, particularly the Urodela (Picheral, 1979).

The 'stellate' variety, another rarity, is espoused by the Crustacea. The sperm is relatively immotile, showing only a convulsive expansion of rays in association with the acrosome reaction, and both the sperm and its reaction have been well described by Barros, Dupre & Viveros (1986).

Development of the acrosome evidently occurred at an early stage and has clearly proven advantageous, being a feature of a wide range of sperms. Variations on the acrosome theme are depicted in Fig. 2.

'Conjugated' sperms represent a variant of a different kind, which exists in varying degrees of complexity and has been amply treated by Afzelius & Dallai (1987). In the oligochaete *Tubifex tubifex*, the male worms release sperm bundles called 'spermatozeugmata', which have a core of normal sperms enclosed

Table 1. *Some features of plant and animal sperms*

	Pauciciliated	Multiciliated	Amoeboid	Spiral	Threadlike	Fusiform	Barrel-shaped	Sphere or disc	Stellate	Conjugated	Undulating membrane	Acrosome present	Extensible perforatorium	Tail with coarse fibres	Indurated nucleus
Protophyta	+														
Algae	+		+												
Ferns		+													
Cycads		+													
Protozoa	+			+											
Porifera	+											+			
Mesozoa			+												
Ctenophora	+											+			
Trematoda					+										
Nematoda			+												
Mollusca	+										+	+	+	+	
Annelida	+							+				+	+	+	
Platyhelminthes						+					+				
Arachnida								+						+	
Crustacea	+		+			+	+	+				+	+		
Ostracoda					+										
Insecta						+	+	+		+		+			
Echinodermata	+											+	+		
Enteropneusta	+											+	+		
Agnatha												+	+	+	
Teleostei	+													+	
Amphibia											+	+		+	
Reptilia				+								+		+	
Aves				+								+		+	
Prototheria				+								+			
Metatheria								+				+		+ +	
Eutheria												+		+ +	+

Lack of space precluded inclusion of 'biflagellate' sperms (mentioned in Chart 1), which are widely distributed, being found in Nematoda, Platyhelminthes, Insecta, Pisces and Amphibia.

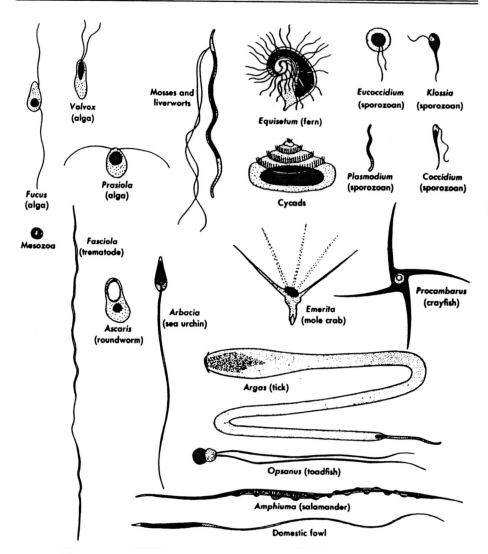

Fig. 1. Sperm forms among non-mammalian species. (From Austin, 1965.)

by several hundred modified sperms with degenerate nuclei; these are joined together to form a continuous outer 'wrapping', which breaks down later to release the normal sperms. Other 'conjugated' systems are simpler: in several families of primitive insects and in American marsupials, the sperms have modified heads, which enable them to be temporarily joined together in pairs, an arrangement that seems greatly to improve their swimming capabilities.

The occurrence of strikingly similar features in spermatozoa of widely divergent animal groups, as particularly with the pauciciliated, amoeboid, spiral and conjugated forms, and those with undulating membranes, underscores the

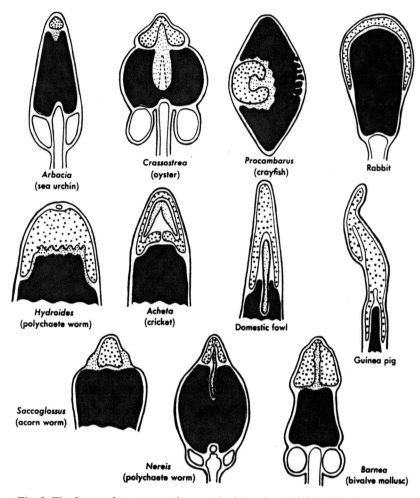

Fig. 2. The forms of acrosomes (heavy stipple) and nuclei (black) in the sperms of
different species. (From Austin, 1965.)

'volatility' of sperm morphology, and the apparent facility with which such
specialized characters can evolve.

Finally, sperms with a compact head, an acrosome associated with the nucleus,
a well-developed mitochondrial sheath and coarse fibres in the tail, are widely
distributed and distinguish the vertebrates listed in Table 1. Amongst these, a
group of more aquatic species have apparently found the extensible perforatorium
biologically advantageous. As a finishing touch, the 'indurated nucleus' evidently
appeared late in evolution, occurring fully developed only in the Eutheria.

Jamieson (1987a) has described several sperm varieties additional to those
mentioned in Table 1. First, there are, in individual annelid species, the
ect-aquasperm which is released into the aqueous environment and fertilizes the

egg there, the *ent-aquasperm* which is also released into the aqueous environment but then passes into the body of the female where fertilization occurs, and the *introsperm* which is passed directly into the female body for fertilization. In addition, certain species within the Oligochaeta, Rotifera, Pogonophora, Hymenoptera and some other groups, have *dimorphic sperms* in the one individual, sometimes described as microsperm and macrosperm, but lacking as yet clearly defined functions. Then there are 'typical' and 'atypical' sperms, and 'eupyrene' and 'apyrene' sperms, the second member of each pair having no nucleus but evidently providing something enabling the first-named to achieve fertilization. Again, there are 'parasperms' of various sizes and shapes, all lacking nuclei, some of which resemble simple cells and others have flagella, including one that has the appearance of a giant sperm; these cells exercise 'nursing' and 'transport' functions for the normal sperms.

Also adopting the electron-microscopic approach, Asa & Phillips (1987) have examined the sperms of birds, finding that these could be grouped under three headings: (a) the sperms of non-passerine birds which have a straight or somewhat curved cylindrical nucleus with perforatorium, a short acrosome, two centrioles in the neck region, and a midpiece which ranges from very short in the crane and the trogon, to long in the dove and pigeon; (b) the sperms of oscine birds, such as the crested tinamou, the white-eyed vireo, house sparrow and red-winged blackbird, which have a helical nucleus without perforatorium, a very long acrosome, only one centriole in the neck region, a midpiece and tail that cannot be separately discerned owing to lack of an annulus, and well-developed coarse fibres; (c) the sperms of sub-oscine birds, such as the great-crested fly-catcher, have some features common to both the preceding groups: for instance, as in non-passerines, the acrosome is shorter than the nucleus and the neck region has two centrioles; as in oscines, the nucleus takes the shape of a helical cylinder and some sections show lateral projections.

Harding, Aplin & Shorey (1987) found ultra-structural studies helpful in reaching conclusions on the phylogeny of Australian marsupials, though in some instances there was distinct conflict with existing ideas on phylogeny. This was especially notable for two genera, *Phascolarctos* and *Tarsipes*, the former genus having a sperm morphology unlike other marsupials and the latter having one that groups it firmly with the dasyurids, from which it clearly differs in general physical characters. The authors conclude that the results of such studies 'should not be adopted uncritically'.

It might have been expected that sperms in the three mammalian groups, Prototheria, Metatheria and Eutheria, would have shown a much greater uniformity than actually exists, as well as characteristics consistent with a possible sequential evolutionary history, but this is far from being the case, and the inference is that deviation of the three lines must have occurred further back than had been thought. The monotreme sperm in fact is much more like those of birds and reptiles than of placental mammals, being vermiform in overall shape, with head, midpiece and tail distinguishable only with difficulty (Fig. 3). The marsupial sperm, too, is 'out of line' from the evolutionary point of view. The head is not a particularly rigid structure and lyses readily when placed on a microscope slide (Figs. 5–9 in Austin, 1976). It lacks the 'stabilized' state of the perforatorium, inner acrosome membrane and nucleus that distinguishes the eutherian sperm head. The zona pellucida of the marsupial egg is much thinner than that of placental mammals, and so offers less of a barrier to sperm penetration; in addition, it is readily soluble in dilute trypsin solution (Bedford, 1990). Despite that, the marsupial acrosome is much more richly endowed with enzymes than the eutherian sperm (Rodger & Young, 1981). The mounting of the sperm head on the tail is quite different from that in placental mammals, not being at the distal end of the head but about half-way along, and having the form of a flexible ball-and-socket joint instead of firm attachment. The acrosome does not form a cap over the anterior part of the nucleus as in eutherians, but takes the form of an oval body adjoined to the side of the nucleus, opposed to the tail attachment.

So much for non-eutherian sperms. Among the placental mammals, sperms also vary greatly in size and form, the larger sperms commonly belonging to the smaller species, and *vice versa* (Bishop & Walton, 1960; Austin, 1976; Setchell, 1982; Cummins, 1983; Dunbar & O'Rand, 1991) (Fig. 3); the human sperm is in the smaller size range. Sperms not only differ between species, but significant differences in both size and functional efficiency have been observed between sub-species or families (Bishop & Walton, 1960; Beatty, 1975). In different strains of mouse, major variations in sperm head shape have been noted by Braden (1959), in the sizes and shapes of the acrosomes by Beatty (1971) and in the frequency of sperm head abnormalities attributable to a Y-linked factor (Krzanowska, 1972). Woolley & Beatty (1967) and Woolley (1970) showed that the midpiece length of mouse sperms could be genetically selected for. Differences also exist in mouse sperm antigenic properties (Snell, 1944). In addition, Friend (1936) has described differences in sperm head length between individual male mice, and indeed he maintained that each species of the Muridae could be identified from sperm head shape alone, and Cohen (1975) described differences in sperm function within individual ejaculates. From these observations it is inferred that many details in the form and function of spermatozoa are determined by their *own* genome, and possibly this is a component of the mechanism whereby speciation is controlled. Among human sperms, those carrying a Y-chromosome (the male-determining spermatozoa) are distinguished by having a fluorescent 'F

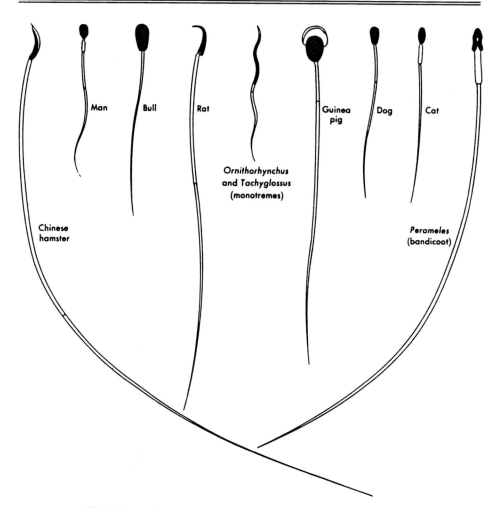

Fig. 3. Sperm forms in mammalian species. (From Austin, 1965.)

body', which is lacking in those with an X-chromosome (Barlow & Vosa, 1970). Differences attributable to the blood-group antigens exist in the sperms of different men (Landsteiner & Levine, 1926). Recently, Cummins (1990) has assembled data supporting the major conclusions that 'most of the sperm phenotype is controlled by the diploid genotype of the male' and that there are 'possible interactions between sperm form and higher order [group selection] phenomena'.

Sperm cladistics

Much time and effort have been expended in the effort to see patterns amongst the multitudinous forms exhibited by sperms, particularly one reflecting evolutionary relationships. A useful contribution to this end has been offered by

CHART 1

A classification of sperms according to systematic order

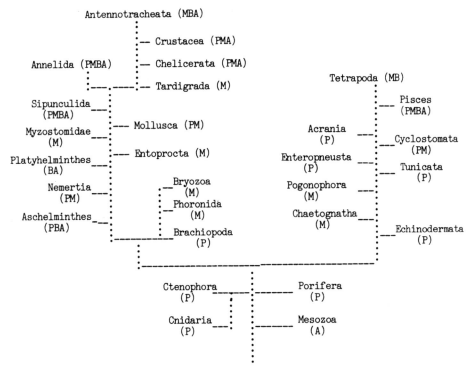

P = primitive; M = modified; B = biflagellate; A = aflagellate

Chart 1. A classification of sperms according to systematic order. P = primitive; M = modified; B = biflagellate; A = aflagellate. (Chart based on Fig. 1 in Baccetti & Afzelius, 1976.)

Baccetti & Afzelius (1976) (Chart 1). In this, just four types of sperms are recognized: (a) primitive (P), (b) modified (M), (c) biflagellate (B) and (d) aflagellate (A), and these are generally clearly identifiable.

'*Primitive*' sperms, such as those of sea urchins and certain other aquatic species, have a rounded head with acrosome, a small number of mitochondria (commonly four) arranged as midpiece just posterior to the head, and a tail consisting of a simple flagellum with a core of microtubules but lacking coarse fibres. Such sperms are generally discharged into the surrounding fluid medium where fertilization occurs. Sperms in the '*modified*' group take part, like mammalian sperms, in internal fertilization; they have a compact head with acrosome, a lengthy midpiece containing numerous mitochondria and a moderately robust tail with a ring of coarse fibres surrounding the microtubule core. In several species, including some insects, molluscs and snakes, the structure of the midpiece and tail is broadly similar to the mammalian, and this may well be related to their need for motility in viscous media. Other species, like the tunicates, exhibiting 'internal' fertilization but where the medium is essentially sea water, have sperms lacking coarse fibres. '*Biflagellate*' sperms resemble the 'primitive' in form except that they have two tails; they are known in the Antennotracheata, Annelida, Platyhelminthes, Aschelminthes, Tetrapoda and Pisces. '*Aflagellate*' sperms as a group show the widest range of morphologies, examples being those of members of the Annelida, Antennotracheata, Crustacea, Chelicerata, Platyhelminthes, Aschelminthes and Pisces.

The scheme put forward by Baccetti & Afzelius (1976) goes a long way to meeting the need. There is by no means a consistent correlation with systematics, but the authors stress that further explanation is necessary. The naming of 'primitive' sperms was introduced by Retzius, famous for his publication, in the first quarter of the century, of the earliest systematic descriptions of spermatozoa from a wide range of organisms. It seemed to be an appropriate name, for these sperms are produced by many relatively simple organisms that release their sperms into the surrounding aqueous medium (usually the sea). (These are not, in fact, the most primitive organisms, for protozoa are allocated a lower level, and as indicated in Fig. 1, their sperms take various unusual forms; then there are the sperms of red algae and the mesozoans, which resemble somatic cells.) However, Baccetti & Afzelius argue that a point of prime importance for evolutionary theory, 'implicit' in their classification, is that organisms producing sperms of the modified variety *cannot be parental* to those with the primitive form, *nor* can those with the biflagellate or aflagellate forms be parental to those with the modified variety of sperm.

Hence the value for cladistics of making detailed studies on sperm morphology by light microscopy. But this is a relatively crude procedure, and so Jamieson (1983, 1987a,b, 1991) has set about gathering evidence by meticulous study of sperm *ultrastructure*. As he points out, the patterns of fine detail thus discernible in sperms are far more abundant than those seen by light microscopy; for instance, in his analysis of the ultrastructure of hexapod spermatozoa (Jamieson, 1987b, Table 20.1), he lists 57 distinctive characters (apomorphies), which enable the construction of a 'family tree' showing likely relationships among the 30 component Orders. The morphological details observable by EM seem to be highly conserved features, which makes them particularly well suited for tracing relationships. Thus, though the Onycophora had been thought related to both the Annelida and Arthropoda (there are embryological similarities with Annelida), they had been placed in the phylum Uniramia, together with the insects. Sperm ultrastructure, however, plainly shows that they have links with Annelida. Again, ultrastructural details have proven invaluable for a more systematic classification of centipedes, as well as certain groups of fish and other lower vertebrates.

Future extensions of cladistic studies along the lines followed so productively by Jamieson could eventually permit recognition of detailed relationships, not only across Genera and Orders, but also across Phyla and Subkingdoms, and in this way the ambition of achieving a logical reconstruction of the possible 'evolutionary' series among the sperms of species all the way from man to protozoa might eventually be realized – a huge undertaking, perhaps even more forbidding than the Human Genome Project in genetics.

Features of the nucleus

The nucleus generally constitutes the major part of the sperm head, and in man and many other mammals, non-primates as well as primates, it takes the form of a somewhat flattened ovoid disc, rather more or rather less elongated in about equal proportions of a sperm population. As noted earlier, the eutherian sperm nucleus is a very rigid structure ('indurated nucleus' in Table 1), apparently attributable to an extremely condensed and tightly packed network of chromatin fibres, with a high degree of disulphide bonding between chromatin molecules (Bedford, 1974; 1991). This strongly contrasts with the nucleus in non-eutherian sperms, where a high degree of plasticity commonly exists. In consequence, the eutherian sperm is able to penetrate the zona pellucida with a steady slicing action. Cells in general characteristically have a bilaminar nuclear envelope, and this is the case also for the sperm, but here the membranes in most species lack pores and cysternae, which exist in other nuclei. However, some pores may be seen in the posterior part of the sperm nucleus in some mammals, amphibians and coleopterans; in several other species, there may even be no distinct nuclear envelope, its place being taken by a fusion product with the cell membrane or by membranes arising from the Golgi apparatus (Baccetti & Afzelius, 1976). Human sperms are exceptional in showing numerous nuclear vacuoles after appropriate treatment, with distinct variations between sperms (Bedford, Bent & Calvin, 1973). Some mammalian species, as among the rodents, have very distinctive hook-shaped sperm heads, the greater part of the shape being attributable to the acrosome rather than the nucleus. In many non-mammals, the highly plastic sperm nucleus undergoes considerable distortion during penetration of the egg investments. In marsupials such as *Perameles*, *Dasyurops*, *Trichosurus* and others, the heads have unique pivoted attachments to the tails.

Acrosome and perforatorium

Accompanying the nucleus in the majority of metazoan species is the sac-like acrosome (the name introduced by Lenhossek, 1898) (Fig. 2). According to Baccetti & Afzelius (1976) and Baccetti (1979), the acrosome is lacking from plant spermatozoids, and from the male germ cells of algae, Protozoa, Mesozoa, Cnidaria and most Porifera. However, in one poriferan, *Oscarella*, a well-formed acrosome was recently discovered (Baccetti, 1987), which makes this the most primitive group to have sperms with acrosomes. In Cnidaria there are Golgi-derived vesicles which could be the antecedents of an acrosome, and consistently these vesicles are lost after penetration into the egg (O'Rand & Miller, 1974). While several species lack an acrosome altogether, in others the acrosome and perforatorium begin to differentiate, but disappear later in spermatogenesis (Baccetti, 1979). Commonly, if the sperm lacks an acrosome, the egg has a micropyle, permitting sperm entry. In man the acrosome is a relatively small crescentic structure moulded over the anterior quarter of the sperm head, but in certain other mammals, notably the rodents, the acrosome has a large and varied form, sometimes larger than the nucleus and reaching perhaps its greatest relative dimensions in the shrew *Suncus murinus* (Cooper & Bedford, 1976).

The contents of the acrosome are largely enzymic in nature, with lytic and hydrolytic actions (consistent with the acrosome being a modified lysosome), which enable sperm passage through egg membranes. The best known of the enzymes is hyaluronidase, which has been demonstrated in the acrosomes of both mammals and birds, and which dissolves the matrix of the cumulus mass surrounding the mammalian egg; there is also the enzyme acrosin which disperses the acrosomal contents, and a membrane-bound protease with its action on the zona pellucida. The quantity of hyaluronidase present varies greatly, the guinea pig sperm having about 50 times the activity of the rat sperm. Of interest, too, is the fact that, while the possum acrosome contains about the same activity of hyaluronidase and acrosin as the rabbit acrosome, it has some 40 times the activity of arylsulphatase and 350 times the activity of N-acetylhexoseaminidase (Rodger & Young, 1981). Yet the marsupial zona is a thin insubstantial structure! Other enzymic agents have also been detected in the eutherian acrosome, including catalase, carbonic anhydrase, lactic dehydrogenase, acid phosphatase, and phospholipase A; specific functions have yet to be convincingly allocated to these.

Recently, the reactivity of the marsupial acrosome has been examined in *Trichosurus vulpecula* and *Macropus eugenii*, in which animals the acrosome is disposed at the tip of the elongated nucleus (Mate & Rodger, 1991). The sperms were subjected to treatments with agents that have been shown to lead to the acrosome reaction in eutherian sperms, namely: calcium ionophore A23187, cyclic nucleotides, phosphoinositide pathway intermediates, lysophospholipids, trypsin, and high ionic-strength media, followed by incubation in bovine serum albumin solution for up to 24 h. A typical eutherian acrosome reaction was not induced, but distinct changes did appear, including many membrane-bound vesicles, which resembled those seen in the acrosomes of *Didelphis virginiana* in sperms traversing the female tract (Rodger & Bedford, 1982).

Breakdown of the acrosome with release of its contents occurs in the acrosome reaction. The event commonly involves fusion between the sperm plasma membrane and the acrosomal membrane, with release of acrosomal contents. In mammals, there is multiple fusion between the two membranes in a process of vesiculation, with consequent escape of acrosomal contents (Barros *et al.*, 1967), and the subacrosomal material plays no obvious role. In many other species, especially among numerous marine invertebrates, such as the echinoderms, bivalve molluscs, annelids, enteropneusts and decapod crustaceans, following membrane fusion at a single location at the tip of the sperm head, the united membranes shrink rapidly back, releasing the contents of the acrosome and exposing the subacrosomal material. This then projects forward in a dramatic fashion, often to a greater distance than the length of the entire sperm. The structure thus formed is referred to as the perforatorium. Exceptionally, as in *Limulus*, the perforatorium is a preformed filament of great length (Andre, 1963). The term perforatorium is also used to identify a structure in rodent sperm heads, in which a relatively rigid (non-extensible) structure apparently provides physical support for the often prominent and asymmetrical acrosome.

Capacitation

In mammals, occurrence of the acrosome reaction depends on the sperm first undergoing capacitation. This change, initially observed in rabbit sperms (Austin, 1951; Chang, 1951), has since been recorded in most other mammals specifically investigated, but its precise nature is poorly understood. Capacitation is considered to involve influx of calcium, which stimulates the enzyme adenylate cyclase and this is followed by increase in cAMP and membrane-associated phospholipases, leading to intrinsic changes in acrosomal membranes (Fraser, 1990). Hyperactivation of the sperm is induced simultaneously with capacitation, as was demonstrated by Yanagimachi (1970), and this too is an essential preliminary to penetration into the egg. Capacitation is not solely a mammalian phenomenon, for a corresponding change has been described in some non-mammalian sperms, namely those of the frog *Rana* (Shivers & James, 1970), the coelenterate *Campanularia* (O'Rand, 1979) and the housefly *Musca* (Leopold & Degrugillier, 1973).

Some other aspects of fertilization, such as the question of specificity, are dealt with in the companion chapter *Evolution of Human Gametes – The Oocyte.*

Are sperms selected for/against in the female tract?

Reproduction in marine invertebrates involves generally the simultaneous release into the environment of untold numbers of sperms and eggs, and a logical explanation for this seemingly wild extravagance is that it provides tolerable chances for the fertilization of every egg. In strong contrast, investigations on fertilization in bees revealed that the queen exerts the utmost economy with the sperm quota she acquired at her only mating ceremony. The huge numbers of sperms ejaculated into the female genital tract in mammals seemed again to be explicable as ensuring high rates of fertilization. But, the female tract greatly reduces the sperm numbers traversing it, and the quota reaching the actual site of fertilization represents in fact a very small fraction of the population originally deposited in the tract. Commonly cited figures for the human subject are: normal semen 20–300 million sperms per ml, ejaculate volume 2–6 ml, resulting in 40–1800 million sperms being deposited in the vagina, the number reaching the site of fertilization being of the order of only 300. So opinions were expressed that the tract exerted a selective action on the sperm population: 'only a small special population achieving the oviducts', data from infertile couples suggesting that selection is antibody-mediated in women (Cohen & Gregson, 1978, and see Cohen & Adeghe, 1987). This notion was strengthened by the observations of Krzanowska (1962), showing that morphologically abnormal sperms tended to be excluded from transport to the site of fertilization.

But this system of ideas clearly needed revision when Ford (1972) produced evidence that the ability of sperms to take part in fertilization was not affected by 'gross unbalance of the genome'. Confirmatory findings were made more recently by Zackowski & Martin-DeLoen (1989), who found that the rates of fertilization by sperms with balanced genomes and those with single or double aneuploidies appeared to take place at rates equivalent to those of their formation. Mortimer (1978) also failed to find any evidence for the existence of mechanisms in the female tract capable of detecting and disposing of faulty spermatozoa, but he adds a rider to the effect that, under the circumstances that exist in the female tract, sperms might be said to 'select themselves'. There are also data to show that abnormal sperms that do reach the site of fertilization are able to penetrate eggs (Olds-Clarke & Becker, 1978). However, two sets of observations strongly support the view that, as with organisms depending on external fertilization, normality of the great majority of mammalian sperms can be inferred. First, the observations on hamsters by Bavister (1979) who obtained high rates of fertilization *in vitro*, and normal subsequent development, in preparations in which the sperm:egg ratio approached unity. Secondly, there are the high rates of fertilization and development achieved with mouse gametes by Lacham *et al.* (1989) and Trounson, Peura & Lacham (1989) following the injection *in vitro* of single sperms into eggs.

The related topic of selectivity in fertilization is discussed in connection with hybridization in the companion chapter '*Evolution of Human Gametes – Oocytes*'.

Summary and conclusions

1. Relics of early sperms are lacking from the fossil record, and so inferences relating to the evolution of spermatozoa have perforce to be based on their current morphology in relation to the taxonomic order of species.

2. Seemingly unlimited variations exist in the size and structure of plant and animal sperms, and numerous attempts have been made to discern pattern in the system, with limited success. That complexity runs parallel in both organism and gamete is broadly correct, animals with internal fertilization possessing the more sophisticated sperms. Eutherian sperms are characterized most plainly by their relatively rigid inner acrosomal and nuclear membranes, their compact and indurated nuclei, and the degree of development and complexity of the tail.

3. There are, however, numerous instances of distinctive morphological features being limited to relatively small groups of animals, suggesting that some of Nature's 'experiments' achieved limited success. Examples of these are the thread-like, barrel-shaped and stellate sperms, those with undulating membranes, and those that adopt the conjugated strategy.

4. Careful study of ultrastructural detail in the sperms of different groups of animals has greatly assisted the development of an improved systematic classification. In this way, it may eventually prove possible to present a tolerable 'reconstruction' of the course of evolution, from protozoan to man, as expressed by spermatozoa.

5. The morphology of eutherian sperms, particularly of their nuclei, varies according to order, genus, species, strain and even to some degree individual, so testifying to the close genetic control of these features. This is also borne out by the success that has been achieved in the experimental selection for various sperm characters.

6. A remarkably wide range of enzymes has been detected in the acrosomes of several species, functions for the majority of which are quite lacking. Possibly the explanation rests with the evolution of the acrosome from the enzyme-rich lysosome, and the proneness of evolutionary relics to persist long after their original function has been lost.

7. The properties of the sperms of the Prototheria, Metatheria and Eutheria, especially those of the nucleus and acrosome, differ quite widely in many respects, supporting the notion that the ancestral stocks of these three groups either separated at long intervals of time or that they arose from distinctly separate reptilian origins.

8. As necessary preliminaries to entry into eggs, the sperms of eutherian mammals particularly, but also some non-eutherian species, must undergo 'capacitation' and 'hyperactivation' in the appropriate environment, both states being considered dependent on calcium entry. Calcium has also been found to stimulate the enzyme adenylate cyclase, which is followed by increase in cAMP and membrane-associated phospholipases, changes that appear to underlie the acrosome reaction.

9. The huge numbers of sperms ejaculated into the female genital tract at coitus in mammals has evoked the proposition that only a small proportion of the sperms is capable of normal fertilization and that these are selected for in the female tract. Experimental evidence, however, involving successful fertilization of eggs by sperms with 'gross unbalance of the genome', and fertilization under conditions in which the sperm-egg ratio approached unity, as well as the practice of fertilizing human eggs by injecting single sperms through the zona pellucida, all point to the great majority of sperms as being capable of taking part in fertilization. The appropriate inference would appear to be that the enormous excess of sperms deposited by the male is an atavistic feature, relevant when fertilization took place in the open environment and persisting with internal fertilization from lack of selection pressure.

References

Afzelius BA, Dallai R. Conjugated spermatozoa. In: Mohri H, ed. *New Horizons in Sperm Cell Research*. Tokyo; Japan Scientific Societies Press and New York, London, Paris, Montreux, Tokyo; Gordon & Breach Science Publishers, 1987; 349–55.

Andre, J. A propos d'une lecon sur la limule. *Ann Fac Sci* 1963; **26**: 27–38.

Asa CS, Phillips DM. Ultrastructure of avian spermatozoa. In: Mohri H, ed. *New Horizons in Sperm Research*. Tokyo; Japan Scientific Societies Press and New York, London, Paris, Montreux, Tokyo; Gordon & Breach Science Publishers, 1987; 365–73.

Austin CR. Observations on the penetration of the sperm into the mammalian egg. *Aust J Sci Res, Ser. B* 1951; **4**: 581–96.

Austin CR. Gametogenesis and fertilization in the Mesozoan *Dicyema aegira*. *Parasitology* 1964; **54**: 597–600.

Austin CR. *Fertilization*. Englewood Cliffs, New Jersey; Prentice-Hall, Inc., 1965.

Austin CR. Specialization of gametes. In: Austin CR, Short RV, eds. *The Evolution of Reproduction*, chap. 5, *Reproduction in Mammals*. Cambridge University Press, 1976; **6**: 149–82.

Baccetti B. Evolution of the acrosomal complex. In: Fawcett DW, Bedford JM, eds. *The Spermatozoon.* Baltimore, Munich; Urban & Schwarzenberg, 1979; 305–29.

Baccetti B. News on phylogenetical and taxonomical spermatology. In: Mohri, H, ed. *New Horizons in Sperm Cell Research.* Tokyo; Japan Scientific Societies Press – New York, London, Paris, Montreux, Tokyo; Gordon and Breach Science Publishers, 1987; 333–48.

Baccetti B, Afzelius BA. *The Biology of the Spern Cell. Monographs in Developmental Biology.* Basel; Karger, 1976.

Barlow P, Vosa CG. The Y chromosome in human spermatozoa. *Nature* 1970; **226**: 961–2.

Barros C, Dupre E, Viveros L. Sperm–egg interactions in the shrimp *Rhynchocinetes typus.* Gam Res, 1986; **14**: 171–80.

Barros C, Bedford JM, Franklin LE, Austin CR. Membrane vesiculation as a feature of the mammalian acrosome reaction. *J Cell Biol* 1967; **34**: C1–C5.

Bavister BD. Fertilization of human eggs *in vitro* at sperm:egg ratios close to unity. *J. Exp. Zool.*, 1979; **210**: 259–64.

Beatty RA. The genetics of size and shape of spermatozoa organelles. In: Beatty RA, Gluecksohn-Waelsch S, eds. *Edinburgh Symposium on the Genetics of the Spermatozoon.* Published by the organizers; Edinburgh, New York, 1971: 97–115.

Beatty RA. Serum diversity within the species. In: BA Afzelius, ed. *The Functional Anatomy of the Spermatozoon.* Oxford, New York, Toronto, Sydney; Pergamon Press, 1975: 319–27.

Bedford JM. Biology of primate spermatozoa. In: Luckett WP, ed. *Reproductive Biology of the Primates. Contributions to Primatology.* Basel; Karger, 1974; **3**: 97–139.

Bedford JM. Fertilization mechanisms in animals and man: current concepts. In: Edwards RG, ed. *Establishing a Successful Human Pregnancy.* New York; Raven Press, 1990: 115–31.

Bedford JM. The coevolution of human gametes. In *A Comparative Overview of Mammal Fertilisation* Eds. Dunbar BS & O'Rand MG, New York; Plenum Press, 1991: 3–35.

Bedford JM, Bent MJ, Calvin HI. Variations in the structural character and stability of the nuclear chromatin in morphologically normal human spermatozoa. *J. Reprod. Fert.* 1973; **33**: 19–29.

Bishop MWH, Walton A. Spermatogenesis and the structure of mammalian spermatozoa. In: Parkes AS, ed. *Marshall's Physiology of Reproduction,* 3rd. edit. London; Longmans, 1960; **1** (2): 1–129.

Braden AWH. Strain differences in the morphology of the gametes of the mouse. *Aust J Biol Sci* 1959; **12**: 65–71.

Chang MC. Fertilizing capacity of spermatozoa deposited into the Fallopian tubes. *Nature* 1951; **168**: 997–8.

Cohen J. Gametic diversity within an ejaculate. In: Afzelius BA, ed. *The Functional Anatomy of the Spermatozoon.* Oxford, New York, Toronto, Sydney, 1975: 329–39.

Cohen J, Adeghe AJ-H. The other spermatozoa: fate and functions. In: Mohri H, ed. *New Horizons in Sperm Cell Research.* Tokyo; Japan Scientific Societies Press – New York, London, Paris, Montreux, Tokyo; Gordon and Breach Science Publishers, 1987: 125–34.

Cohen J, Gregson SH. Antibodies and sperm survival in the female genital tract. In: Cohen J, Hendry WF, eds. *Spermatozoa, Antibodies and Fertility;* chap. 3: *Proceedings of a Symposium on Immunological Infertility, London.* Oxford, London, Edinburgh, Melbourne; Blackwell Scientific Publications, 1978: 17–29.

Cooper GW, Bedford JM. Asymmetry of spermiation and sperm surface charge patterns over the giant acrosome in the Musk Shrew *Suncus murinus. J. Cell Biol.,* 1976; **69**: 415–28.

18 C. R. Austin

Cummins JM. Sperm size, body mass and reproduction in mammals. In: Andre J, ed. *The Sperm Cell*. The Hague; Martinmans Nijhoff, 1983: 395–8.

Cummins JM. Evolution of sperm form: levels of control and competition. In: Bavister BD, Cummins J, Roldan ERS, eds. *Fertilization in Mammals*, Norwell, Massachusetts; Serono Symposia, USA, 1990: 51–64.

Dunbar BS, O'Rand MG 1991. *A Comparative Overview of Mammalian Fertilisation*, Plenum Press New York 457.

Ford CE. Gross genome unbalance in mouse spermatozoa: does it influence the capacity to fertilize? In: Beatty RA, Glueksohn-Waelsch S, eds. *The Genetics of the Spermatozoon*. Edinburgh, New York, 1972: 359–69.

Fraser LR. Sperm capacitation and its modulation. In: Bavister BD, Cummins J, Roldan ERS, eds. *Fertilization in Mammals*. Norwell, Massachusetts; Serono Symposia, USA, 1990: 141–53.

Friend GF. The sperms of the British Muridae. *Quart. J. Micr. Sci.* 1936; **78**: 419–43.

Harding HR, Aplin K, Shorey CD. Parsimony analysis of marsupial sperm structure: a preliminary report. In: Mohri, H, ed. *New Horizons in Sperm Cell Research*. Tokyo; Japan Scientific Societies Press: New York, London, Paris, Montreux, Tokyo; Gordon and Breach Science Publishers, 1987: 375–85.

Hendelberg J. On the development of different types of spermatozoa from spermatids with two flagella in the Turbullaria with remarks on the ultrastructure of the flagella. *Zool Bidr Uppsala*, 1969; **38**: 2–45.

Holmes S. *Henderson's Dictionary of Biological Terms*, 9th edn. London, New York; Longmans, 1979.

Jamieson BGM. Spermatozoal ultrastructure: evolution and congruence with a holomorphological phylogeny of the Oligochaeta (Annelida). *Zool Scripta*, 1983; **12**: 107–14.

Jamieson BGM. A biological classification of sperm types, with special reference to annelids and molluscs, and an example of spermiocladistics. In: Mohri H, ed. *New Horizons in Sperm Cell Research*. Tokyo; Japan Scientific Societies Press, and New York, London, Paris, Montreux, Tokyo; Gordon and Breach Science Publishers, 1987a: 311–32.

Jamieson BGM. *The Ultrastructure and Phylogeny of Insect Spermatozoa*. Cambridge; Cambridge University Press, 1987b.

Jamieson BGM. *Fish Evolution and Systematics: Evidence from Spermatozoa*. Cambridge; Cambridge University Press, 1991.

Krzanowska H. Sperm quality and quantity in inbred lines of mice and their crosses. *Acta Biol. Cracov. (Ser. Zool.)* 1962; **5**: 279–90.

Krzanowska H. Influence of Y chromosome on fertility in mice. In: Beatty RA, Glueksohn-Waelsch S. eds, *The Genetics of the Spermatozoon*, 1972: 370–86.

Lacham O, Trounson A, Holden C, Mann J, Sathananthan H. Fertilization and development of mouse eggs injected under the zona pellucida with single spermatozoa treated to induce the acrosome reaction. *Gam Res* 1989; **23**: 1–11.

Landsteiner K, Levine P. On blood group substances in human spermatozoa. *J Immunol* 1926; **12**: 415–27.

Lenhossek MV. Untersuchungen uber Spermatogenese. *Arch Mikr Anat* 1898; **51**: 215–318.

Leopold RA, Degrugillier ME. Sperm penetration of housefly eggs: evidence of involvement of a female accessory secretion. *Science* 1973; **181**: 555–7.

Marshall FHA. *The Physiology of Reproduction*, 2nd edn. London: Longmans, Green & Co., 1992: 641.

Mate KE, Rodger JC. Stability of the acrosome of the brush-tailed possum (*Trichosurus vulpecula*) and tammar wallaby (*Macropus eugenii*) *in vitro* and after exposure to conditions and agents known to cause capacitation or acrosome reaction of eutherian spermatozoa. *J. Reprod. Fert.* 1991; **91**: 41–8.

Mortimer D. Selectivity of sperm transport in the female genital tract. In: Cohen J, Hendry WF, eds. *Spermatozoa, Antibodies and Infertility*, chap. 5. Oxford, London, Edinburgh, Melbourne; Blackwell Scientific Publications, 1978: 37–53.

Olds-Clarke P, Becker A. The effect of the *T/t* locus on sperm penetration *in vivo* in the house mouse. *Biol. Reprod.* 1978; **18**: 132–40.

O'Rand MG. Changes in sperm surface properties correlated with capacitation. In: Fawcett DW, Bedford JM, eds. *The Spermatozoon*. Baltimore-Munich: Urban & Schwarzenberg; 1979: 195–204.

O'Rand M, Miller RL. Spermatozoan vesicle loss during penetration of the female gonangium in the hydroid, *Campanularia flexuosa*. *J. Exp. Zool.*, 1974; **188**: 179–95.

Picheral B. Structural, comparative and functional aspects of spermatozoa in urodeles. In: Fawcett DW, Bedford JM, eds. *The Spermatozoon: Maturation, Motility, Surface Properties and Comparative Aspects*. Baltimore-Munich; Urban & Schwarzenberg, 1979: 267–87.

Rodger JC, Bedford JM. Separation of sperm pairs and sperm-egg interaction in the opossum, *Didelphis virginiana*. *J Reprod Fert* 1982; **64**: 171–9.

Rodger JC, Young RJ. Glucosidase and cumulus dispersal activities of acrosomal extracts from opossum (marsupial) and rabbit (eutheria) spermatozoa. *Gam Res* 1981; **4**: 507–14.

Setchell BP. *Spermatogenesia and spermatozoa*. In: Austin CR, Short RV, eds. *Reproduction in Mammals*, vol. 1, chap. 4. Cambridge; Cambridge University Press, 1982; vol. 1, chap. 4: 63–101.

Shivers CA, James JM. Capacitation of frog sperm. *Nature* 1970; **227**: 183–4.

Snell GD. Antigenic differences between the sperm of different inbred strains of mice. *Science* 1944; **100**: 272–3.

Trounson A, Peura A, Lahcam O. Fertilization of mouse and human eggs by microinjection of single spermatozoa under the zona pellucida. *J Reprod Fert* 1989; **38**: 145–52.

Walter MR, Buick R, Dunlop ISR. Stromatolites 3400 to 3500 Myr. old from the North Pole area, Western Australia. *Nature (Lond)* 1980; **284**: 443–5.

Woolley DM. Selection for the length of the spermatozoon midpiece in the mouse. *Genet Res Camb* 1970; **16**: 261–75.

Woolley DM, Beatty RA. Inheritance of midpiece length in mouse spermatozoa. *Nature (Lond)* 1967; **215**: 94–5.

Yanagimachi R. The movement of golden hamster spermatozoa before and after capacitation. *J Reprod Fert* 1970; **23**: 193–6.

Yanagimachi R. Specificity of sperm-egg interaction. In: Edidin M, Johnson MH, eds. *Immunobiology of Gametes*. Cambridge: Cambridge University Press, 1977: 255–89.

Zackowski JL, Martin-DeLeon PA. Segregation products of male mice doubly heterozygous for the TB(6.16) and RB(16.17) translocations: influence of sperm karyotype on fertilization compared under varying mating frequencies. *Gam Res* 1989; **22**: 93–107.

2

The mammalian sperm surface: molecular and cellular aspects

C. D. THALER and R. A. CARDULLO

Introduction

Successful fertilization is a result of complex molecular events that ultimately enable the sperm to recognize, bind, and fuse with the egg (Fig. 1). In order to achieve this goal the mammalian sperm undergoes a plethora of cell surface modifications throughout its development from spermatogenesis to fertilization. These developmental changes are largely the result of three different mechanisms: (1) the biosynthetic capabilities of the germ cells prior to meiosis, (2) direct contact with Sertoli cells (during spermatogenesis) and eggs (during fertilization) and (3) exposure to ever-changing extracellular fluids in the male and female reproductive tracts, primarily through the processes of epididymal maturation and capacitation.

During spermatogenesis the Sertoli cells are in direct contact with the developing spermatogonia, spermatocytes, and spermatids during an active period of macromolecular biosynthesis. Subsequent to this, the spermatozoon undergoes a series of morphological transformations during spermiogenesis which ultimately leads to the formation of a well-defined head, containing the haploid nucleus and acrosome, the midpiece and the principal piece. These major morphological demarcations are easily resolved in the light microscope and as the sperm enters the caput epididymis it is clearly recognizable as the male gamete although it is still incapable of motility or of fertilization. Within the epididymis a number of cell surface modifications occur including redistributions of macromolecules from one morphological region to another, addition of new macromolecules secreted from the epididymal epithelia, post-translational modifications of membrane proteins, and the sloughing off of a cytoplasmic droplet. These alterations are coincident with the acquisition of motility competence in the cauda epididymis but the ability to fertilize the egg is achieved only after additional changes have

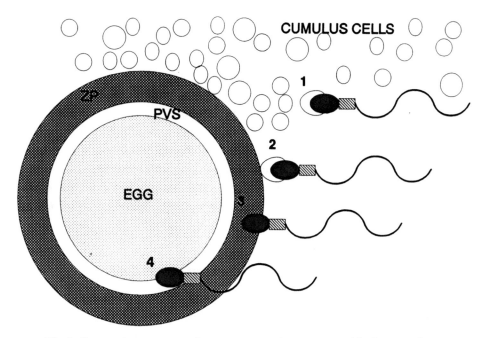

Fig. 1. Progression events as the sperm comes into contact with the egg prior to fertilization. **1** After passing through the cumulus cells the acrosome intact sperm arrives at the zona pellucida (ZP). **2** At the zona pellucida, specific receptors on the sperm surface recognize and bind to the complementary zone ligand ZP3. The identity and biochemical nature of these zona adhesion molecules on the sperm surface is still an active area of investigation. In addition to its role as an adhesion molecule, ZP3 also serves as an agonist for acrosomal exocytosis. **3** After the acrosome reaction is completed, the sperm can then negotiate its way through the zona pellucida. During this stage it has been postulated that the sperm interacts with another zona pellucida glycoprotein, ZP2. **4** Once through the zona pellucida and the perivitelline space (PVS), the fusion between the sperm plasma membrane and egg plasma membrane is mediated by another set of specific egg and sperm associated fusion molecules. See text for details.

occurred within the female reproductive tract. As a result of these cell surface modifications, the mature sperm emerges as a highly polarized and differentiated cell which shares some cell surface similarities with only other highly differentiated cell types such as epithelia, photoreceptors, and neurons.

In this chapter we will discuss some of the key molecules that are involved in the differentiation of the sperm plasma membrane and focus on how these molecules become involved in the fertilization process through sperm–zona adhesion, initiation of signal transduction pathways resulting in acrosomal exocytosis, and the fusion of the sperm and egg membranes.

Biophysical and biochemical properties of the developing sperm plasma membrane

Before discussing the characteristics and physiological role of particular molecules on the mammalian sperm surface, it is instructive to look at the basic properties of this unique cell surface. Like many cells ultimately involved in recognition, binding, and signalling events, the mammalian sperm is a highly differentiated cell exhibiting a high degree of molecular mosaicism on its surface. Interestingly, this mosaicism applies not only to membrane proteins but to the lipid environment as well. In this section we will discuss the general biophysical and biochemical properties of sperm lipids and proteins during spermatogenesis and epididymal maturation.

Characteristics of some sperm membrane lipids

A number of fluorescent lipid analogues have served as useful probes to investigate the nature of the spermatozoa membrane during development. Using the technique of fluorescence recovery after photobleaching (FRAP), a spectroscopic technique that follows molecular motions on cellular surfaces, Wolf and colleagues have shown that a number of fluorescent lipid analogues (e.g. $C_n$diIs) exhibit differential solubility and mobility on the mammalian sperm surface (for reviews see Wolf, 1986; Cardullo & Wolf, 1991). In somatic tissues, nearly 100% of a cell's lipid is free to diffuse within the plane of the membrane. However, in this respect, mature sperm are remarkably different: a large fraction of the lipid appears to be immobilized with typically only 50% to 70% of the membrane lipids freely diffusing (Wolf, Lipscomb & Maynard, 1988). FRAP experiments on mouse pachytene spermatocytes showed that these cells have lipid environments which resemble most somatic cells. However, as spermatogenic cells progress through development to round spermatids, condensing spermatids, and testicular sperm there is an increasing fraction of immobile lipid. These findings have prompted Wolf to propose that, during development, lipid domains (on the order of a micron or less in diameter) are established within the membrane of mammalian sperm (Wolf, 1986).

Further evidence that the mammalian sperm surface is organized into lipid domains and is significantly different from somatic cells comes from experiments using differential scanning calorimetry on mature ram sperm (Wolf et al., 1990). Using this technique, it is possible to establish the presence of gel-to-fluid transitions as the temperature is changed. Whereas lipids extracted from most somatic cell membranes exhibit little, or no, detectable phase transitions, the ram sperm plasma membrane isolated from the anterior head possesses two: one extending between 12 °C and 39 °C and a second that extends between 48 °C and 74 °C. As with the FRAP experiments, the appearance of phase transitions demonstrates that the mammalian sperm surface is separated into both fluid (mobile) and gel (immobile) domains. Of particular interest is the first phase transition which may be physiologically relevant as sperm pass from the relatively low temperature environment of the cauda epididymis (30 °C–33 °C) to the much warmer environment within the female reproductive tract (37 °C–39 °C). It is entirely possible that this abrupt temperature increase upon ejaculation could act as a 'thermodynamic trigger' driving an immobile, inactive sperm membrane fraction into a dynamic and activated state which is requisite for fertilization.

Extensive biochemical studies have shown that sperm contain some unique lipids in relatively high concentrations. Spermatozoa have high levels of ether-linked lipids and highly unsaturated fatty acyl groups such as docosahexaenoyl (22:6) (Parks & Hammerstedt, 1985). Further studies revealed that the major plasma membrane lipid on sperm was 1-alkenyl- or 1 alkyl-2-actyl-*sn*-glycero-phosphocholine (Wolf *et al.*, 1990). Although sperm have lost the ability to synthesize new lipids after spermatogenesis, significant modifications of sperm membrane lipids do occur during epididymal maturation and capacitation. In particular, it has been shown that cholesterol/phospholipid changes occur during capacitation in the female reproductive tract suggesting a possible mechanism for capacitation (Langlais *et al.*, 1988). These findings are intriguing but more work needs to be performed before physiologically relevant information can be gleaned from it.

Characteristics of some sperm membrane proteins

Like sperm surface lipids, most sperm plasma membrane proteins also reveal a high degree of mosaicism. Using immunofluorescence microscopy a number of investigators have shown that antigens can be localized to isolated regions of the sperm head, midpiece, or flagellum (for a review see Cardullo & Wolf, 1991). Of particular interest to researchers studying fertilization are antigens that are localized to the sperm head since these may ultimately be involved in sperm–egg recognition events (e.g. sperm–zona adhesion, induction of the acrosome reaction, and sperm–egg fusion – see pp. 26ff.). An interesting feature of many of these membrane proteins is their ability to change their cellular localization abruptly in response to a variety of immunological and physiological stimuli. Three sperm membrane proteins which all undergo these types of redistributions but have different biochemical and molecular properties are PH-20 (guinea pig) (Myles & Primakoff, 1991), M-42 (mouse) (Lakoski *et al.*, 1988*a*; Lakoski, Williams & Saling, 1988*b*), and ESA-152 (ram) (McKinnon *et al.*, 1991).

PH-20 is an antigen that is localized to the posterior head of mature, acrosome intact, guinea pig sperm. As will be discussed later in this review, PH-20 is of particular interest during fertilization since it has been implicated in sperm–zona adhesion. PH-20 is synthesized during spermatogenesis and first appears in the Golgi apparatus of round spermatids (Phelps & Myles, 1987). It next appears on the membranes of the developing acrosome and subsequent to this a second population appears to be directly inserted into the plasma membrane. During epididymal maturation the plasma membrane population becomes localized to the posterior head (hence the designation PH) while the acrosomal population of PH-20 is localized to the inner acrosomal membrane. Two molecular isoforms, affinity purified from a single monoclonal antibody (PH-22), of the PH-20 antigen have been identified, a major form with an M_r of 66 kD and a minor form with an M_r of 56 kD (Phelps & Myles, 1987). It is not yet known whether these two isoforms represent the two distinct populations found on the plasma membrane and the inner acrosomal membrane although the minor 56 kD form appears to be related to the major form of cauda sperm. Interestingly, when the acrosome reaction is induced in guinea pig sperm, the PH-20 population that originally resided on the posterior head completely joins the second population residing on the inner acrosomal membrane which becomes the new exposed sperm surface facing the zona pellucida (Cowan, Primalkoff & Myles, 1986). This redistribution from the posterior head to the anterior head is indicative of many sperm membrane proteins to be discussed in this chapter and has important biophysical and physiological implications in fertilization.

Biophysical determinations of PH-20 mobility using FRAP (Myles, Primakoff & Keppel, 1984; Cowan et al., 1986; Cowan, Myles & Koppel, 1987) have revealed that PH-20 localized to the posterior head of acrosome intact sperm exhibits diffusion coefficients similar to membrane proteins on somatic cells ($D = 1.8 \times 10^{-10}$ cm^2/s, 75% recovery). However, when this population migrates to the inner acrosomal membrane after acrosome reaction is induced, the PH-20 antigen displays rapid movement characterized by 'lipid-like' diffusion properties ($D = 10^{-9}$ cm^2/s, 80% recovery). In contrast, PH-20 on testicular sperm is much more restricted and displays much lower diffusion coefficients of the order of 10^{-11} cm^2/s. These results are particularly interesting since it has been shown that PH-20 is not a classical integral membrane protein, rather, PH-20 is linked to a membrane lipid via a glycosylphosphatidylinositol (GPI) linkage (Phelps et al., 1988). Hence, in addition to the progressive localized distribution of PH-20 during spermatogenesis and epididymal maturation, there is an increase in the mobility of this antigen as sperm acquire fertilization competence.

M-42 is a mouse sperm antigen that, like the guinea pig sperm antigen PH-20, is produced by spermatogenic cells. It is apparently synthesized as a large membrane protein ($M_r > 300$ kD) which undergoes significant post-translational modifications in the epididymis (Lakoski *et al.*, 1988*a,b*). In the different regions of the epididymis M42 exists as a doublet (as resolved by SDS–PAGE and Western Blotting) with molecular weights of 280/260 kD in the caput, 260/240 kD in the corpus, and 240/220 kD in the cauda. It is not known whether these changes represent a reduction in the polypeptide backbone or in the degree of glycosylation of this protein.

Initial reports on the cellular localization of the M42 antigen revealed that it was on the plasma membrane overlying the acrosome (Lakoski *et al.*, 1988*a*). However, subsequent studies showed that this redistribution may have been an artefact of cross-linking by a bivalent IgG (Wolf *et al.*, 1992). Use of an anti-M42 monovalent Fab fragment showed that the initial distribution of the M42 antigen was on the posterior head of capacitated mouse sperm. Such antibody induced redistributions are apparently not uncommon for mouse sperm head antigens as they have also been reported for the M5 antigen (Wolf *et al.*, 1992) and sperm surface galactosyltransferase (Cardullo & Wolf, 1994).

M42 also has a high diffusion coefficient ($3-8 \times 10^{-9}$ cm^2/s) but unlike the guinea pig sperm antigen, PH-20, only about 25% of the antigen is free to diffuse and there have been no reports that M42 is GPI linked. In fact, lage diffusion coefficients appear to be the rule, rather than the exception for many sperm surface antigens. This may reflect the absence of a significant cytoskeleton or extracellular matrix which is primarily responsible for retarding the motion of membrane macromolecules in somatic cells.

Another membrane protein of interest is the ram sperm antigen ESA-152 (Wolf *et al.*, 1986; McKinnon *et al.*, 1991). Unlike PH-20 or M42, ESA-152 is not synthesized by spermatogenic cells in the testis. Rather, ESA-12, a highly hydrophobic 18 kD M_r sialoglycoprotein, is synthesized by the proximal cauda epididymis and appears on the sperm surface within the cauda epididymis (Weaver *et al.*, 1993). ESA-152 is a highly hydrophobic sialoglycoprotein with an M_r of 18 kD. Immunofluorescence studies have revealed that the antigen is adsorbed to the entire surface of the sperm including the head, tail, and midpiece although the most intense labelling is over the posterior region of the ram sperm head. Similar to both PH-20 and M42, ESA-152 exhibits a rapid, lipid-like, diffiusion coefficient (Wolf *et al.*, 1986). Interestingly, inducing the acrosome reaction with the calcium ionophore A23187 results in the redistribution of the ESA-152 antigen from the posterior to the anterior head. In addition, both the redistribution and the acrosome reaction can be initiated by bivalent ESA-152 IgG antibodies but not by their monovalent Fab fragments. These observations suggest that ESA-152 may be involved in the introduction of the acrosome reaction but its direct role is still unclear at this time.

Table 1. *Differential effects of bivalent antibodies on three different sperm surface antigens*

Name	Species	Localization on acrosome intact sperm	Localization on acrosome reacted sperm	Redistribution induced by antibody?	Acrosome reaction induced by antibody?
PH-20	Guinea pig	PH and IAM	IAM	No	No
M42	Mouse	PH	AH	Yes	No
ESA-152	Ram	PH	AH	Yes	Yes

Antibodies can lead to a number of physiological transformations on the sperm cell surface including redistribution of antigen from one domain to another and induction of the acrosome reaction. AH = anterior head, PH = posterior head, IAM = inner acrosomal membrane.

The three proteins described above, PH-20, M-42, and ESA-152, share similar biophysical properties (highly mosaic distributions, rapid diffusion coefficients) but are dramatically different in their sites of synthesis, association with the sperm plasma membrane, and putative function. In addition, these three proteins have all been probed with antibodies and these antibodies have differential effects on the antigens they recognize (Table 1). In cases where an antibody induces a redistribution of the antigen from one portion of the cell to the other, one must ask whether this represents a physiologically relevant (or related) event or whether it reflects an artefact of antibody-induced cross-linking. Indeed, many biophysical properties can be altered when attaching a large antibody (or Fab fragment) to the antigen of interest. For that reason, it would be desirable to use the native ligand (if one exists) or a small molecular weight probe when studying protein dynamics and relating it to function.

The mammalian sperm surface and its role in fertilization

After the many molecular and membrane modifications that occur in the testis, epididymis, and oviduct, the mammalian sperm is capable of fertilizing the egg. At the cellular level, the sperm undergoes a number of physiologically distinct steps after traversing the female reproductive tract and the cumulus cells surrounding the oocyte (Fig. 1). The zona pellucida, an acellular coat that surrounds the egg, is the site of initial adhesion between the two gametes and also contains the agonist for the acrosome reaction. After acrosomal exocytosis is initiated, sperm can negotiate the zona pellucida and fuse with the egg plasma membrane. The three processes of sperm–zona adhesion, induction of the acrosome reaction, and sperm–egg fusion will be addressed separately.

Molecules involved in sperm adhesion to the zona pellucida

Biochemical and molecular aspects of the zona pellucida have been studied most extensively in the mouse and primarily by Wassarman and colleagues (for a review, see Wassarman, 1988). The zona pellucida is composed of three glycoproteins and the polypeptide chains are highly conserved among mammals. The mouse zona pellucida components, designated ZP1, ZP2, and ZP3 based on their relative electrophoretic mobility on SDS PAGE, have average molecular masses of approximately 200 kD, 120 kD, and 83 kD, respectively. All three are heavily glycosylated polypeptides containing both N- and O-linked oligo-saccharidde chains. The 83 kD glycoprotein, ZP3, is the bioactive component which is responsible for both initial sperm–egg binding and induction of the acrosome reaction. Studies have shown that O-linked oligosaccharides are responsible for specific binding activity (Florman & Wassarman, 1985; Bleil & Wassarman, 1988), but suggest that binding of these oligosaccharides alone is not sufficient to induce the acrosome reaction. Moreover, proteolygically derived ZP3 glycopeptides retain sperm binding activity but do not induce acrosomal exocytosis (Florman & Wassarman, 1985). Antibody cross-linking of the ZP3 glycopeptides resulted in apparent dimerization of sperm ZP3 binding sites inducing the acrosome reaction (Leyton & Saling, 1989a). Based on experiments such as these, in which aggregation of sperm surface components induces the acrosome reaction, several researchers have suggested that cross-linking of receptors subsequent to binding may be required for signal transduction resulting in the acrosome reaction.

Putative zona receptors with associated enzymatic activities

A number of investigators have identified putative ZP3 receptors using several different strategies. By far, the most studied putative receptor is a cell surface β-1,4-galactosyltransferase (GalTase) that has been exhaustively characterized by Shur and colleagues using biochemical, cell biological, and immunological approaches (for review see Shur, 1991). This molecule is thought to act as a receptor, rather than an enzyme on the cell surface interacting only with its acceptor site and leaving its donor site unoccupied. Experiments using a polyclonal antibody against a bovine milk soluble GalTase demonstrated that sperm surface GalTase is localized to the plasma membrane early in spermatogenesis, coalesces to a region over the acrosomal crescent on condensing spermatids and maintains this distribution until the acrosome reaction (Scully, Shaper & Shur, 1987). GalTase has been postulated to be involved in recognition and binding to the zona pellucida based on the observations that sperm–zona adhesion is inhibited by a number of substrates specific for GalTase (UDP-Gal, GlcNAc, lactosaminoglycan, α-lactalbumin), antibodies against GalTase, and competition with a bovine milk-soluble GalTase (Shur & Hall, 1982). Recently, Miller, Macek & Shur (1992) demonstrated that ZP3 can act as a substrate for GalTase under enzymatic conditions. This membrane-bound sperm surface GalTase galactosylates ZP3 but not the other zona pellucida glucoproteins, ZP1 and ZP2 (Miller *et al.*, 1992). In contrast, the milk-soluble GalTase galactosylated all three zona pellucida glycoproteins indicating that lack of galactosylation of ZP1 and ZP2 by the sperm GalTase is not due to an absence of terminal N-acetylglucosamine residues but may indicate a restricted specificity of sperm surface GalTase reflecting its specialized function of sperm–zona binding (Miller *et al.*, 1992). Similar to previously reported experiments employing UDP-galactose to disrupt sperm–egg binding, removing or blocking the terminal N-acetyl-glucosamine residues on solubilized ZP3 resulted in a reduction of ZP3 inhibition of sperm–egg binding in a standard competitive binding assay (Miller *et al.*, 1992). The notion of a glycosyltransferase being involved in zona recognition is indeed an attractive one since the zona pellucida is itself a glycoprotein matrix that may contain potential carbohydrate acceptors for these molecules.

In addition to GalTase, a cell surface fucosyltransferase (FucTase) has also been implicated in zona recognition by sperm although the evidence is less compelling (Cardullo *et al.*, 1989). The sperm surface FucTase is localized to the cell surface during spermatogenesis and is present only on the head by the time epididymal maturation is complete. Further, substrates for FucTase (GDP-fucose and asialofetuin) inhibit sperm–zona binding in an *in vitro* fertilization assay. However, data showing that zone constituents can act as enzymatic or binding substrates are still lacking.

Another sperm-associated enzymatic molecule that may be involved in sperm–zona binding is a sperm surface α-D-mannosidase that has been identified by Tulsiani, Skudlarek & Orgebin-Crist (1989). Initial experiments revealed that inhibitors of mouse sperm surface α-D-mannosidase led to a corresponding decrease in sperm–egg zona binding *in vitro* (Cornwall, Tulsiani & Orgebin-Crist, 1991). Subsequent studies demonstrated that rat epididymal fluid contained a 460 kD soluble form of α-D-mannosidase and that polyclonal antibodies raised against this soluble form cross-reacted with a component from detergent extracted mouse and rat sperm (Tulsiani *et al.*, 1993), suggesting that the soluble and sperm membrane molecules may be molecular isoforms. Interestingly, these investigators have shown that both ZP2 and ZP3 have a high mannose content suggesting that the sperm surface α-D-mannosidase may interact with the zona both before and after the acrosome reaction (Tulsiani *et al.*, 1992).

Several additional putative receptors with associated enzymatic activities have been identified on the basis of their ability to interact with the zona pellucida. One such sperm component was identified by the disruption of its binding capacity by inhibitors of trypsin-like proteases (Saling, 1981; Benau & Storey, 1987). Addition of soy bean trypsin inhibitor blocked binding of sperm to zonae *in vitro*, suggesting that the sperm zona pellucida receptor contained a binding site similar in structure to the active site of serine proteases such as trypsin. Despite several reports of tryspin inhibitors blocking sperm–zona interactions, the sperm component responsible for this behaviour has not been characterized further.

Another serine protease that may function as a zona is acrosin. Acrosin resides either within the acrosomal vesicle or on the inner acrosomal membrane as proacrosin prior to the acrosome reaction. Since soy bean trypsin inhibitor disrupts continued binding to the zona pellucida by acrosome reacted sperm (Bleil, Greve & Wassarman, 1988), it has been suggested that some protease, perhaps acrosin, may function as a ZP2 receptor. However, any role for acrosin, as well as any of the putative receptors with associated enzymatic activity, awaits direct observation of zone constituent binding with these molecules.

Sperm membrane proteins that directly recognize ZP3

A more direct approach for identifying putative zona pellucida receptors on sperm has been to demonstrate direct binding to different zona glycoproteins. At this time two major proteins have emerged from two different research groups: a 56 kD M_r protein identified by Bleil and Wassarman (1990) and a 95 kD M_r protein identified by Leyton and Saling (1989b). Interestingly, the two proteins appear to be subject to rather stringent conditions since neither group has identified the other's protein.

The mouse sperm protein, sp56, was identified as a ZP3 binding component using the Denny–Jaffe heterobifunctional crosslinking reagent. sp56 has also been proposed as a signalling molecule for initiation of the acrosome reaction although this has not yet been directly demonstrated. The ZP3 binding component, as localized by covalent linkage of ZP3 to sperm using the Denny–Jaffe reagent, is present on the head of acrosome intact but not acrosome reacted sperm and does not localize to the midpiece or tail of mouse sperm. A polypeptide of similar molecular weight (i.e. 56 kD) displays high affinity binding to a ZP3 affinity column but not to a ZP2 affinity column. These characteristics are consistent with a ZP3 binding protein, but further studies investigating the role of the sperm sp56 have not appeared. Another sperm component, an approximately 40 kD M_r polypeptide, binds to the ZP3 affinity column with relatively high affinity but is presumed by the authors to be actin and therefore non-specific. Thus, the role of the sp56 in sperm–egg binding and signalling of the acrosome reaction remains unclear and awaits further characterization.

In contrast, Leyton and Saling (1989b) have demonstrated that a 95 kD M_r component directly binds to ZP3. In this procedure, sperm were first dissolved in SDS and were separated electrophoretically on polyacrylamide gels. Two components, of M_rs 95 kD and 42 kD were identified by a protein blot technique using [^{125}I]-labelled ZP2 showed no reactivity toward any sperm components under identical conditions. In a separate experiment, these authors demonstrated that three proteins from capacitated mouse sperm, with M_rs of 52, 75, and 95 kD, were recognized by an anti-phosphotyrosine antibody in a Western blot assay. The authors therefore argued that the 95 kD protein recognized by both ZP3 and the anti-phosphotyrosine antibodies functioned as both a zona receptor and as a signalling molecule important in the induction of the acrosome reaction (see section below). Further, the antiphosphotyrosine antibodies were used to localize the phosphorylated components on permeabilized and fixed mouse sperm using immunofluorescence microscopy. These studies revealed that the phosphorylated tyrosines were localized to the acrosomal region suggesting that the p95 protein (as well, presumably as the p52 and p75) were present only on the region of the sperm that binds to the zona. Taken together, these studies suggested that the p95 resides on the head of mouse sperm and functions as both the ZP3 receptor and as a signalling molecule involved in the induction of the acrosome reaction. It has not yet been demonstrated whether the 42 kD binding component is the same component as the 40 kD component identified by Bleil and Wassarman (1988) or if the phosphorylated p52 and p75 proteins play any significant role in sperm–egg interaction.

Identification of putative sperm–zona receptors using immunological approaches

A number of putative zona pellucida receptors have also been identified using a number of antibodies directed against membrane proteins that block zona binding or fertilization. Three molecules of particular note are the GalTase (Scully et al., 1987) and M42 (Lakoski et al., 1988a) antigens on mouse sperm and the PH-20 (Phelps and Myles, 1987) antigen on guinea pig sperm. All of these antigens are localized to the head of the appropriate sperm. It should be noted that antibody inhibition does not, by itself, implicate a membrane protein as a zona receptor. Indeed, it is possible that antibodies block fertilization through other mechanisms including antibody-induced patching and capping or steric hindrance with other critical molecules. Table 2 presents a range of effects on cellular localization of an antigen and the initiation of the acrosome reaction when sperm are incubated in the presence of specific bivalent antibodies.

Table 2. *Sperm surface molecules putatively involved in adhesion to the zona pellucida*

Name[a]	M_r	Association with ZP3?	Comments
PH-20 (guinea pig)	62 kD	None shown	Implicated using different antibodies in fertilization assays
GalTase (mouse)	60 kD	Galactosylates ZP3 when enzymatic activity is initiated	Blocks to fertilization using enzymatic substrates and a monospecific polyconal antibody
FucTase (mouse)	unknown	None shown	Enzymatic substrates block fertilization
Mannosidase (rat)	460 kD[b]	None shown	ZP2 and ZP3 have high levels of mannose
Trypsin-inhibitor insensitive site (mouse)	unknown	None shown	Zona binding blocked by enzymatic substrates
p95 (mouse)	95 kD	Protein blotting	Identified as a receptor tyrosine kinase that becomes activated after associating with ZP3
sp56 (mouse)	56 kD	ZP3 affinity chromatograph and chemical cross-linking	Some minor proteins are also recognized under these conditions

Some molecules which have been implicated in sperm–zona adhesion. Molecules are identified primarily by three different methods, by inhibiting binding by initiating an intrinsic enzymatic activity, by blocking the adhesion site using an antibody, or by showing some direct association with ZP3.
[a]Species in parentheses represent where most information is known.
[b]Molecular weight of soluble epididymal form.

As discussed earlier, PH-20 is a guinea pig sperm surface molecule that is synthesized during the round spermatid stage and is localized to the head region upon entering the epididymis (see pp. 23–26). Investigations have shown that both acrosome intact and acrosome-reacted sperm will bind to the zona pellucida. Using both polyclonal and monoclonal antibodies, Cowan and colleagues (1986) have shown that the PH-20 antigen is localized to the posterior head of acrosome intact sperm and to the inner acrosomal membrane on the anterior head of acrosome reacted sperm. Three monoclonal antibodies of subclass IgG_1 (PH-20, PH-21, and PH-22) were used to localize the cell surface antigen of M_r 62 kD. Interestingly, PH-20 inhibits zona binding 80–90% whereas PH-22 has no effect on zona binding and PH-21 inhibits zona binding at an intermediate level. Presumably this difference in zona binding inhibition is due to recognition of different epitopes on the mature 62 kD membrane protein; however, no direct evidence yet exists for a binding domain on the membrane protein.

Antibodies to both GalTase (Shur, 1991) and M42 (Lakoski *et al.*, 1988*a,b*) will reduce sperm–zona binding *in vitro*. Although in the case of GalTase it is not clear whether the block to fertilization by intact bivalent IgGs is due to blocking a zone recognition epitope or is a result of prematurely firing the acrosome reaction (Macek, Lopez & Shur, 1991, see pp. 33–35). Both M42 and GalTase appear to undergo a gross redistribution from the posterior head to the anterior head upon cross-linking by bivalent IgG antibodies (Wolf *et al.*, 1992; Cardullo & Wolf, 1994) similar to that seen with the ESA-152 antibody on ram sperm (McKinnon *et al.*, 1991). In general, immunological studies are inconclusive until peptide directed antibodies can be made against known, or putative, binding domains for a given zona receptor.

Molecules involved in acrosomal exocytosis

Sperm–zona binding and induction of the acrosome reaction are essential prerequisites for fertilization and the signal transduction pathway involved in binding and induction of acrosomal exocytosis have been investigated extensively. Signalling is initiated by a ligand binding to a receptor, usually on the cell surface. This binding event transduces a signal to the interior of the cell by a ligand induced conformational change in the receptor. In the case of sperm–egg binding and induction of the acrosome reaction, the zona pellucida component ZP3 is the ligand (Bleil & Wassarman, 1980*a,b*; Florman & Wassarman, 1985) which binds to a sperm plasma membrane receptor initiating a cascade of signalling events culminating in the acrosome reaction. The ligand bound receptor activates effectors such as heterotrimeric G-proteins, tyrosine kinases or phosphatases. The activation or mobilization of these components ultimately activates other components (second messengers) which carry out the cell's response to the signal. Although there is substantial evidence that ZP3 is the *in vivo* ligand, the sperm receptor and subsequent signalling mechanisms in this process are not well understood. Fig. 2 shows the key steps involved in the signal transduction events leading from the initial binding of ZP3 to a complementary receptor to the activation of effector molecules which, in turn, activate second messenger systems which are requisite for the onset of exocytosis. In this vein, the molecular players

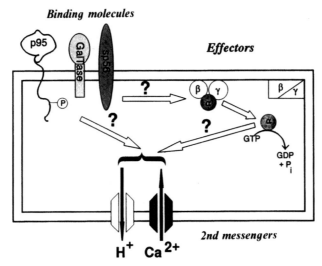

Fig. 2. Molecular players implicated in ZP3-induced acrosomal exocytosis. One or more binding molecules comes into contact with ZP3 and a complex series of molecular events is initiated, ultimately leading to the acrosome reaction. Three of the putative binding molecules that have been shown to recognize ZP3 are p95, a sperm surface β-1,4 galactosyltransferase (GalTase), and sp56. These molecules must either interact with, or contain, a signalling domain which initiates downstream signal transduction pathways. However, only one of these three binding molecules, p95, has been shown to contain a signalling domain that becomes activated upon binding ZP3. One of the effectors which has been shown to be present activated after ZP3 binding is a G_i protein although no receptor has been identified for its activation. Finally, ionic regulators such as Ca^{2+} and H^+ have been shown to be involved in the final stages of the acrosome reaction. Precise molecular details relating binding to the activation of signal transduction pathways and acrosomal exocytosis are still forthcoming. See text for details.

shown in Fig. 2 represent a 'best guess' based on current data for mouse fertilization.

Signalling domains within putative zona receptors

Many putative receptors on sperm have been identified by their ZP3 binding ability, but none have yet been definitively characterized as having both ZP3 binding and signal transducing components. As discussed previously (see pp. 29–30), the mouse sperm component p95, is a 95 kD polypeptide that is tyrosine phosphorylated and binds to ZP3 on protein blots of whole sperm (Leyton & Saling, 1989*b*). p95 maintains basal levels of tyrosine phosphorylation in both epididymal and capacitated sperm and tyrosine phosphorylation of p95 increases in response to incubation of sperm with solubilized zonae or purified ZP3 whereas similar increases in phosphorylation of other sperm components containing phosphotyrosine residues (p75 and p52) are not observed in response to treatment with zona glycoproteins. These data suggest that p95 may be involved in signalling the acrosome reaction upon ZP3 binding by sperm (Leyton & Saling, 1989b).

A large family of signal transducing receptors are protein tyrosine kinases (PTKs) which possess intrinsic tyrosine kinase activity and undergo auto-phosphorylation of specific highly conserved tyrosine residues in response to ligand binding. The receptor PTKs subsequently phosphorylate other cellular components to propagate the signal. Further studies have shown that p95 possesses intrinsic tyrosine kinase activity which can be stimulated by ZP3 and inhibited by tyrphostins or by genistein (Leyton et al., 1992), inhibitors that are relatively specific for tyrosine kinase activities. These chemicals also inhibit the acrosome reaction and Leyton et al. (1992) suggest that tyrosine phosphorylation of p95 is required for acrosomal exocytosis. Their data indicate, however, that treatment of sperm with tyrphostins inhibits phosphorylation of several poly-peptides in addition to the p95. These polypeptides are not recognized by the anti-phosphotyrosine antibody despite the fact that their phosphorylation is inhibited by the tyrphostins. The authors suggest that these data are consistent with activation of multiple kinases by the initial tyrosine kinase p95, and may indicate that additional phosphorylation events are necessary for signalling of the acrosome reaction (Leyton et al., 1992). Alternatively, the kinase inhibitors may have broader or more non-specific effects in this system than previously documented for somatic cells.

In guinea pig sperm, the GPI-linked membrane component, PH-20, is thought to function in sperm-zona adhesion since removal of 50% of the PH-20 by treatment of sperm with phosphatidylinositol specific-phospholipase C (PI-PLC) also reduces the ability of acrosome reacted sperm to bind to the zona pellucida by 50–60%. Since these experiments were performed on acrosome reacted sperm, the role of PH-20 in initial sperm–zona binding or in signalling the acrosome reaction was not addressed (Phelps et al., 1988). Any role of PH-20 in signalling is not clear since GPI-linked proteins have no intracellular domain and are thought to be incapable of transducing a signal directly. However, GPI-linked proteins have been associated with changes in tyrosine kinase activity and using co-immunoprecipitation assays have been shown to interact with protein tyrosine kinases after binding of ligand by the GPI-linked protein (Stefanova et al., 1991). Experiments addressing this possible mechanism in the case of PH-20 have not been reported. Further, a recent report demonstrates that PH-20 shares considerable DNA sequence homology with a bee venom hyaluronidase (Gmachl & Kreil, 1993). Direct evidence that PH-20 actually possesses hyaluronidase activity has not yet been reported, but hyaluronidase activity of this protein might suggest that its primary function may be in penetration of the cumulus oophorus surrounding the egg and not in zona binding.

Sperm surface GalTase has been implicated in adhesion to the zona based on a variety of biochemical and cell biological experiments (see pp. 27–29). In addition, sperm surface GalTase has also been implicated as a direct initiator of the acrosome reaction. Cross-linking and aggregation of sperm surface GalTase by an antibody against bovine milk GalTase will induce the acrosome reaction in mouse sperm (Macek *et al.*, 1991). It has been suggested therefore that the initial sperm–egg binding is mediated by sperm surface GalTase and subsequent to binding that aggregation of the GalTase initiates the acrosome reaction. However, as discussed above for PH-20, galactosyltransferases have never been shown to be signal transducing molecules, and neither the mechanism by which aggregation of a non-signalling molecule could induce the acrosome reaction, nor its possible physiological relevance, have been elucidated.

Use of a heterobifunctional crosslinking reagent, the Denny–Jaffe reagent, to identify ZP3 binding components resulted in the identification of a single sperm surface 56 kD polypeptide (sp56). The sp56 binds tightly to a ZP3 affinity column, but not to a ZP2 affinity column, suggesting that the interaction with ZP3 is specific (Bleil & Wassarman, 1990). Further characterization of the sp56 following this initial report has not appeared and, thus, its role in sperm–zona binding or in signal transduction leading to the acrosome reaction has not been clarified.

G proteins and other effectors of signal transduction pathways leading to the acrosome reaction

Despite the lack of definitive evidence identifying particular sperm surface components to which ZP3 binds, it is clear that binding does occur and that this binding ultimately results in the acrosome reaction (Wassarman, 1990'). Signal transduction components downstream of the receptor have also been studied. The most extensively characterized effectors important for acrosomal exocytosis are the G_i-proteins. The acrosome reaction can be inhibited by pertussis toxin (PT) (Endo, Lee & Kopf, 1987, 1988), a bacterial polypeptide which inactivates the $G_{i\alpha}$ subunit of inhibitory heterotrimeric G-proteins by ADP-ribosylation of that subunit. In contrast, the acrosome reaction is not inhibited by cholera toxin which inactivates the $G_{s\alpha}$ subunit of stimulatory G-proteins (Endo *et al.*, 1988). These initial data suggested that the activity of an inhibitory G-protein is essential for the acrosome reaction. Indeed, a 41 kD polypeptide of mouse sperm has been found to be a substrate for PT-mediated ADP-ribosylation (Endo *et al.*, 1987; Glassner *et al.*, 1991; Ward, Storey & Kopf, 1992). In addition, immunofluorescence microscopy has revealed that $G_{i\alpha}$ subunits are localized to the acrosomal region of intact sperm in mouse, guinea pig (Glassner *et al.*, 1991) and human sperm (Lee, Check & Kopf, 1992).

Searches for other classes of G-proteins in mature sperm have been fruitless. $G_{o\alpha}$ subunits, which modulate the activity of a variety of ion channels, have been immunolocalized in some early developmental stages of spermatogenic cells, but were not found in mature sperm (Karnik *et al.*, 1992). The $G_{z\alpha}$ subunit occurs in the post-acrosomal head region of mature sperm, but does not appear to be a major component of the sperm (Glassner *et al.*, 1991). The $G_{s\alpha}$ subunit does not appear to occur in developing or in mature sperm (Glassner *et al.*, 1991; Karnik *et al.*, 1992). Thus, the major sperm G-proteins are G_i-proteins.

G_i-protein involvement in the acrosome reaction is demonstrated by the fact that solubilized ZPs stimulate GTPase activity and $GRP\gamma[^{34}S]$ binding activity in mouse sperm membrane fractions (Ward *et al.*, 1992). Stimulation of the GTPase activity also protects against ADP-ribosylation of a 40–41 kD polypeptide by PT (Ward *et al.*, 1992), as would be predicted for G-proteins, which are only susceptible to ADP-ribosylation while inactive. The authors have suggested that these data may indicate the presence of a G-protein coupled ZP3 receptor. Treatment of the membrane fraction with mastoparan, a wasp venom derived peptide that activates G-proteins directly, confirmed the activation of GTPase activity and $GTP\gamma[^{35}S]$ binding. In addition, mastoparan will induce the acrosome reaction in intact sperm, suggesting that G-protein activation is sufficient to stimulate exocytosis of acrosomal contents (Ward *et al.*, 1992).

G-protein coupled receptors comprise a highly conserved family of receptors including the adrenergic, serotonergic, dopaminergic and cholinergic receptors. These receptors are characterized by seven conserved transmembrane domains and are often referred to as the serpentine receptors (Probst *et al.*, 1992). Earlier reports have indicated that the acrosome reaction in mouse sperm can be inhibited by 3-quinuclidinyl benzilate (QNB), an antagonist of the muscarinic subclass of cholinergic receptors (Florman & Storey, 1981). This antagonist is correlated with a block in the rise of intracellular free Ca^{2+} normally associated with the acrosome reaction (Storey, Houranic & Kim, 1992). If QNB is acting at the level of a serpentine receptor, such a receptor would be a good candidate for a G_i-protein coupled sperm receptor for ZP3. Recently, an mRNA from a novel member of the serpentine receptor family has been identified by screening of a rat testis cDNA library (Meyerhof, Muller-Brechlin & Richter, 1991). This mRNA is expressed only in the testis and only in sexually mature males. *In situ* hybridization revealed that the message is expressed in cells lining the seminiferous tubules, possibly developing spermatids (Meyerhof *et al.*, 1991). More recently, a G-protein receptor mRNA specifically expressed in human testis has been cloned and shows typical structural features of serpentine type receptors (Parmentier *et al.*, 1992). At present, no protein products from either of these genes have been isolated and the expression of the receptors, localization to specific cell types of the testis including sperm, and function during development or fertilization remain for future studies. Currently, there are essentially no data to identify the sperm components with which the G_i-protein may interact in downstream steps of this signalling pathway.

Tyrosine kinase activity in the form of the p95 sperm ZP3 binding protein is also a possible effector in signalling of the acrosome reaction (Leyton & Saling, 1989*b*; Leyton *et al.*, 1992). As noted previously, inhibition of tyrosine phosphorylation will inhibit the acrosome reaction and phosphorylation not only of the p95, but of several other polypeptides as well. This observation suggests the possibility of a cascade of phosphorylations subsequent to initial activation of the receptor tyrosine kinase activity upon binding ZP3 (Leyton *et al.*, 1992). The possibility of multiple kinases in signalling of the acrosome reaction and the identity or function of possible substrates of the p95 sperm PTK have not been reported.

The identification of G-proteins and of tyrosine kinase activity in signalling during induction of acrosomal exocytosis would appear to be in conflict with previously characterized signalling pathways. G-proteins are generally coupled to serpentine receptors and PTK receptors are generally coupled to a completely different class of G-protein, the small G-proteins. Small G-proteins are monomeric proteins with molecular weights in the range of 20–23 kD. One such small G-protein is the proto-oncogene product *ras*. Recently, *ras* has been localized to the head of human sperm using a monoclonal antibody (Naz, Ahmad & Kaplan, 1992). This same antibody was shown to reduce the fraction of sperm undergoing the acrosome reaction, suggesting that the *ras* protein may function in signalling acrosomal exocytosis. Further studies will be needed to determine the role of *ras* in signalling events during mammalian fertilization. Recently, several reports linking PTK receptors to heterotrimeric G-proteins have been published, suggesting that there is, in fact, cross-talk between these two signalling pathways (Ward & Kopf, 1993). Thus, the current data could represent components of independent and redundant pathways or of a single integrated pathway for induction of the acrosome reaction.

The acrosome reaction in mammalian sperm is Ca^{2+} dependent (see pp. 45–69) and recent studies using phorbol esters to activate the Ca^{2+}/phospholipid-dependent kinase, protein kinase C (PKC), in bull sperm have shown that phorbol ester treatment results in an increase in acrosome reacted sperm (Breitbart *et al.*, 1992). PKC was localized immunologically to the post-acrosomal region of the sperm and staurosporine, an inhibitor of PKC, inhibited the phorbol ester induced increase in acrosome reactions (Breitbart *et al.*, 1992). Following this initial report, further studies will be needed to evaluate role of PKC as an effector in signalling acrosomal exocytosis.

In sperm of the sea urchin *Arbacia ounctulata*, the receptor and effector for signalling the acrosome reaction are in fact the same component, a membrane bound guanylate cyclase receptor (Shimomura, Dangott & Garbets, 1986). Binding of the peptide ligand by the receptor activates its cyclase activity, resulting in production of the second messenger cGMP. Guanylate cyclase receptor proteins are also widespread among vertebrates, and are currently the only example in which a receptor directly generates production of a second messenger (Schulz, Chinkers & Garbers, 1989). To date, however, cGMP has not been implicated in the signal transduction pathway leading to acrosomal exocytosis in mammalian sperm.

Second messengers

The requirement for increased intracellular free Ca^{2+} in signalling of the acrosome reaction has been extensively documented and appears to depend on extracellular sources of Ca^{2+} implying the presence of at least one type of ion channel. Entry of extracellular Ca^{2+} requires the activation of Ca^{2+} channels which could be ligand gated, voltage gated, or G-protein coupled. The absence in mature sperm of G_o-proteins (Karnik *et al.*, 1992) which are found to modulate G-protein coupled as well as voltage-gated channels in some somatic cells would suggest that a 'classical' G-protein modulated channel is not used in this signalling pathway. However, Florman *et al.* (1989) show that PT inhibition of the acrosome reaction also inhibited elevations of intracellular Ca^{2+} and pH, suggesting that these changes may, in fact, be coupled to a G-protein regulated signalling pathway. Depolarization of the sperm plasma membrane, treatment with gramidicin, or treatment with the Ca^{2+} ionophore A23187, is sufficient to induce the acrosome reaction in the absence of ZP3 even after treatment with PT. This observation suggests that the action of the sperm G_i-protein is upstream of the Ca^{2+} influx in this signalling pathway (Florman *et al.*, 1989, 1992). In addition, a voltage gated Ca^{2+} channel has been identified in mammalian sperm using both electrophysiological (Cox & Peterson, 1989) and pharmacological (Babcock & Pfeiffer, 1987) approaches. Activation of this channel is required for acrosomal exocytosis, since pharmacological Ca^{2+} channel blockers inhibit the ZP3-induced acrosome reaction (Babcock & Pfeiffer, 1987; Florman *et al.*, 1989). The intracellular targets of Ca^{2+} and the possible mediation of its action by calmodulin have not been elucidated.

In addition to the influx of Ca^{2+} in response to ZP3, the physiological agonist for acrosomal exocytosis, an efflux of H^+ ions resulting in increased internal pH (pH_i) accompanies ZP3 binding (Babcock & Pfeiffer, 1987; Florman *et al.*, 1989). This increase in pH_i appears to be independent of Ca^{2+} influx since the change in pH_i can occur in the absence of external Ca^{2+}, and Cs^+/valinomycin induced membrane depolarization effectively increases pH_i, but only slightly affects internal Ca^{2+} levels (Babcock & Pfeiffer, 1987). The H^+ efflux is not attributable to a Na^+/H^+ exchange protein since treatment of sperm with amiloride, a compound that blocks Na^+/H^+ exchangers, did not inhibit alkalinization of treated sperm. It is possible, however, that sperm have a unique mechanism for K^+ induced alkalinization (Babcock & Pfeiffer, 1987).

Among the multitude of other second messengers, none has been actively investigated for a possible role in induction of acrosomal exocytosis. The report of protein kinase C (PKC) involvement in acrosomal exocytosis (Breitbart *et al.*, 1992) would suggest the involvement of diacylglycerol (DAG) in addition to Ca^{2+}, but this has yet to be shown directly. Cyclic nucleotides (cAMP and cGMP) have not been implicated in acrosome reactions in mammalian sperm, and the major focus of research in this area appears to be centered on changes in membrane potential leading to increased intracellular free Ca^{2+} and pH_i. Ca^{2+} remains the most downstream component identified in this signalling pathway, and appears to be both necessary and sufficient for acrosomal exocytosis since calcium ionophores result in acrosomal exocytosis. However, the exact role that calcium plays in inducing exocytosis remains to be elucidated in future studies.

Molecules involved in sperm-egg fusion

Following completion of the acrosome reaction, sperm are capable of penetrating the zona pellucida and binding to and fusing with the egg plasma membrane. Sperm–egg fusion is the final step that completes the process of fertilization. The fusion event allows entry of the male pronucleus into the egg and signals the egg to activate its developmental programme.

Fusion with the egg plasma membrane occurs along the equatorial region of the sperm head. Any sperm plasma membrane components involved in sperm–egg binding and fusion would have to be present on the sperm in this region. Several sperm surface components have been investigated for potential roles in sperm–egg fusion. The majority of these components have been identified by immunological methods in which antibodies against sperm surface antigens were shown to specifically inhibit sperm–egg fusion and not prior steps in fertilization (Myles, 1993).

Extensive characterization of one of these antigens, PH-30, in guinea pig sperm has revealed two motifs that may be essential for the binding and fusogenic properties of this protein (Blobel *et al.*, 1992). PH-30 contains a region shared by integrin binding proteins, or disintegrins, which could be used for recognition and binding of the egg plasma membrane. The recognition sequence for integrin binding proteins contains the conserved tripeptide RGD (arginine–glycine–aspartic acid). In PH-30 this peptide has been replaced by TDE (threonine–aspartic acid–glutamic acid) (Blobel *et al.*, 1992). None the less, preliminary experiments indicate that peptides containing this sequence can prevent sperm–egg fusion (Myles, 1993). In addition, PH-30 contains a region homologous to viral fusion peptides that can be modelled as a sided α-helix with most of the bulky, hydrophobic residues on one side. This region of PH-30 could confer the fusogenic properties of this protein (Blobel *et al.*, 1992).

Studies in other species of mammals have identified antigens that appear to be required for proper sperm–egg fusion because fusion is inhibited in the presence of antibodies against the test antigen. To date, none of these sperm surface antigens has been characterized other than by molecular weight (Myles, 1993). Thus, the fusogenic properties of these antigens is only implied by indirect evidence, and the actual structural role of the proteins in sperm–egg fusion remains for further study.

Conclusions

The mammalian sperm cell surface undergoes constant transformation from spermatogenesis through fertilization. In this short review we have shown that both sperm membrane lipids and proteins exhibit a high degree of mosaicism with unique biochemical and biophysical properties. Identification of a variety of proteins have allowed investigators to study the complex series of molecular events that ultimately leads to the syngamy of sperm and egg. However, the synergistic and concerted fusion in which these molecules interact with one another, and with egg associated macromolecules, is still poorly understood. Recent advances in biochemistry, molecular biology, and pharmacology will aid greatly in determining the correct sequence of molecular events leading to sperm–zona adhesion, induction of the acrosome reaction, and sperm–egg plasma membrane fusion.

References

Babcock DF, Pfeiffer, DR. Independent elevation of cytosolic [Ca^{2+}] and pH of mammalian sperm by voltage-dependent and pH-sensitive mechanisms. *J Biol Chem* 1987; **262**: 15041–7.

Benau DA, Storey BT. Characterization of the mouse sperm plasma membrane zona-binding site sensitive to trypsin inhibitors. *Biol Reprod* 1987; **36**: 282–92.

Bleil JD, Greve JM, Wassarman PM. Identification of a secondary sperm receptor in the mouse egg zona pellucida: role in maintenance of binding of acrosome-reacted sperm to eggs. *Devel Biol* 1988; **128**: 376–85.

Bleil JD, Wassarman PM. Structure and function of the zona pellucida: identification and characterization of the proteins of the mouse oocyte's zona pellucida. *Devel Biol* 1980*a*; **76**: 185–202.

Bleil JD, Wassarman PM. Mammalian sperm–egg interaction: identification of a glycoprotein in mouse egg zonae pellucidae possessing receptor activity for sperm. *Cell* 1980*b*; **20**: 873–82.

Bleil JD, Wassarman PM. Galactose at the nonreducing terminus of O-linked oligosaccharides of mouse egg zona pellucida glycoprotein ZP3 is essential for the glycoprotein's sperm receptor activity. *Proc Natl Acad Sci, USA* 1988; **85**: 6778–82.

Bleil JD, Wassarman PM. Identification of a ZP3-binding protein on acrosome-intact mouse sperm by photoaffinity crosslinking. *Proc Natl Acad Sci, USA* 1990: **87**: 5563–7.

Blobel CP, Wolfsberg TG, Turck CW, Myles DG, Primakoff P, White JM. A potential fusion peptide and an integrin ligand domain in a protein active in sperm–egg fusion. *Nature* 1992; **356**: 248–52.

Breitbart H, Lax J, Rotem R, Naor Z. Role of protein kinase C in the acrosome reaction of mammalian spermatozoa. *Biochem J* 1992; **281**: 473–6.

Cardullo RA, Armant DR, Millette CF. Characterization of a fucosyltransferase activity during mouse spermatogenesis: evidence for a cell surface fucosyltransferase. *Biochemistry* 1989; **28**: 1611–17.

Cardullo RA, Wolf DE. The sperm plasma membrane. A little more than mosaic, a little less than fluid. In: RA Bloodgood, ed *Ciliary and Flagellar Membranes* Plenum Press, New York, 1991: 305–36.

Cardullo RA, Wolf DE. Crosslinking mouse sperm galactosyltransferase induces its redistribution but not the acrosome reaction. *Dev Biol* 1994; In Press.

Cornwall GA, Tulsiani DR, Orgebin-Crist MC. Inhibition of the mouse sperm surface alpha-D-mannosidase inhibits sperm–egg binding *in vitro*. *Biol Reprod* 1991; **44**: 913–21.

Cowan AE, Primakoff P, Myles DG. Sperm exocytosis increases the amount of PH-20 antigen on the surface of guinea pig sperm. *J Cell Biol* 1986; **103**: 1289–97.

Cowan AE, Myles DG, Koppel DE. Lateral diffusion of the PH-20 protein on guinea pig sperm: evidence that barriers to diffusion maintain plasma membrane domains in mammalian sperm. *J Cell Biol* 1987; **104**: 917–23.

Cox T, Peterson RN. Identification of calcium conducting channels in isolated boar sperm plasma membranes. *Biochem Biophys Res Comm* 1989; **161**: 162–8.

Endo Y, Lee MA, Kopf GS. Evidence for the role of a guanine nucleotide-binding regulatory protein in the zona pellucida-induced mouse sperm acrosome reaction. *Devel Biol* 1987; **119**: 210–26.

Endo Y, Lee MA, Kopf GS. Characterization of an islet activating protein sensitive site in mouse sperm that is involved in the zona pellucida-induced acrosome reaction. *Devel Biol* 1988; **129**: 12–24.

Florman HM, Corron ME, Kim TD-H, Babcock DF. Activation of Ca^{2+} dependent calcium channels of mammalian sperm is required for zone pellucida-induced acrosomal exocytosis. *Devel Biol* 1992; **152**: 304–14.

Florman HM, Tombes RM, First NL, Babock DF. An adhesion-associated agonist from the zona pellucida activates G protein-promoted elevations of internal Ca^{2+} and pH that mediate mammalian sperm acrosomal exocytosis. *Devel Biol* 1989; **135**: 133–46.

Florman HM, Storey BT. Inhibition of *in vitro* fertilization of mouse eggs: 3-quinuclidinyl benzilate specifically blocks penetration of zonae pellucidae by mouse spermatozoa. *J Exp Zool* 1981; **216**: 159–67.

Florman HM, Wassarman PM. O-linked oligosaccharides of mouse egg ZP3 account for its sperm receptor activity. *Cell* 1985; **41**: 313–24.

Glassner M, Jones J, Kligman I, Woolkalis MJ, Gerton GL, Kopf GS. Immunocytochemical and biochemical characterization of guanine nucleotide-binding regulatory proteins in mammalian spermatozoa. *Devel Biol* 1991; **146**: 438–50.

Gmachl M, Kreil G. Bee venom hyaluronidase is homologous to a membrane protein of mammalian sperm. *Proc Natl Acad Sci, USA* 1993; **90**: 3569–73.

Karnik NS, Newman S, Kopf GS, Gerton GL. Developmental expression of G protein α subunits in mouse spermatogenic cells: evidence that $G_{\alpha i}$ is associated with the developing acrosome. *Devel Biol* 1992; **152**: 393–402.

Lakoski KA, Carron CP, Cabot CL, Saling PM. Epididymal maturation and the acrosome reaction in mouse sperm: response to the zona pellucida develops coincident with modification of M42 antigen. *Biol Reprod* 1988a; **38**: 221–37.

Lakoski KA, Williams C, Saling, PM. Epididymal maturation and the acrosome reaction in mouse sperm: immunological probes reveal post-testicular modifications. *Gamete Res* 1988b; **23**: 21–37.

Langlais J, Kan FW, Granger L, Raymond L, Bleau G, Roberts KD. Identification of sterol acceptors that stimulate cholesterol efflux from human spermatozoa during *in vitro* capacitation. *Gamete Res* 1988; **20**: 185–201.

Lee MA, Check JH, Kopf GS. A guanine nucleotide-binding regulatory protein in human sperm mediates acrosomal exocytosis induced by the human zona pellucida. *Mol Reprod Devel* 1992; **31**: 78–86.

Leyton L, LeGuen P, Bunch D, Saling PM. Regulation of mouse gamete interaction by a sperm tyrosine kinase. *Proc Natl Acad Sci, USA* 1992; **89**: 11692–5.

Leyton L, Saling PM. Evidence that aggregation of mouse sperm receptors by ZP3 triggers the acrosome reaction. *J Cell Biol* 1989a; **108**: 2136–68.

Leyton L, Saling PM. 95 kD sperm proteins bind ZP3 and serve as tyrosine kinase substrates in response to zona binding. *Cell* 1989b; **57**: 1123–30.

Macek MB, Lopez LC, Shur BD. Aggregation of beta-1,4-galactosyltransferase on mouse sperm induces the acrosome reaction. *Devel Biol* 1991; **147**: 440–4.

McKinnon CA, Weaver FE, Yoder JA, Fairbanks G, Wolf DE. Cross-linking a maturation dependent ram sperm plasma membrane antigen induces the acrosome reaction. *Molec Reprod Devel* 1991; **29**: 200–7.

Meyerhof W, Muller-Brechlin R, Richeter D. Molecular cloning of a novel putative G-protein coupled receptor expressed during rat spermiogenesis. *FEBS Lett* 1991; **284**: 155–60.

Miller DJ, Macek MB, Shur BD. Complementarity between sperm surface beta-1,4-galactosyl-transferase and egg-coat ZP3 mediates sperm binding. *Nature (Lond)* 1992; **357**: 589–93.

Myles DG. Molecular mechanisms of sperm–egg membrane binding and fusion in mammals. *Devel Biol* 1993; **158**: 35–45.

Myles DG, Primakoff P, Koppel DE. A localized sperm surface protein of guinea pig sperm exhibits free diffusion in its domain. *J Cell Biol* 1984; **98**: 1905–9.

Myles DG, Primakoff P. Sperm proteins that serve as receptors for the zona pellucida and their post-testicular modification. *Ann NY Acad Sci* 1991; **30**: 486–93.

Naz RK, Ahmad K, Kaplan P. Expression and function of ras proto-oncogene proteins in human sperm cells. *J Cell Sci* 1992; **102**: 487–94.

Parmentier M, Libert F, Schurmans S, Schiffmann S, Lefort A, Eggerickx D, Ledent C, Mollereau C, Gerard C, Perret J, Grootegoed A, Vassart G. Expression of members of the putative olfactory receptor gene family in mammalian germ cells.*Nature (Lond)* 1992; **355**: 453–5.

Phelps BM, Myles DG. The guinea pig sperm plasma membrane protein, PH-20, reaches the surface via two transport pathways and becomes localized to a domain after an initial uniform distribution. *Dev Biol* 1987; **123**: 63–72.

Phelps BM, Primakoff P, Koppel DE, Low MG, Myles DG. Restricted lateral diffusion of PH-20, a PI-anchored sperm membrane protein. *Science* 1988; **240**: 1780–2.

Probst WC, Snyder LA, Schustrr DI, Brosius J, Sealfon SC. Sequence alignment of the G-Protein coupled receptor superfamily. *DNA and Cell Biol* 1992; **11**: 1–20.

Saling PM. Involvement of trypsin-like activity in binding of mouse spermatozoa to zonae pellucidae. *Proc Natl Acad Sci, USA* 1981; **78**: 6231–5.

Schulz S, Chinkers M, Garbers DL. The guanylate cyclase/receptor family of proteins. *FASEB J* 1989; **3**: 2026–35.

Scully NF, Shaper JH, Shur BD. Spatial and temporal expression of cell surface galactosyltransferase during mouse spermatogenesis and epididymal maturation. *Dev Biol* 1987; **124**: 111–24.

Shimomura HL, Dangott LJ, Garbers DL. Covalent coupling of a resact analogue to guanulate cyclase. *J Biol Chem* 1986; **261**: 15778–82.

Shur BD. Cell surface β-1,4 galactosyltransferase: twenty years later. *Glycobiology* 1991; **1**: 563–75.

Shur BD, Hall NG. A role for mouse surface galactosyltransferase in sperm binding to the egg zona pellucida. *J Cell Biol* 1982; **95**: 574–9.

Stefanova I, Horejsi V, Ansotegui IJ, Knapp W, Stockinger H. GPI-anchored cell-surface molecules complexed to protein tyrosine kinases. *Science* 1991; **254**: 1016–19.

Storey BT, Hourani CL, Kim JB. A transient rise in intracellular Ca^{2+} is a precursor reaction to the zona pelluica-induced acrosome reaction in mouse sperm and is blocked by the induced acrosome reaction inhibitor 3-quinuclidinyl benzilate. *Mol Reprod Devel* 1992; **32**: 41–50.

Tulsiani DRP, Skudlarek MD, Orgebin-Crist MC. Novel alpha-D-mannosidase of rat sperm plasma membranes: characterization and potential role in sperm-egg interactions. *J Cell Biol* 1989; **109**: 1257–67.

Tulsiani DR, Nagdas SK, Cornwall GA, Orgebin-Crist MC. Evidence for the presence of high-mannose/hybrid oligosaccharide chain(s) on the mouse ZP2 and ZP3. *Biol Reprod* 1992; **46**: 93–100.

Tulsiani DR, Skudlarek MD, Nagdas SK, Orgebin-Crist MC. Purification and characterization of rat epididymal-fluid alpha-D-mannosidase: similarities to sperm plasma-membrane alpha-D-mannosidase. *Biochem J* 1993; **290**: 427–36.

Ward CR, Kopf GS. Molecular events mediating sperm activation. *Devel Biol* 1993; **158**: 9–34.

Ward CR, Storey BT, Kopf GS. Activation of a G_i protein in mouse sperm membranes by solubilized proteins of the zona pellucida, the egg's extracellular matrix. *J Biol Chem* 1992; **267**: 14016–67.

Wassarman PM. Zona pellucida glycoproteins. *Ann Rev Biochem* 1988; **57**: 415–42.

Wassarman PM. Profile of a mammalian sperm receptor. *Development* 1990; **108**: 1–17.

Weaver FE, Dino JE, Germain BJ, Wolf DE, Fairbanks G. Biochemical characterization and epididymal localization of the maturation-dependent ram sperm surface antigen ESA152. *Molec Reprod Devel* 1993; **35**: 293–301.

Wolf DE. Overcoming random diffusion in polarized cells – coralling the drunken beggar. *Bioassays* 1986; **6**: 116–21.

Wolf DE, Hagopian SS, Lewis RG, Voglmayr JL, Fairbanks G. Lateral diffusion and distribution of a maturation-dependent antigen in the ram sperm plasma membrane. *J Cell Biol* 1986; **102**: 1826–31.

Wolf DE, Lipscomb AC, Maynard VM. Causes of nondiffusing lipid in the plasma membrane of mammalian spermatozoa. *Biochemistry* 1988; **27**: 860–5.

Wolf DE, Maynard VM, McKinnon CA, Melchior DL. Lipid domains in the ram sperm plasma membrane demonstrated by differential scanning calorimetry. *Proc Natl Acad Sci USA* 1990; **87**: 6893–6.

Wolf DE, McKinnon CA, Leyton L, Lakoski-Loveland K, Saling PM. Protein dynamics in sperm membranes: implications for sperm function during gamete interaction. *Molec Reprod Devel* 1992; **33**: 228–34.

3

Sperm structure and function

M. R. CURRY AND P. F. WATSON

Introduction

The primary function of the spermatozoon is to provide the male pronucleus for the fertilized egg. Creation of a new diploid individual critically requires the contribution of both the male and the female haploid pronuclei. The success of this primary function is dependent upon the outcome of a series of secondary processes, the spermatozoon must conserve its DNA, transport it to the site of fertilization and be able to recognize and fuse with the receptive egg. In the higher vertebrates the complexity of this task has been vastly increased both by the advent of internal fertilization and by structural and functional adaptations of the oocyte vestments. The human spermatozoon must make its way from the vagina, the site of semen deposition, to the ampulla of the Fallopian tube, where fertilization will take place, a complex journey through a foreign and potentially hostile environment. Furthermore, during the course of its passage the spermatozoon must complete a process of functional maturation, termed capacitation. Capacitation, simultaneously but independently first identified by Austin and Chang in 1951, is actually an highly ordered series of events, involving reorganization of cell surface components and changes in cell metabolism and motility patterns, and is a prerequisite for sperm penetration of the formidable egg vestments and for fusion with the oocyte. Hence, for fertilization to take place, passage of the spermatozoon through the female reproductive tract and the capacitation process must be coordinated, together with ovulation, in such a way that spermatozoon and oocyte are brought together in a receptive condition within the ampulla of the Fallopian tube.

To enable it to perform these multifarious functions, the spermatozoon has developed a highly specialized morphology with its various structural components elegantly tailored to specific aspects of function. The general appearance of the spermatozoon was first described more than 300 years ago. Using a microscope, consisting of a single highly convex lens, van Leeuwenhoek in 1677 was able to describe the basic structure and swimming behaviour of the spermatozoon. Progressive advances in light microscopy, particularly with the development of the compound microscope, and improvements in resolving power, during the nineteenth century, really only amplified van Leeuwenhoek's description of the external features of the spermatozoon and it was not until the development of transmission electron microscopy in the 1950s that any progress was made in elucidating the complex internal structure of the sperm cell. The spermatozoon can be divided into two major parts, the flagellum concerned with energy production and the initiation and maintenance of motility, and the head containing the all important DNA and the mechanisms for zona recognition and for sperm–egg fusion. Both these two major regions can be further subdivided into a number of cellular compartments each with their own functional correlates. This compartmentalism is a critically important feature of the sperm structure enabling the cell to perform the variety of tasks it must undertake. The structural characteristics of the different cell compartments will be described and will, wherever possible, be related to their functional significance in the overall process of fertilization (for reviews dealing particularly with sperm function see Yanagimachi, 1988; Bavister, Cummins & Roldan, 1990). The role of the various cell membranes will also be examined in an attempt to show how they can complement the underlying compartmented structure of the cell.

Flagellum

The flagellar region is concerned with sperm motility containing both the site of energy production and the propulsive apparatus for the cell. Motility is an essential requirement for fertilization to take place. Spermatozoa first become fully motile on ejaculation and the need for motility is evidenced from the earliest stages of the post-ejaculatory life history; active motility is required to traverse the cervical mucus, to cross the utero-tubal junction and to penetrate the egg vestments.

Fundamental understanding of the mechanisms governing sperm movement has come from study of the flagellar structure and motion of numerous invertebrate species. However, although the basic principles are common to all, the higher vertebrates show a tendency towards increased complexity in their flagellar organization, with the presence of a number of additional structures not seen in the invertebrate models. The flagellum of the human spermatozoon may be divided into four major regions, a short connecting piece, the midpiece, the principal piece and the terminal piece. Each of these regions has a distinct anatomy which is directly related to its function. The four regions will each be considered in turn, together with two structures, the axoneme and the outer dense fibres, which are common to more than one region and will therefore be described separately.

Axoneme

The axoneme or axial filament stretches the full length of the flagellum, through all four regions, and constitutes the motor apparatus of the sperm tail. The organization of the axoneme is similar to that seen in the cilia and flagella of all eukaryotic cells, with two central microtubules surrounded by nine evenly spaced microtubular doublets, the classic $9+2$ pattern (Figs. 1 and 4). Based on this similarity, much of the early understanding of sperm movement came from examining the flagellar structure of lower organisms. The nine peripheral doublets are numbered 1 to 9 in a clockwise direction with 1 being the only doublet situated on a plane perpendicular to that of the two central microtubules (Fig. 1). Each doublet consists of an A subunit forming a complete microtubule, 26 nm in diameter, and a B subunit which is an incomplete microtubule (C-shaped in cross-section) attached by its free edges to the A tubule. The main structural component of these microtubules is tubulin, a protein also linked with a wide range of somatic cell functions (Farrell, 1982). Tubulin molecules are arranged in rows to form protofilaments which are then aligned side by side to form the microtubule walls. The A tubule is composed of 13 protofilaments, as are each of the two central microtubules, the incomplete B tubule is made up of 10 protofilaments. Tubulin is present in two forms, alpha and beta, within protofilaments and differences in electrophoretic mobility, amino acid composition and phosphorylation sites between the two forms results in a high degree of heterogeneity both within and between microtubules. Extending from each A tubule towards the B tubule of the adjacent doublet are pairs of projections, or 'arms', sited at 24 nm intervals and designated by their position as either 'inner' or 'outer'. These arms play a crucial role in flagellar movement as the mechanism by which the chemical energy generated by the mitochondria is translated into the kinetic energy of cell movement. The principal component of the arms is a Ca^{2+} Mg^{2+} dependent ATPase isomer of the protein, dynein. It is the dynein arms that enable adjacent doublets to slide relative to one another, in a system analogous to the sliding filaments seen in muscle contraction, and it is this doublet sliding that generates the flagellar movement. The nine peripheral doublets are each connected to their immediate neighbour by links composed of the protein, nexin (Fig. 1). The nexin links are situated at 96 nm intervals along the length of the doublets and are thought to act as elastic elements regulating the extent of sheer forces during doublet sliding, and retaining the symmetry of the axoneme

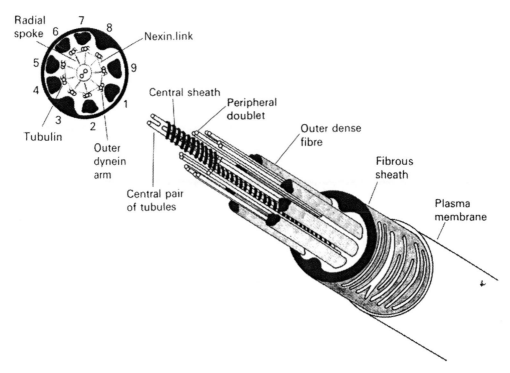

Fig. 1. Diagrammatic representation of the tail elements at the level of the principal piece.

structure. The two central microtubules are interconnected by a series of regularly spaced linkages and are surrounded by a pair of spiral fibres attached to the microtubules at the levels of the connecting links. These two spiral fibres form the central sheath from which a series of radial spokes go out to the A subunit of each doublet (Fig. 4). The function of the central pair of microtubules and of the associated central sheath and radial spokes is unclear; it has been suggested that each of the two fibres of the central sheath supports spokes going to opposing peripheral doublets and that the central complex may in some way initiate an asynchronous sliding of the doublets resulting in the flagellar beat (Pederson, 1970). However, the mechanism by which any such asynchronous activation might be achieved is at present unknown.

Connecting piece

The connecting piece forms a short linking segment (0.5 μ in length) between the flagellum and the sperm head. Its major components are the capitulum, a dense dome-shaped fibrous structure and the segmented columns (Fig. 2). The head–tail

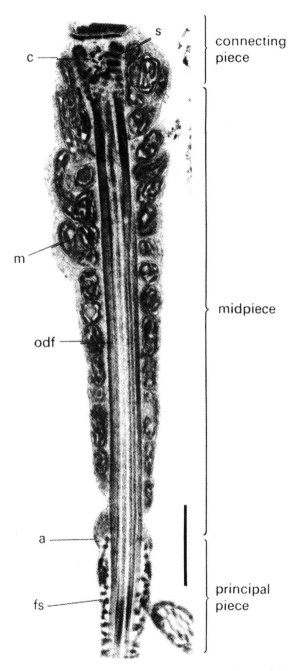

Fig. 2. Longitudinal section through the proximal regions of the flagellum:
a annulus, **c** proximal centriole, **odf** outer dense fibre, **fs** fibrous sheath, **m**
mitochondria, **s** segmented column. (Bar = 500 nm.)

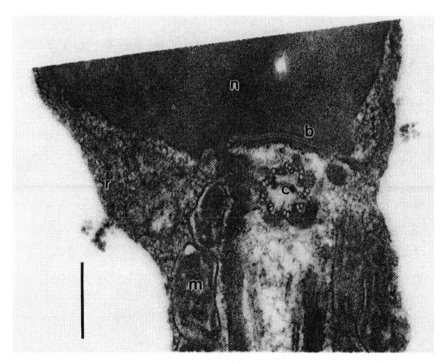

Fig. 3. Longitudinal section through connecting piece: **b** basal plate of nucleus,
c proximal centriole, **m** mitochondrion, **n** nucleus, **r** fold of redundant nuclear
membrane enclosing chromatin-free nuclear space. (Bar = 250 nm.)

connection is mediated by a series of fine proteinaceous filaments between the
capitulum in the connecting piece and the basal plate lying at the caudal surface
of the nucleus. Proximally two pairs of segmented columns fuse to give two major
and five minor columns implanted into the capitulum while distally the nine
columns each overlap and attach to an outer dense fibre in the midpiece (Fig.
2). Although the segmented columns are attached to the outer dense fibres in the
mature spermatozoon, the two arise quite separately and only become linked at
a comparatively late stage in spermiogenesis. The columns are cross-striated, with
a periodicity of 6.5 nm between segments, each segment having nine or ten
horizontal striations. No function, beyond that of a simple structural connection,
has been confirmed for the apparently complex organization of the segmented
columns. However, it is possible that the columns are articulated, thus giving
flexibility to the neck region to allow bending without placing stress on the
capitulum–basal plate link.

The capitulum is also the site of the proximal centriole, positioned at right
angles to the axis of the flagellum (Fig. 3). The proximal centriole is the single
remainder of the pair of centrioles since the distal centriole disintegrates during

the later stages of spermiogenesis. The centrioles play an important role in the construction of the axoneme during spermiogenesis, but do not appear to be essential for its proper functioning in the adult spermatozoon (Woolley & Fawcett, 1973). The centrioles have a similar structure to that of the axoneme but lack the central pair of microtubules and have peripheral triplets rather than the axonemal tubular doublets. The proximal centriole marks the origin of the pair of central microtubules of the axoneme with the peripheral doublets arising more distally.

Outer dense fibres

The axoneme of the eutherian spermatozoon is surrounded by complex accessory structures, not seen in the simpler invertebrate flagella, termed the outer dense fibres. Each of the microtubule doublets is associated with an outer dense fibre arising at the distal end of the segmented columns and terminating at some variable along the principal piece. Individual fibres, numbered by their association with particular axonemal doublets, have a characteristic shape in cross-section although all are approximately teardrop shaped with the rounded edge outermost and tapering towards the axoneme (Fig. 4). Size and thickness varies with species, those of the human spermatozoon being relatively small. Each fibre is composed of a dense core or medulla surrounded by an incomplete cortex which covers the abaxial surface but is absent from the surface adjacent to the microtubule doublet. The medulla is highly stabilized, composed of a keratin-like protein rich in cysteine and with extensive disulphide cross-linkages. The cortex is less stabilized than

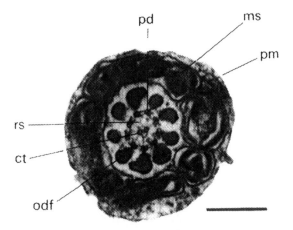

Fig. 4. Cross-section of flagellum through midpiece: **ct** central pair of tubules, **ms** mitochondrial sheath, **odf** outer dense fibre, **pm** plasma membrane, **pd** peripheral doublet, **rs** radial spoke. (Bar = 250 nm.)

the medulla and is soluble with SDS treatment. Surface replicas of the cortex show striations with a periodicity of 40 nm at an angle of 60–80° to the axis of the fibre. The striations appear to be composed of a double line of 6–8 nm diameter globular subunits. In human spermatozoa, it is claimed that this substructure also exists in the medulla (Pedersen, 1972a). The outer dense fibres are not all of equal length; in the human flagellum they extend along 60% of the principal piece and can be divided into three groups, two short fibres, numbers 3 and 8 (6 μm), three medium fibres, numbers 2, 4 and 7 (17–21 μm), and four long fibres, numbers 1, 5, 6 and 9 (31–35 μm). Although fibre lengths may vary between spermatozoa the order of termination is constant (Serres, Escalier & David, 1983).

The close association of the outer dense fibres with the axoneme together with the complexity of their structure has resulted in a range of suggestions, but no clear consensus as to their function. The fibres have no contractile proteins but may have ATPase (Baccetti, Pallini & Burrini, 1973) and or calcium-binding properties which might indicate a role in the control of motility. In invertebrate species, devoid of outer dense fibres, maximum curvature of the tail is achieved only a short distance from the head, whereas in the human sperm maximum curvature is seen only in that region of the principal piece marked by the progressive disappearance of the outer dense fibres (Serres *et al.*, 1983). Thus, the fibres appear to act as stiffening rods within the tail. Furthermore, there is a clear correlation between the size of the outer dense fibres and the degree of curvature of the flagellum in different species; human sperm, with relatively small outer dense fibres, having a comparatively flexible flagellum. The asymmetrical disappearance of the outer dense fibres may result in unequal constraints on different sides of the axoneme that could influence the plane of the flagellar beat. A stiffening function for the outer dense fibres must, however, be reconciled with the exaggerated curvature of the flagellar beat seen during phases of hyperactivated motility.

Midpiece

The midpiece of the flagellum (3.5 μ in length) stretches from the distal end of the connecting piece to the annulus, a circumferential band marking the junction of the midpiece and the principal piece. The major distinguishing characteristic of the midpiece is the presence of the mitochondrial sheath consisting of a species-specific number of mitochondria lying end to end in a helical arrangement around the underlying axoneme. The human spermatozoon has a helix composed of 11–15 gyres (Fig. 2), with on average two mitochondria to each gyre; junctions between mitochondria are situated randomly, although in some other species mitochrondrial junctions may be aligned in register along the length of the sheath

(Phillips, 1970). In fact, the mitochondrial sheath of the human spermatozoon often has a rather disorganized appearance in contrast to the highly regular arrangement seen in other mammalian species. The internal mitochondrial structure is similar to that seen in other cell-types, however, sperm mitochondria are unusual in the great stability of their outer membranes. This high degree of stability is evidenced by mitochondrial resistance to osmotic changes (Keyhani & Storey, 1973) and to detergent treatments (Bedford & Calvin, 1974), and may be related to the ordered particular arrays seen in freeze–etch preparations of sperm mitochondrial membranes (Friend & Heuser, 1981), or to the presence of disulphide bonds (Wallace, Cooper & Calvin, 1983). The functional significance of a highly stabilized mitochrondrial membrane is unclear; one suggestion is that it may serve to resist alternate stretching and compression of the mitochondria during the flagellar beat. The mitochondrial inner membrane is the site of energy production for the spermatozoon and the position of the mitochondria surrounding the root of the flagellum, favours the ready supply of ATP to the axoneme for sperm motility. However, many invertebrate sperm have very few mitochondria to maintain cell motility and the requirement for such a relatively large mitochondrial sheath in the eutherian species is as yet unexplained, but may reflect a greater energy requirement generated by the need for prolonged motility associated with the complexities of internal fertilization (Favard & Andre, 1970).

Principal piece

The principal piece, as it name suggests, is the longest segment of the flagellum extending from the annulus to the proximal end of the short terminal piece, a length of approximately 55 μm. The principal piece is characterized by the presence of the fibrous sheath, a cytoskeletal structure surrounding the axoneme and the outer dense fibres (Figs. 1 and 6). The sheath consists of two peripheral longitudinal columns, positioned in the plane of the central microtubule pair, which are connected together round the circumference of the tail by a series of ribs composed of closely packed filaments. In the human spermatozoon the ribs are 10–20 nm apart and approximately 50 nm thick. The longitudinal columns overlie and are fused with the two short outer dense fibres (3 and 8), and beyond the termination of these fibres the columns continue attached to their underlying microtubule doublets. The constituent proteins of the fibrous sheath have extensive disulphide bonding making the whole structure extremely stable. The function of the fibrous sheath would appear to be similar or complimentary to that proposed for the outer dense fibres acing as an elastic 'corset' restricting and controlling flagellar movement. The fact that pathological human specimens with

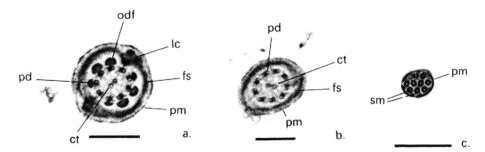

Fig. 5. Cross-sections of flagellum through (*a*) proximal and (*b*) distal principal piece and through (*c*) terminal piece: **fs** fibrous sheath, **lc** longitudinal column of fibrous sheath, **odf** outer dense fibre (longitudinal columns have replaced fibres 3 and 8 in (*a*), all outer dense fibres have terminated in (*b*)), **pd** peripheral doublets, **pm** plasma membrane, **sm** single 'A' tubule. (Bars = 250 nm.)

a disorganized fibrous sheath show severely disrupted motility indicates the importance of the sheath to normal motility patterns.

Terminal piece

Beyond the distal end of the fibrous sheath is the short (3 μm) terminal piece of the flagellum. The microtubular elements of the axoneme terminate in this region, in general following a regular pattern although variations are not uncommon. First, the dynein arms disappear and the A subunit takes on an 'hollow' appearance (Pedersen, 1972*a*). The central pair of microtubules terminate and two of the outer doublets move to the centre to be surrounded by seven unevenly spaced doublets. The doublets separate and the open B tubules successively disappear leaving a circle of single microtubules usually surrounding a single central tubule and bounded by the plasma membrane (Fig. 5(*c*)). There is successive termination of the remaining tubules as the tip of the flagellum is reached. In some invertebrate species, this region has been shown to be incapable of active bending, merely tailing the rest of the flagellar beat.

Head

The functions of the sperm head are to contain and conserve the cell DNA and to deliver it at the time of fertilization by fusing with the egg. To achieve this, the DNA must be held in a stable form until required for formation of the male pronucleus, the spermatozoon must be able to penetrate the extensive egg vestments to reach the oocyte surface, there must be some mechanism for species-specific sperm–egg recognition, and there must be the capability for

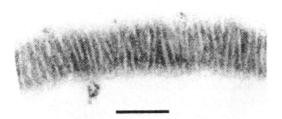

Fig. 6. Tangential longitudinal section through fibrous sheath showing circumferential ribs. (Bar = 250 nm.)

membrane fusion. The sperm head contains a very limited range of structures with which to perform these functions; apart from the nucleus the only major organelles in the head region are the acrosome and the post-acrosomal sheath (Fig. 7). Sperm–egg recognition is primarily a function of the head plasma membrane as described below. The basic organization of the sperm head is common to all mammalian sperm but the size and shape of both the nucleus and the acrosome, and therefore of the head itself, are extremely variable and highly species specific. For human spermatozoa, the head shape is described as pleomorphic, presenting a very heterogeneous range of appearances, and making the definition of a 'normal' shape and size extremely difficult (Fig. 6). Nevertheless, the normal sperm head is considered to be about 4.5 μm in length and about 3 μm at its widest point. It is slightly bilaterally flattened but much less so than those of ungulate species.

Acromsome

The acrosome or literally terminal body, is a membrane-bound vesicle forming a cap-like covering over the anterior part of the nucleus. In the human spermatozoon the acrosome is relatively small, covering approximately two-thirds of the nucleus but not extending much beyond its anterior edge (Fig, 7). The outer acrosomal membrane lies directly beneath the plasma membrane and is continuous at the posterior margins of the cap with the inner acrosomal membrane which overlays the nuclear envelope. The two membranes are broadly parallel enclosing a narrow space filled by the acrosomal matrix. The matrix consists of a number of different hydrolytic enzymes packed in an ordered paracrystalline array. The two major, and best characterized, enzymes are hyaluronidase and acrosin, a trypsin-like proteinase present in an inactive zymogen form as proacrosin; human spermatozoa also contain a second zymogen called sperminogen (Siegel *et al.*, 1987). The inactive state of these zymogens may be

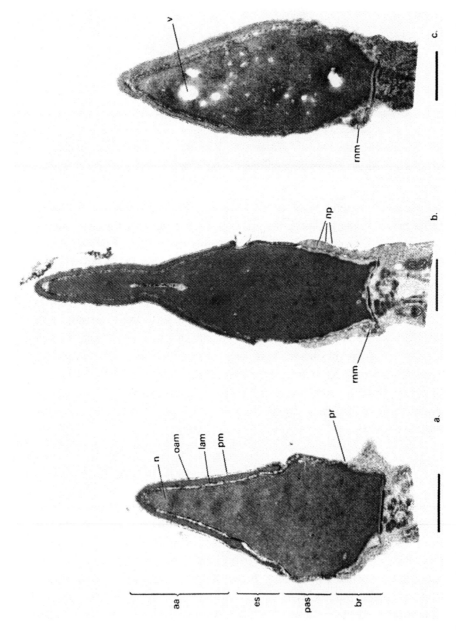

Fig. 7. Longitudinal sections through sperm heads: **aa** anterior acrosome, **br** basal region, **es** equatorial segment, **iam** inner asrosomal membrane, **n** nucleus, **np** nuclear membrane pores, **oas** outer acrosomal membrane, **pas** post-acrosomal sheath, **pm** plasma membrane, **pr** posterior ring, **rnm** redundant nuclear membrane, **v** nuclear vacuole. (Bars = 250 nm.)

promoted by complexing with specific inhibitors within the acrosomal matrix (Zaneveld, Polarkoski & Williams, 1973). Other enzymes present include acid phosphatase, phospholipases, N-acetylglucosaminidase and collaginase, the matrix is also rich in carbohydrates. There is evidence, from some animal species, that the various enzymes may not be randomly distributed throughout the acrosome but packaged so as to allow sequential activation and release of different emzymes (Holt, 1979). Enzymes are released in the course of the acrosome reaction, a major exocytotic event in the life history of the spermatozoon (see below).

A unique feature of eutherian spermatozoa is the presence of a stable region situated at the posterior border of the acrosomal cap, termed the equatorial segment. In the human spermatozoon the equatorial segment is crescent shaped and extends, at its widest point, to approximately one-quarter of the total acrosome length, it can be identified in cross-section by an abrupt narrowing of the acrosomal space to 40–45 nm in width compared to 70–80 nm in the anterior region (Fig. 7). The acrosomal membranes of the equatorial segment are lined with an electron dense material giving a pentalaminar appearance in thin section with electron dense septa or cross bridges between the membranes. Surface replicas of the outer membranes show rows of evenly spaced, hexagonally packed membrane particles. The enzyme-rich matrix present in the anterior acrosome is absent from the equatorial region. The equatorial segment is also a site of veimentin accumulation in the human spermatozoon (Virtanen *et al.*, 1984). These features suggest a very stable membrane structure probably with extensive interactions with cytoskeletal elements. The equatorial segment remains intact following the acrosome reaction and it is at the border between the anterior acrosome and the equatorial segment that the outer acrosomal membrane fuses with the plasma membrane to maintain cell integrity after loss of the acrosomal cap (see below). The plasma membrane domain overlying the equatorial segment is the site of sperm–egg recognition and ultimately of membrane fusion. The equatorial segment of the acrosome is therefore well placed to stabilize this critical membrane region, particularly during the penetration of the zona pellucida following the acrosome reaction.

Whilst much has been learned concerning the structure of the acrosome and of the mechanisms controlling the acrosome reaction, its precise function in the process of fertilization remains unclear. The necessity for the acrosome reaction to take place is well established, and it has been generally accepted that the hydrolytic enzymes released serve to assist the spermatozoon in its passage through the extensive cumulus mass and in its penetration of a formidable zona pellucida. However, there are a number of evident anomalies when considering this proposition. If the contents of the acrosome are dispersed so as to act on the cumulus matrix during sperm passage to the zona surface no enzyme will remain to facilitate zona penetration. To overcome this problem, the presence of acrosin bound to the inner acrosomal membrane has been postulated, but careful examination of acrosome-reacted spermatozoa from animal species has so far failed to detect any such bound enzyme (Harrison, 1982). Furthermore, acrosome intact sperm are apparently fully able to traverse the cumulus mass and reach the zona surface. A number of egg-related putative inducers of the acrosome reaction have been demonstrated including follicular fluid, zona proteins and progesterone, but the precise site of the normal acrosome reaction *in vivo* remains ill defined. The role of acrosomal enzymes in zona penetration is also confused; the very narrow, sharply defined penetration slit created by the spermatozoon does not seem consistent with an enzymic digestion of the zona. It has been suggested that the great stability of the membrane systems, and in the nucleus itself, argue for a mechanical penetration with the spermatozoon forcing its way through the zona perhaps utilizing the greater force generated by the hyperactivated motility pattern. However, evidence suggests spermatozoa are unable to penetrate the zona by force alone and a combination of thrust and soluble enzyme leading to a strain induced proteolysis and hence to formation of the penetration slit has been proposed (Green, 1988).

Perinuclear material

Directly beneath the acrosome and separating it from the nucleus is a thin layer of perinuclear material. Stabilized by disulphide bridges, the perinuclear material forms a continuous layer coating the nucleus and appears to act as a 'cement-like' substance between the acrosome and the nucleus. The human spermatozoon does not appear to have any specialized spical projection that would correspond to the perforatorium prominent in the spermatozoa of rodents and some other mammalian species (Olson, Hamilton & Fawcett, 1976). Posteriorly to the acrosome, this material forms the post-acrosomal sheath. Longitudinal sections through the sperm head show the post-acrosomal sheath to be composed of two distinct regions separated by a shallow groove in the plasma membrane. The anterior region of the sheath consists of a homogeneous layer of electron dense material lying parallel to the plasma membrane and separated from it by approximately 20 nm. Along this layer are a series of rounded projections extending towards the plasma membrane with a separation of 12 nm between them (Pedersen, 1972*b*). This pattern seen only in longitudinal section suggests a series of regularly spaced ridges arranged circumferentially around the sperm head. Freeze–etched preparations show the surface of the anterior region to be rather featureless (Fig. 7), with no surface structures corresponding to the ridges seen in section. The posterior region of the sheath is composed of granular material with no particular features seen in longitudinal section but with a series of obliquely oriented cordlike structures visible in freeze-etched preparations (Koehler, 1972). Despite its apparently rather complex structure, no functional significance has yet been assigned to the post-acrosomal sheath.

Nucleus

The chromatin of the sperm nucleus consists of DNA complexed with highly basic proteins termed protamines, rich in arginine and cysteine. Unlike the histones of somatic nuclei which are highly conserved, sperm nucleoproteins show considerable differences between species. Most mammalian species have a single predominant protamine but human and mouse spermatozoa have been shown to contain two (Kolk & Samuel, 1975). The basic character of the protamines is sufficient to neutralize the charge of the phosphate–ester backbone in the DNA and to allow the very close packing of the chromatin. The high cysteine content of the protamines allows the formation of disulphide cross bridges between free thiols. This cross linking, which gives the nucleus its highly stable keratinoid nature, begins during the later stages of spermiogenesis but is mainly accomplished during passage through the epididymis. The great stability of the nucleus, and consequently the severe treatments required to disrupt it, has made the arrangement of the chromatin packing difficult to uncover. Sperm DNA exists in beta form, probably in the highly folded configuration favoured by neutralization of its negative charge through complexing with protamines. The most probable arrangement appears to be in tightly packed nucleoprotein cords in an hexagonal array consistent with the lamellar appearance seen in some freeze–fracture preparations (Balhorn, 1982).

The nucleus contains the haploid chromosome number, one half of each chromosome pair, and the DNA is completely inactive and does not replicate until the protamines are displaced after sperm entry into the egg.

Nuclear shape is highly species specific, determined by the sperm genotype and most species show a very high degree of uniformity. Human spermatozoa are an exception to this rule exhibiting a great variety of nuclear shapes ranging from elongate tapering forms to short rounded nuclei (Fig. 7). Previously it has even been thought that the population was dimorphic representing male and female spermatozoa, but this is obviously not the case. However, the range of nuclear shape does make it difficult to define a morphologically 'normal' oval-shaped human sperm nucleus. The heterogeneity in nuclear shape may be linked to heterogeneity in chromatin condensation, many nuclei having numerous vacuoles and areas of poorly condensed chromatin (Fig. 7(c)). It is not known whether these vacuoles and other condensation defects adversely affect the fertility of the spermatozoa.

The posterior ring, or striated band, is a circumferential junction between the plasma membrane and the nuclear envelope composed of a series of fine cords or striations made up of small membrane particles (Pedersen, 1972b). The posterior ring, like the annulus of the flagellum, is a physical barrier between membrane domains; it acts as a major dividing point separating the sperm flagellum and head regions.

The nuclear envelope anterior to the striated band has a narrow apposition of its inner and outer laminae and a complete absence of nuclear pores (Bedford & Hoskins, 1990). These unusual features probably reflect the inert nature of the sperm nucleus with its highly condensed chromatin and lack of any synthetic function. Caudal to the striated band the nuclear envelope forms folds of apparently redundant membrane enclosing a variable amount of posterior nuclear space empty of any chromatin (Figs. 3, 7(b),(c)). These folds of membrane have a wider apposition between their laminae, and have numerous densely packed nuclear pores in a regular hexagonal arrangement. This portion of the membrane appears to be a remnant from an early stage in spermiogenesis when nucleo-cytoplasmic interaction is involved in shaping the sperm nucleus. At the base of the nucleus, the envelope has a specialized structure forming the surface of the implantation fossa for the sperm tail. The narrow space between the inner and outer laminae is traversed by regular periodic densities 60 nm apart; these interlaminar bridges have an important role in maintaining the head-tail connection. The outer lamina of the fossa is covered by a layer of electron dense material forming the basal plate which constitutes an anchor point for fibres passing to the capitulum of the connecting piece of the tail. The implantation fossa of the human spermatozoon is much flatter and less developed than the concave structure seen in other mammalian species (Bedford, 1967).

Cytoplasmic droplet

The cytoplasmic droplet consists of the remains of the residual cytoplasm made redundant after the morphological reshaping of the cell during spermiogenesis. In the majority of animal species the droplet moves distally along the flagellum during passage through the epididymis, and is shed during ejaculation. However, human spermatozoa frequently retain a voluminous droplet in the form of a cytoplasmic collar around the connecting/midpiece of the flagellum. The droplet often contains numerous redundant organelles including ribosomes and mito-chrondria. The presence of the cytoplasmic droplet is not considered to be pathological in human spermatozoa and there is no evidence that its presence in any way compromises the normal functioning of the cell.

Plasma membrane

As with other cell types, the sperm plasma membrane serves as a continuous limiting cell boundary, maintaining cell integrity and forming a dynamic interface between the cell and its immediate environment. However, unlike many other cell types, both the structure and function of the sperm plasma membrane are highly heterogeneous, with a number of sharply defined membrane domains. This regional specialization, is evidenced by physical, chemical and immunological parameters and reflects both the surface properties and the three-dimensional architecture of the membrane. Furthermore, the components and pattern of membrane domains established during passage through the male reproductive tract are not fixed but undergo reorganization during the capacitation process within the female tract.

The sperm surface has five major membrane domains, each closely associated with an underlying cell compartment and each involved with different aspects of cell function. The flagellum has distinct domains over the midpiece and the principal piece, and the head has three major domains covering the acrosome, the equatorial region and the post-acrosomal region. These various membrane areas differ in their binding affinity for plant lectins (Koehler, 1981), reflecting differences in the extent and make up of their glycocalyx. There are differences in membrane fluidity and in lipid composition revealed by various molecular probes (Friend, 1982). Freeze–fracture and freeze–etch preparations (Fig. 8) show differences in intramembranous particle distributions (Friend, 1982). Different domains show different binding patterns for specific monoclonal antibodies (Villarroya & Scholler, 1986), and there are differences in the membrane surface charge (Yanagimachi *et al.*, 1972). This regional membrane specialization allows the underlying cellular compartments to interact independently with their external environment, thereby enabling the efficient performance of the various tasks necessary for successful fertilization.

The mechanisms by which characteristic membrane domains are established and maintained in what is theoretically a fluid membrane are not fully understood. Clear boundary structures exist between some domains, e.g. the annulus and the posterior ring, but other regions show restricted mobility of membrane components in the absence of any apparent physical barrier, or may restrict certain antigens and not others, or restrict antigens at certain stages of development only. There is evidence for a complementary regional specialization of cytoskeletal elements underlying the plasma membrane which may serve to maintain the boundaries of separate domains. The distribution of actin, spectrin and vimentin can be correlated with the different membrane domains, the anterior acrosome and principal piece are sites of actin and spectrin (spectrin appears to be the major calmodulin binding protein in spermatozoa) whilst vimentin is restricted to the

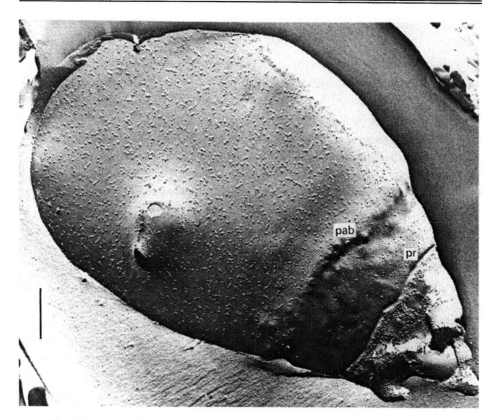

Fig. 8. Freeze–etching showing plasma membrane of sperm head in face view: **pab** posterior border of acrosome, **pr** posterior ring. (Bar = 500 nm.) (Reprinted from Koehler JK. *J Ultrastruct. Res* 1972; **39**: 520–39. With permission of Academic Press and the author.)

equatorial segment (Virtanen *et al.*, 1984). Alternatively, membrane domains may be maintained by association with their particular underlying organelles such as the acrosome in the head or the fibrous sheath of the flagellum. These mechanisms do not, however, explain the dynamic nature of the domain structure which changes over the life span of the spermatozoon. The fact that cell death is accompanied by loss of domain structure indicates that the maintenance of membrane domains is, at least in part, an active process within the cell. The unique regional membrane composition facilitates the simultaneous achievement of a number of cell processes, e.g. capacitation and motility.

Midpiece region

The midpiece plasma membrane must permit the passage of substrates to the mitochrondrial sheath, and it seems likely that important changes in cell metabolism during capacitation are mediated via changes in the midpiece plasma membrane. The membrane overlying the mitochondrial sheath contains chains of intramembranous particles that follow the underlying mitochondrial helix and which are absent from the interstices between mitochondria. In these regions the membrane is found to be very closely applied to the mitochondrial sheath. These particles were first recognized, and are especially apparent, in the guinea pig spermatozoon (Friend & Fawcett, 1974) but in other species, areas of hexagonally packed particles are seen which similarly follow the helix of the mitochondria. This arrangement of particles bears a similarity to the 'necklace' of somatic cell cilia and flagella, consisting of strands of membrane particles surrounding the axoneme adjacent to the basal plate (Gilula & Satir, 1972). It has been suggested that the necklace is situated in an energy transducing region of the cilium, probably mediated via Ca^{2+} influx, and that its function is to control local membrane permeability. However, although the ciliary necklace, like the $9+2$ axoneme structure, appears to be universally present in somatic cell cilia and flagella, the sperm flagellum appears to lack the typical necklace structure. This may reflect the greater complexity of the sperm flagellum and/or differences in the mechanisms regulating flagellar movement.

Principal piece region

The principal piece generates the motive force for sperm movement and, for it to function efficiently, the axonemal complex must be attached to the plasma membrane, rather than beat within an unattached membrane envelope. This attachment can be seen in the so-called 'zipper', a longitudinal double row of staggered intramembranous particles overlying outer dense fibre number 1 (Friend & Fawcett, 1974). These particles traverse the membrane and their appearance in freeze–etched preparations suggests that, as well as forming a mechanical attachment, they may have a role in controlling axonemal functions, such as the changing pattern of flagellar beat seen during capacitation. However, zipper particles attach to the ribs of the fibrous sheath, the presence of the sheath and of the outer dense fibres between the particles and the axoneme argues against a regulatory function.

The membrane domains of the midpiece and the principal piece are separated by the annulus, a fibrous ring underlying the plasma membrane and attached to it by circumferential strands of intramembranous particles. The annulus appears to act as a physical barrier restricting the movement of membrane particles between the two domains, although at least in the guinea pig, antigens are able to cross the annulus from principle to midpiece after capacitation. This easing of the barrier between membrane domains may be related to the functional changes in motility (hyperactivation) occurring during capacitation.

Anterior acrosomal region

The plasma membrane covering the anterior portion of the sperm head is involved in two major processes, the initial recognition and binding to the zona pellucida, and fusion with the underlying outer acrosomal membrane in the exocytotic acrosome reaction. Both these functions can be related to changes in particular aspects of membrane structure occurring with capacitation. Zona-binding is probably mediated by complex glycoconjugates present in the membrane glycocalyx which is extensive in this region. The composition of the glycocalyx, as revealed by lectin binding patterns, established on ejaculation undergoes extensive reorganization and loss during capacitation prior to zona attachment (Cross & Overstreet, 1987). The potential fusogenic nature of the membrane is reflected by changes in membrane fluidity, patchy clearance of intramembranous particles and by changes in the membrane lipid composition (Flechon, 1985). These various changes together result in a destabilized region of plasma membrane able to fuse with the outer acrosomal membrane on initiation of the acrosome reaction. The first observable change after the initiation of the acrosome reaction is the decondensation and swelling of the matrix resulting in a wave-like appearance of the outer acrosomal membrane, rapidly followed by the appearance of point fusions between the plasma membrane and the outer acrosomal membrane. This initial fusion is a process of fenestration creating a series of holes in the plasma membrane and the outer acrosomal membrane (Fig. 9). Under *in vitro* conditions, after approximately 20 seconds fenestration is complete, and the point fusions have coalesced resulting in the surface of the acrosome being covered with hybrid vesicles (Fig. 9), composed of both plasma membrane and outer acrosomal membranes (Yudin, Gottlieb & Meizel, 1988). These vesicles are mostly spherical and of varying sizes. The acrosomal matrix is relatively undispersed at this stage although it is no longer confined within the membranes. By three minutes the matrix is almost fully lost, membrane vesicles are still present and undergo only a gradual dispersion with time. At this point the inner acrosomal membrane has become the limiting membrane in the anterior region of the head. There have been reports that the human sperm acrosome reaction differs from this pattern, which has been established for a number of mammalian species. It has been suggested that, at least initially, vesicle formation results from invagination of the outer acrosomal membrane producing homogeneous vesicles, and that fusion only occurs after vesicle formation is complete (Nagae *et al.*, 1986). However, the most recent descriptions of the human acrosome reaction appear to support the generally held model (Fig. 10).

Before the acrosome reaction can be initiated, the spermatozoon must undergo capacitation involving the changes in the plasma membrane previously described

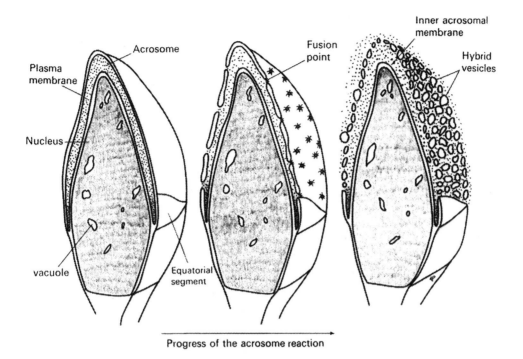

Fig. 9. Diagram showing the progress of the acrosome reaction which involves point fusions of the outer acrosomal membrane and the overlying plasma membrane, point fusions coalesce leaving hybrid vesicles and releasing acrosomal contents. The equatorial segment remains intact.

and also important changes in the acrosomal membranes. Like the plasma membrane the acrosomal membranes are of a heterogeneous nature with marked differences between the inner and outer membranes, differences which reflect their respective roles in the acrosome reaction and subsequent zona penetration. After capacitation the outer acrosomal membrane is unstable and easily disrupted by mild detergent treatments, the inner membrane is by contrast highly stable and quite unaffected by similar treatments. The instability of the outer membrane is consistent with the requirement that it fuse with the plasma membrane whilst the stability of the inner membrane is important for its role as limiting cell membrane, particularly during penetration of the zone when the membrane may come under considerable stress as the sperm head forces its way through the zona pellucida. The basis of the inner acrosomal membrane's greater stability is unclear, it may be associated with the characteristic crystalline arrangement of its intramembranous particles or it may depend on underlying cytoskeletal elements present in the perinuclear material (Huang & Yanagimachi, 1985).s

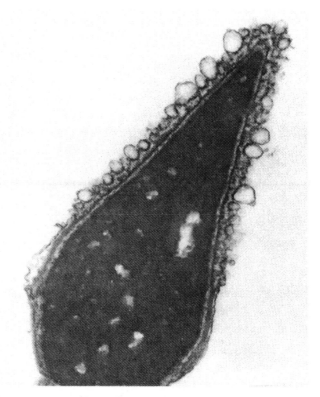

Fig. 10. Electron micrograph showing the acrosome reaction. (Reprinted from Yudin *et al. Gam Res* 1988; **20**: 11–24, with the permission of the copyright owner, © Wiley-Liss, a division of John Wiley & Sons Inc, and the authors.)

Equatorial region

The equatorial segment is the ultimate site of membrane fusion with the oocyte. However, sperm–egg fusion can only occur after the acrosome reaction has been completed (Yanagimachi, 1988). This would seem to indicate that an important physiological membrane change is occurring in the equatorial region at or around the time of the acrosome reaction but no major structural changes to the membrane in this region have been identified to account for this. The membrane of the equatorial region is highly stable and probably acts as a barrier preventing diffusion of intramembranous particles between the anterior and post-acrosomal membrane domains.

Post-acrosomal region

Freeze–fracture preparations show this region to have a denser population of intramembranous particles than the anterior acrosomal membrane, with apparent cords or bands of particles running away from the posterior ring (Koehler, 1972). These cords may be considered homologous to the much more obvious and elaborate 'basal striations' seen in the larger sperm heads of species such as the bull and the rabbit. These species all display a distinct anterior 'bumpy' domain and a posterior structurally more complex domain in the post-acrosomal region. This clear division is not present in the human spermatozoon which has only indistinct basal striations posteriorly and an anterior domain consisting of an irregular smooth ridge around the base of the acrosome.

Conclusion

Consideration of the detailed cellular anatomy of the spermatozoon reinforces the view that function determines structure. While this is clearly apposite for many features of the spermatozoon, there are some which do not support this thesis, e.g. the particular shape of the nucleus and the acrosome. Whether this is due to as yet inadequate understanding of the function remains to be elucidated. A proper hesitation is appropriate in ascribing particular functions in view of changes in understanding as knowledge has increased. In evidence for this is the putative role(s) of the acrosomal enzymes, whose precise function is as yet uncertain, in spite of confident assertions in the past.

There can be little doubt that the highly specialized sperm cell still represents a considerable intellectual challenge to the cell biologist, and whose secrets will yield stimulating rewards for persistent and perceptive study.

Acknowledgements

The authors acknowledge the support of the Medical Research Council (Research Grant No. G8912737SB).

References

Baccetti B, Pallini V, Burrini AG. The accessory fibres of the sperm tail. 1. Structure and chemical composition of the bull coarse fibres. *J Submicrosc Cytol* 1973; **5**: 237–56.

Balhorn R. A model for the structure of chromatin in mammalian sperm. *J Cell Biol* 1982; **93**: 298–305.

Bavister BD, Cummins J, Roldan RS (eds.). *Fertilization in Mammals.* Norwell, Mass.: Serono Symposia, 1990. 469 pp.

Bedford JM. Observations on the fine structure of spermatozoa of the Bush Baby (*Galago senegalensis*), the African Green Monkey (*Cercopithecus aethiops*) and Man. *Am J Anat* 1967; **121**: 443–60.

Bedford JM, Calvin HI. Changes in –S–S– linked structures of the sperm tail during epididymal maturation with comparative observations in sub-mammalian species. *J Exp Zool* 1974; **187**: 181–204.

Bedford JM, Hoskins DD. The mammalian spermatozoon: morphology, biochemistry and physology. In: Lamming GE, ed. *Marshall's Physiology of Reproduction*, 4th ed. Vol. II. Edingurgh: Churchill Livingstone, 1990: 379–568.

Cross NL, Overstreet JW. Glycoconjugates of the human sperm surface: distribution and alterations that accompany capacitation *in vitro*. *Gam Res* 1987; **16**: 23–35.

Farrell KW. Purification and reassembly of tubulin from outer doublet microtubules. *Methods Cell Biol* 1982; **24**: 61–78.

Favard P, Andre J. The mitochondria of spermatozoa. In: Baccetti B, ed. *Comparative Spermatology*. New York: Academic Press, 1970: 415–29.

Fawcett DW. The mammalian spermatozoon. *Dev Biol* 1975; **44**: 394–436.

Flechon J. Sperm surface changes during the acrosome reaction as observed by freeze fracture. *Am J Anat* 1985; **174**: 239–48.

Friend DS, Fawcett DW. Membrane differentiation in freeze–fracture mammalian sperm. *J Cell Biol* 1974; **63**: 641–64.

Friend DS, Heuser JE. Orderly particle arrays on the mitochondrial outer membrane in rapidly frozen sperm. *Anat Rec* 1981; **199**: 159–75.

Friend DS. Plasma membrane diversity in a highly polarized cell. *J Cell Biol* 1982; **93**: 243–9.

Gilula NB, Satir P. The ciliary necklace. A ciliary membrane specialization. *J Cell Biol* 1972; **53**: 494–509.

Green DPL. Sperm thrusts and the problem of penetration. *Biol Rev Camb Phil Soc* 1988; **63**: 79–105.

Harrison RAP. The location of acrosin and proacrosin in ram spermatozoa. *J Reprod Fertil* 1982; **66**: 349–58.

Holt WV. Development and maturation of the mammalian acrosome. A cytochemical study using phosphotungstic acid staining. *J Ultrastruct Res* 1979; **68**: 58–71.

Huang TTF, Yanagimachi R. Inner acrosomal membrane of mammalian spermatozoa; its properties and possible functions in fertilization. *Am J Anat* 1985; **174**: 249–68.

Keyhani E, Storey BR. Oxidation rates of Krebs cycle carboxylic acids by the mitochondria of hypotonically treated rabbit epididymal spermatozoa. *Fertil Steril* 1973; **24**: 864–71.

Koehler JK. Human sperm head ultrastructure: a freeze–etching study. *J Ultrastruct Res* 1972; **39**: 520–39.

Koehler JK. Lectins as probes of the spermatozoon surface. *Arch Androl* 1981; **6**: 197–217.

Kolk AHJ, Samuel T. Isolation, chemical and immunological characterization of two strongly basic nuclear proteins from human spermatozoa. *Biochim Biophys Acta* 1975; **393**: 307–19.

Nagae T, Yanagimachi R, Srivastava PN, Yanagimachi H. Acrosome reaction in human spermatozoa. *Fertil Steril* 1986; **45**: 701–7.

Olson GE, Hamilton DW, Fawcett DW. Isolation and characterization of the perforatorium of rat spermatozoa. *J Reprod Fertil* 1976; **47**: 293–7.

Pedersen H. Observations on the axial filament complex of the human spermatozoon. *J Ultrastruct Res* 1970; **33**: 451–62.

Pedersen H. Further observations on the fine structure of the human spermatozoon. *Z. Zelforsch* 1972a; **123**: 305–15.

Pedersen H. The postacrosomal region of the spermatozoa of man and *Macaca arctoides*. *J Ultrastruct Res* 1972b; **40**: 366–77.

Phillips DM. Mitochondrial disposition in mammalian spermatozoa. *J Ultrastruct Res* 1970; **58**: 144–54.

Serres C, Escalier D, David G. Ultrastructural morphometry of human spermatozoa flagellum with a sterological analysis of the lengths of the dense fibres. *Biol Cell* 1983; **49**: 153–62.

Siegel MS, Bechtold DS, Willard JC, Polakoski KL. Partial characterization and purification of human sperminogen. *Biol Reprod* 1987; **36**: 1063–8.

van Leeuwenhoek A. Observations de Anthonü Lewenhoeck, de natis e semine genitali animalculis. *Phil Trans Roy Soc*, 1678; **12**: 1040–3.

Villarroya S, Scholler R. Regional heterogeneity of human spermatozoa detected with monoclonal antibodies. *J Reprod Fertil* 1986; **76**: 435–47.

Virtanen I, Bradley RA, Paasivuo R, Lehto V-P. Distinct cytoskeletal domains revealed in sperm cells. *J Cell Biol* 1984; **99**: 1983–91.

Wallace E, Cooper GW, Calvin HI. Effects of selenium deficiency on the shape and arrangement of rodent sperm mitochondria. *Gam Res* 1983; **7**: 389–99.

Woolley DM, Fawcett DW. The degeneration and disappearance of the centroiles during the development of the rat spermatozoon. *Anat Rec* 1973; **177**: 289–302.

Yanagimachi R. Mammalian fertilization. In: Knobil E, Neill JD *et al.*, eds. *The Physiology of Reproduction*. New York: Raven Press Ltd. 1972: 135–84.

Yanagimachi R Mammalian fertilization. In: Knobil E, Neill J *et al.*, eds. *The Physiology of Reproduction*. New York: Raven Press, 1988: 135–85.

Yanagimachi R, Noda YD, Fujimoto M, Nicholson G. The distribution of negative surface charges on mammalian spermatozoa. *Am J Anat* 1972; **135**: 497–520.

Yudin AI, Gottlieb W, Meizel S. Ultrastructural studies of the early events of the human sperm acrosome reaction is initiated by human follicular fluid. *Gam Res* 1988; **20**: 11–24.

Zaneveld LJD, Polarkoski KL, Williams WL. A proteinase and proteinase inhibitor of mammalian sperm acrosomes. *Biol Reprod* 1973; **9**: 219–25.

4

Tests of sperm function

J. M. CUMMINS

Introduction

The past decade has seen rapid changes in the treatment and understanding of male infertility. Assisted conception techniques such *in vitro* fertilization (IVF), aspiration of spermatozoa from blocked epididymides and micromanipulation of sperm and ova give men with semen of very poor quality, or even total azoospermia, the opportunity to procreate. This is so even when we do not understand the underlying cause of the problem. These techniques are expensive, invasive and sometimes hazardous to the female partner, therefore we need to establish more accurate tests of the fertilizing potential of semen and to evaluate those tests in a critical and constructive manner. In this review I will argue that we must base effective functional tests of spermatozoa *in vitro* firmly on an understanding of the challenges faced by the sperm cell *in vivo*.

How do we define infertility?

One central problem in assessing any test of sperm function is that it is extremely difficult to assign an exact fertility status to any individual man. Is a man fertile if, at some stage in his life, he has initiated a pregnancy? This is not very realistic, as we know that fertility declines with age. In the classic series of studies that established 'normal' limits for semen, many of which are unchanged today Macleod, in his classic series of studies in the 1950s, defined men as fertile if their partners were pregnant at the time of testing. However, this definition did not take account of pregnancy outcome, and the paternal contribution to early pregnancy failure. The most rigorous definition of male *in*fertility is probably the demonstration of repeated fertilization failure in IVF, with no defects in the oocytes of the partner. To be absolutely sure that the oocytes are indeed normal, one must simultaneously demonstrate fertilization and normal embryogenesis with fertile donor spermatozoa at the same time, but this can pose ethical and legal problems. Without such unequivocal evidence the best assessments of fertility or infertility in the general population will come from prospective long-term follow-up studies. As some men can achieve pregnancy through assisted reproduction but not through natural conception the term 'subfertile' is used for this group.

How do we assess tests of sperm fertilizing ability?

Boyers, Davis & Katz (1989) have stated, concerning tests of sperm function and their relation to fertility, 'Criteria that predict success *in vitro* should be regarded as necessary but not sufficient for predictive fertility following coitus or artificial insemination'. As it is difficult to define male fertility and infertility with precision, we must apply a high degree of rigour to evaluating any test that purports to predict fertilization outcome. A variety of statistical approaches have been applied to the problem including non-parametric approaches, logistic regression models, multivariate analysis and more recently multivariate analysis coupled with three-dimensional data plotting or the use of star plots (also called radar plots) to display complex sets of variables.

In real life, the distributions of semen parameters for fertile and infertile men overlap considerably and in addition are usually skewed or otherwise vary widely from the normal distribution, as seen in Fig. 1 (Boyers *et al.*, 1989).

The value of a predictive test can be assessed by comparing the distribution of normal and abnormal individuals for the parameter being measured (Fig. 2). Here the analogy that infertility is a disease state or affliction can be used, and the test has an arbitrary cut-off point that is varied in trying to discriminate between the afflicted and the non-afflicted groups. Thus a 'positive' test identifies

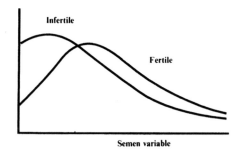

Fig. 1. Typical distribution of a semen parameter (in this case, sperm count) for fertile and infertile men. (Adapted from Boyers *et al.*, 1989 from data of Macleod, 1951.)

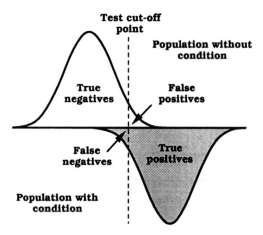

Fig. 2. This demonstrates the near inevitable overlap that occurs in the incidence of a clinical condition, such as infertility, when one applies a given test to a single measure of the condition.

those who exceed the cut-off point: these may be really afflicted ('true positives') or they may be normal, wrongly characterized as afflicted ('false positives').

From Fig. 2 five major descriptors of the test's effectiveness can be derived as shown in Table 1.

No cut-off for any such test can obviously ever perfectly distinguish between the two groups. The fertile and infertile populations generally overlap in any measured parameter (e.g. sperm count, percentage 'normal' forms). Therefore the aim must be to derive the maximum discriminating power by minimizing both false negatives and false positives. A powerful way of demonstrating this is by using 'receiver–operator–characteristic' curves in which we plot sensitivity against false positive rate. Sensitivity and specificity are the most stable attributes of a diagnostic test, as they do not change when the group sizes studied differ. However, as different cut-off values are used, they fluctuate against each other, and the receiver-operator curve is one way of plotting this. A useful test shows high true positive rates while false positive rates are minimal. This is illustrated in Fig. 3.

Treatment of male infertiliby by assisted reproductive technology

Under normal circumstances, semen is deposited in the upper vagina and sperm make their way through the female tract to contact the oocyte (Chapter 8). In sub-fertile men the sperm are deficient in number and/or inherent quality, and the changes of successful fertilization are accordingly reduced or negligible. *In vitro* fertilization (IVF), by bringing the gametes into close apposition, improves the chances of successful reproduction for these men. This was recognized a

Table 1. *Derivations of terms to define a clinical test*

Descriptor	Formula	What does it describe?
Sensitivty (true positive rate)	TP/(TP + FN)	Proportion of afflicted individuals correctly identified as such
False positive rate (= 1-Specificity)	FP/(TN + FP)	Proportion of normal individuals incorrectly identified as afflicted
Specificity	TN/(TN + FP)	Proportion of normal population correctly identified as affliction-free
Predictive value	TN/(TN + FN)	Proportion of population with a normal (negative) test who are actually not afflicted
Accuracy	(TP + TN)/ (TP + TN + FP + FN)	Overall performance of the test in correct identification of the problem

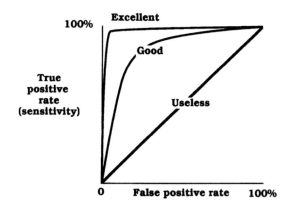

Fig. 3. Derivation of the receiver–operator–characteristic curve.

decade ago and now many men are requesting IVF whereas in previous times they may have been resigned to donor insemination or for the option, now remote, of adoption. This shift in attitude is part of the increased public awareness of reproductive technology and its positive and negative ramifications.

While IVF certainly improves the probability of fertilization, fertilization rates can be disappointing for men with extremely low sperm counts, poor sperm motility or elevated levels of abnormal forms of spermatozoa. Results are particularly bad if all three forms of semen defect are present, or if there are anti-sperm antibodies in the semen. In addition, poor embryo growth rates and quality are observed following the use of low fertility semen. One likely cause of this is the increased probability that, even if fertilization occurs, it will be late in the fertile life of the oocytes. However, genetic factors may well contribute, as spermatozoa that have been exposed to high levels of free radicals may show increased DNA damage. This is consistent with observations which show that, where embryos are genetically defective, faults due to chromosome breakage largely originate in the spermatozoa whereas gross chromosomal rearrangements are more likely to arise in the oocyte.

The use of metabolic enhancers such as pentoxifylline can improve the chances of fertilization for sub-fertile men, but the long-term genetic consequences of this, while unlikely to be deleterious, are unknown. Other approaches to the management of sub-fertility include increasing the chances of gamete collision by culturing in micro-droplets or capillary tubes. Many IVF groups are now turning to various forms of micromanipulation to enhance fertilization rates (Ng, 1990). This can take the form of drilling or cutting holes in the zona pellucida to enhance the likelihood of poorly motile sperm entering, micro injection of spermatozoa into the perivitelline space, or even injection of spermatozoa directly into the oocyte cytoplasm (Palermo *et al.*, 1993). While there has not yet been any controlled study comparing the use of simple metabolic enhancement with micromanipulation, combinations of the two approaches are being attempted. Some laboratories are starting to use combinations of micromanipulation with metabolic enhancement, coupled with electroporation, to promote acrosome reactions and gamete fusion.

It is hard to predict limits to the possibilities of assisted reproduction. We already know that fertilization can be accomplished with entirely immotile spermatozoa or spermatozoa lacking an acrosome (Aitken, 1990), and there is no theoretical reason why even demembranated sperm nuclei could not be used to generate living embryos. Work from Yanagimachi's group in Hawaii has shown that the nuclei of mammalian spermatozoa are remarkably tough. Isolated nuclei from human, hamster and mouse spermatozoa injected into zona-free hamster eggs can develop into normal-looking pronuclei even after 30 minutes at 90 °C! It is thus entirely possible that isolated sperm nuclei could be stored for long periods without the need for cyropreservation.

The sperm life history

After ejaculation, the spermatozoon passes through a number of distinct phases while interacting with the female tract and preparing for fertilization. Many aspects of this life history are difficult to study *in vivo*, especially in humans, and so we have to extrapolate from studies *in vitro* and from animal models. Fertilization occurs *in vitro* with fairly simple culture media. Thus interaction with the female tract is not obligatory for capacitation. Nevertheless, full understanding of sperm function requires that we recognize that spermatozoa have been shaped by complex evolutionary pressures including sperm competition in the female tract (Cummins, 1990).

Broadly speaking, sperm movement through the tract involves both passive and active transport phases, during which they enter the cervical mucus and pass into the uterus and then the Fallopian tube. While immotile sperm in some species can pass very rapidly through the tract, it is generally assumed that sperm motility is an important component in both establishing reservoirs of viable sperm in the tract (for example, in the cervix and the uterotubal junction) and in penetrating the various barriers to fertilization. This aspect of sperm function is covered elsewhere in this series. Three ideas are central to the present chapter. These are as follows:

1. Sperm selection occurs at many sites consecutively through the tract, so that the population that reaches the fertilization arena is an 'elite' subset of the original;
2. Tests of sperm function should centre on these selection processes, as they are likely to reveal more about fertilizing potential than simple mensuration of factors in the original unselected population, such as sperm concentration or viability.
3. Several steps in the sequence can be bypassed *in vitro* (e.g. the need to penetrate cervical mucus) but nevertheless can form the basis for useful tests of sperm competence.

Sperm undergo post-ejaculatory changes, collectively known as capacitation, which *in vivo* force a lag phase between insemination and fertilization (Yanagimachi, 1988a). Capacitation includes a range of poorly understood processes that do not alter the ultrastructure of the cell but change its potential for fertilization. Changes include sperm surface alterations including the removal of inhibitory 'decapacitation' factors, alterations to sperm intramembranous molecular arrangements, and metabolic changes reflected in a shift to a 'hyperactivated' motility pattern (qv). Some of these surface alterations, for example the binding of Ca^{2+}-conjugated chlortetracycline, can be used to monitor the state of capacitation. They may be useful clinically (see below). The timing of capacitation is variable between species, between individuals within a species and even between spermatozoa within the same ejaculate. It can also be modified by varying experimental conditions. In hamsters, for example, capacitation times can be modulated by elevating the temperature of the sperm store in the cauda epididymis, thus giving some evidence to the idea that capacitation involves a reversal or an 'escape' from the stable state imposed by prolonged epididymal storage.

Even fertile men show variations in capacitation rates *in vitro* as measured by the penetration of zona-free hamster ova with time. These variations are not normally taken into account when preparing sperm for IVF, but perhaps they should be. The major obstacle to doing so is the lack, so far, of any simple and inexpensive method of assessing capacitation rate *in vitro* prospectively, but perhaps the tests of motility or surface changes described below will open up this area.

Hyperactivation

As competent sperm become capacitated they may enter a high-energy phase of exaggerated motility, known as hyperactivation to distinguish it from the *activation* of motility that occurs at ejaculation or when epididymal sperm are experimentally diluted with culture media (Yanagimachi, 1981). This phase of movement has high-amplitude asymmetric flagellation, increased tail curvature and energy output and low linearity in culture medium (Burkman, 1990). Individual spermatozoa can move in and out of hyperactivation if observed over time, but we know little of the energetics or metabolic control of this phenomenon. Presumably hyperactivation assists sperm *in vivo* in swimming through the complex environment of the Fallopian tube and the cumulus matrix. In hamsters, spermatozoa probably use linear motion to pass through the utero-tubal junction and then switch to hyperactivation motility as they enter the ampulla. *In vitro* modelling using hamster sperm exposed to high viscosity medium supports the idea that hyperactivated motility conveys a selective advantage (Suarez *et al.*, 1991). Hyperactivation enabled sperm to generate greater forces in viscous as compared with non viscous media, whereas non-hyperactivated sperm showed similar force output at all viscosities.

The acrosome reaction

The acrosome reaction of the fertilizing spermatozoon, in most species that have been studied, occurs very close to, or on, the zona pellucida. There is some variation in this, however. Guinea pig spermatozoa can only penetrate the cumulus oophorus after they have completed the acrosome reaction. Hamster spermatozoa appear to be limited in their ability to enter the cumulus, to a brief period of capacitation just before the acrosome reaction *per se* (which occurs spontaneously in most sperm after about 4 hours of culture *in vitro*). The evidence for human spermatozoa is equivocal, as a low rate of spontaneous reactions is seen in free-swimming capacitated spermatozoa. However, most authorities agree that there is probably a need for close synchrony between cumulus penetration,

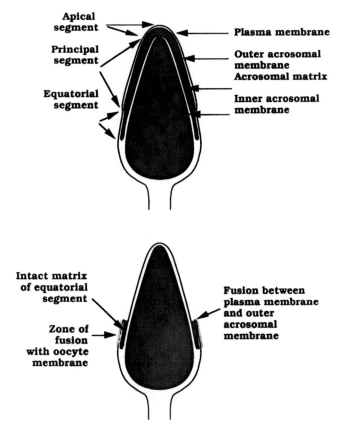

Fig. 4. General features of the human sperm acrosome before and after the acrosome reaction.

approach to the zona pellucida, and completion of the acrosome reaction. Sperm need to be capacitated to achieve this. The biochemical control of the reaction has been best characterized using mouse gametes, where there is a clear distinction between the 'spontaneous' and the 'physiological' (i.e. normal) reaction on the zona pellucida (Storey, 1991). A specific protein component of the zona (ZP3) is responsible for binding the spermatozoon and initiating the acrosome reaction. This is covered in detail below in the section dealing with sperm–zona binding. The binding event probably triggers a membrane fusion cascade involving Ca^{2+} influx, guanine nucleotide-binding ('G') proteins, protein kinase C and phospholipase C. The consequence of this is a process of point fusions between the plasma membrane and the outer acrosomal membrane resulting in pores that permit the acrosomal contents to escape. These processes are summarized in Figs. 4 and 5.

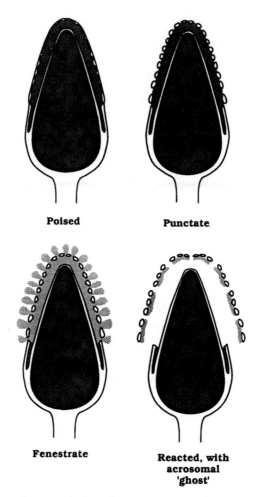

Poised   **Punctate**

Fenestrate   **Reacted, with
                              acrosomal
                              'ghost'**

Fig. 5. Sequence of events during the acrosome reaction (after Storey, 1991
and others).

The acrosomal matrix contains a number of enzymes of which probably the
most important is the serine protease acrosin (packaged as the inactive precursor
proacrosin). Other hydrolytic enzymes include hyaluronidase, neuraminidase, acid
phosphateses and esterases.

In the physiological acrosome reaction, membrane fusion only occurs over the
principal and apical segments, and the equatorial segment remains intact. At least
five separate steps can be dissected out based on chlortetracycline binding patterns
in mouse spermatozoa (Storey, 1991) and these are illustrated in Fig. 5. Fusion
between the outer acrosomal membrane and the plasma membrane around the
head in this region assures cell integrity. From a point of understanding sperm
function in fertility and infertility, the following points are important.

1. The physiological acrosome reaction only occurs in capacitated spermatozoa upon binding to a suitable ligand. In the mouse this is ZP3, but in other species a variety of alternative ligands can elicit a reaction, including progesterone, follicular fluid, and a variety of glycosaminoglycans such as heparin. The proportion of spermatozoa that can respond to a ligand varies widely according to the species, to the individual, and to the capacitation culture conditions. I will argue below that variation in this proportion is the basis for differences in fertilizing capacity between different sperm populations.

2. In capacitated human spermatozoa a reaction can be induced by treating with divalent cation ionophores such as A23187 or ionomycin. Again, wide differences between individuals in the proportion of spermatozoa that can respond indicate that this may be one cause of fertilization failure, and I describe below a test of human sperm function based on this.

3. Physiologically, the relevance of the acrosome reaction is that it permits normal penetration of the zona pellucida. It also exposes or activates binding sites to the egg surface over the postacrosomal head region (Yanagimachi, 1988*b*).

Penetration of the zona pellucida

The zona pellucida is one of the most important barriers faced by the fertilizing spermatozoon. The zona is a biochemically complex structure which in the mouse (the best studied model) consists of three acidic glycoproteins, ZP1 (200 kD), ZP2 (120 kD) and ZP3 (83 kD) arranged in a complex three-dimensional matrix. ZP2 and ZP3 are filamentous molecules cross-linked by the globular ZP1. A class of O-linked oligosaccharides on ZP3 may act as the primary receptors for the fertilizing spermatozoon and thereby induce the acrosome reaction through activation of sperm G proteins, phospholipase C and protein kinase C (Wassarman, 1991). There is increasing evidence (in the mouse) that sperm surface molecule that recognizes ZP3 receptors is a species-specific glycoside transferase enzyme that recognizes the binding oligosaccharides on ZP3. Almost certainly the oligosaccharides will give sperm–zona binding its specificity. In human fertilization binding appears to be mediated by D-mannose. The plasma membrane contains D-mannosidase and sperm of fertile men cultured under capacitating conditions show a characteristic increase in D-mannose binding activity and pattern that is not seen in infertile men (Tesarik, Mendoza & Carreras, 1991).

Following attachment, the acrosome-reacted spermatozoon remains bound to the zona pellucida, by specific receptors to ZP2 localized on the inner acrosomal membrane. Penetration of the zona matrix by the fertilizing sperm is not well understood. Only a narrow penetration slit is formed. It presumably involves a combination of physical forces driven by the hyperactivated motility of the sperm flagellum acting through the sharp edge of the tip of the head, and limited proteolytic cleavage (Oehninger, 1992). Following successful fertilization, release of cortical granule proteases from the activated oocyte (the cortical reaction) results in inactivation of the sperm receptor and acrosome reaction-inducing properties of ZP3. Proteolytic changes occur in ZP2 and the zona pellucida 'hardens'.

This secondary block to polyspermic fertilization (the primary one being at the oocyte surface) is an essential component to maximize the chances of normal syngamy. Not surprisingly, the zona pellucida in most cases has a high degree of species-specificity for sperm binding and penetration. While commonly cited as being a barrier to inter-species fertilization, this specificity is probably more a result of drifting molecular mechanisms, in response to the intense sexual selection pressures on fertilization mechanisms. Inter-species mating leading to gamete interaction is not common (Cummins, 1990). The human zona pellucida also contains a group of three glycoproteins, although the role of ZP3 in particular in inducing the acrosome reaction is not as clear-cut as it is in the mouse. Human sperm acrosome reactions can be induced by a wide variety of the molecules likely to be in close vicinity to the oocyte including follicular fluid, progesterone and components of the cumulus matrix as well as by the zona pellucida. In addition, of course, human spermatozoa cultured under capacitating conditions will show a relatively steady rate of spontaneous acrosome reactions, the level of which is only poorly related to fertile status (Cummins *et al.*, 1991).

Sperm subsets

There is good evidence that spermatozoa fall into a number of population subsets, with different potential for fertility. Conventional approaches to IVF tacitly assume this point, and there is extensive literature on techniques for separating 'good' from 'bad' spermatozoa. There are four basic approaches which Mortimer (Mortimer, 1990) has described in detail. These are simple dilution and washing; sperm migration 'swim up' or 'swim down' techniques relying on inherent motility; selective washing techniques based on density-gradient centrifugation; and selective adherence or filtration techniques such as the use of glass wool or Sephadex®. Several commercially available systems such as the SpermPrep Sephadex columns are now available. For most practical purposes in IVF a simple 'swim up' technique suffices. For poor quality semen, discontinuous Percoll gradients or continuous Nycodenz gradients give superior results. Any technique used should minimize shear forces that can result in free radical release and lipid peroxidation, and in addition should aim at separating the 'best' sperm rapidly from seminal leukocytes. Activated leukocytes are a potent source of radicals

(Aitken *et al.*, 1992*b*; Kessopoulou *et al.*, 1992) and can markedly reduce fertilization rates *in vitro*.

Ideas on subsets in the sperm population have been around for a number of years. Twenty years ago Cohen even suggested that the great majority of mammalian sperm may be dysfunctional through meiotic errors and that the female tract acts to select against all but an 'elite' sub-population that is permitted to reach the site of fertilization. The means of such selection are not clear, but may be immunological. Certainly the numbers reaching the ova are very low: in the hamster, for example, eggs *outnumber* sperms in the ampulla during the early phases of fertilization and similar low gamete ratios exist in other mammalian species. Experiments using IVF with very low sperm–egg ratios or even micro-insemination with operator-selected single spermatozoa have seriously challenged Cohen's hypothesis, and recently Ivani and Seidel (Ivani & Seidel, 1991) have shown that around 50% of capacitated motile mouse sperm chosen at random by micromanipulation can fertilize zone-free oocytes. Conversely, it could be argued that 50% of sperm are *incapable* of fertilizing! Cohen's arguments on genetically programmed dysfunction may be difficult to disprove, but they have been remarkably successful in forcing us to think about the nature of the sperm population and its interaction with the female reproductive system. One must recognize that evolutionary pressures, such as sperm competition between males, drive the form and function of the sperm cell and much of this is still obscure (Cummins, 1990). Recently Eisenbach and Ralt (Eisenbach & Ralt, 1992) have suggested that there is a turnover of fertilizing spermatozoa in the female tract so that at any given moments only a small percentage are able to fertilize. They couple this idea with the possibility that the egg might emit attractants, but the evidence for true chemotaxis in mammalian spermatozoa (as opposed to chemokinesis or 'trapping' by changes in linearity of motion) is not very convincing.

Evidence accumulating from a number of areas, therefore, suggests that only a sub-set of human sperm is fertile, and that many sperm are dysfunctional. The differences between fertile and infertile men may thus lie in the relative proportions of functional versus dysfunctional spermatozoa that can be produced, and tests of sperm function are likely to be most helpful if they are aimed at elucidating this proportion. This idea is summarized in Fig. 6. Man may indeed be fertile, despite very low sperm counts, provided the sperm that are produced are fully competent. This is typically seen in men with gonadotrophin deficiency when testicular function is rescued with exogenous hormone treatment. Thus research on the inductibility of the acrosome reaction referred to below indicates that in subfertile men few or none of spermatozoa cultured under capacitating conditions can respond to calcium influx by undergoing the acrosome reaction (Cummins

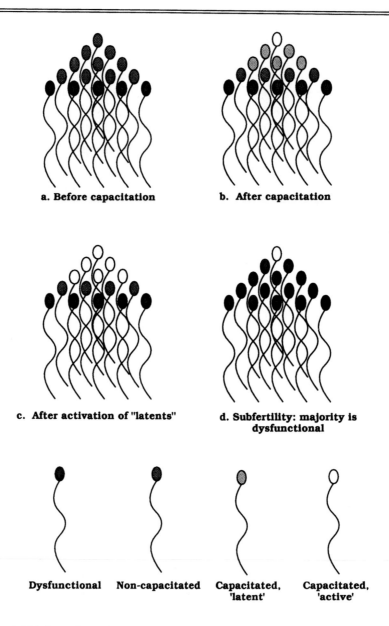

a. Before capacitation   b. After capacitation

c. After activation of "latents"   d. Subfertility: majority is
                                            dysfunctional

Dysfunctional   Non-capacitated   Capacitated,   Capacitated,
                                      'latent'   'active'

Fig. 6. This is a schematic depiction of the idea of sperm subsets, in fertility and
infertility. Dead spermatozoa are not considered here. In (a) the sperm population
consists of a mixture of dysfunctional and non-capacitated cells. In (b) a period
of capacitation with a fertile population results in a mix of non-capacitated and
capacitated spermatozoa. Of the capacitated set, only a few are 'active' in that
they exhibit hyperactivation and (possibly) spontaneous acrosome reactions: the
rest are capacitated but 'latent', awaiting a suitable stimulus. In (c) a stimulus
(such as A23187) has been applied, exposing the total 'latent' population. I suggest
that, in the case of a subfertile man, the majority of sperm are dysfunctional and
cannot even enter the 'latent' phase of capacitation. This results in (d).

et al., 1991). Likewise, work on the distribution of creating kinase isoforms in human spermatozoa demonstrates a strong association between the immature B-form and infertility (Huszar, Vigue & Morshedi, 1992). The presence of this enzyme isoform may be a marker for residual sperm cytoplasm resulting from imperfect spermiation, and such abnormal sperm forms, along with seminal leucocytes, are more likely to release the damaging reactive oxygen species that are thought to be implicated in poor sperm function.

The idea of subsets opens the way to sperm separation. Sample enrichment could be based on expression of a surface marker, or specific pattern of a marker for capacitation such as chlortetracycline (below). In animal breeding, preliminary reports show that flow cytometry can successfully identify sub-populations, monitor changes in semen quality and separate sexed sperm for IVF or artificial insemination (Morrell, 1991). Human sperm sex chromatin can be detected in decondensed nuclei using fluorescence *in situ* hybridization with a DNA probe specific for the Y chromosome. It has not yet been possible to apply such probes to living, condensed nuclei but the eventual application of similar techniques to human reproduction seems certain.

Indirect tests of sperm function

Conventional semen parameters

While I have argued above that conventional sperm counts are of limited value in predictive fertility, there is no doubt that good semen analysis, and investigation of any possible underlying disorder, must be performed as part of routine investigation. The nature of routine semen analysis is covered by exhaustive reviews elsewhere (Mortimer, 1990) and need not be repeated in detail here. However, at minimum it should include observation of physical parameters such as liquefaction, pH and volume together with cell concentration, morphology and viability (WHO, 1987; 1992). In addition, the laboratory should assess the presence of auto immune antibodies to spermatozoa, in both male and female partners. These have the potential to inhibit fertilization possibly by inhibiting the acrosome reaction. However, the role of antibodies in IVF failure is complicated. Major antigenic differences may exist between capacitated and non-capacitated spermatozoa, as cases are known where women have developed antibodies against the former but not the latter.

Nuclear decondensation **in vitro**

Under normal circumstances the sperm nuclei become condensed during the final stages of spermatogenesis. Cysteine-rich protamines replace histones. Further hardening of the nuclear matrix, as well as alterations to the cytoskeletal elements of the flagellum, occurs by increasing disulphide bonding during epididymal maturation. However, the transit time for sperm through the human epididymis is enormously variable and may be indeed only a few days in men with concurrently impaired spermatogenesis (Johnson & Varner, 1988). Variations in the degree of nuclear condensation can be evaluated by acridine orange fluorescence staining which identifies 'immature' or imperfectly condensed DNA. The use of acridine orange staining to evaluate human spermatozoa clinically shows a high level of correlation between normal DNA and 'normal' morphology, but strict morphological assessment would appear to be a better predictor of fertilization *in vitro*.

It is essential that rapid nuclear decondensation occurs following sperm entry to the oocyte, otherwise correct syngamy will fail. Human sperm heads can be decondensed *in vitro* relatively simply using combinations of detergents and disulphide bond reducing agents such as dithiothreitol. At least one report has suggested that this propensity is linked to fertility and thus could serve as a simple predictive laboratory test (Chan & Tredway, 1992) similar to the hypoosmotic swelling test described below.

Hypoosmotic swelling test

Living sperm normally actively exclude water by osmoregulation, but if suspended in hyopoosmotic solutions this capacity is overcome and they will undergo swelling of the tail membrane. This is reversible provided only the principal piece and not the midpiece is involved. The hypoosmotic swelling test exploits this capacity (Jeyendran *et al.*, 1984) and in essence evaluates the functional integrity of the sperm membrane. The correlation between hypoosmotic swelling and fertilizing capacity is not especially good but the technique is simple and easy to quantitate and it has been used in combination with tests of acrosomal function to combine information about capacitation status and viability simultaneously.

Axonemal ultrastructure

Poor sperm motility is undoubtedly associated with infertility, and motility defects have been linked with underlying abnormalities in axonemal structure (Serres, Feneux & Jouannet, 1986). Even fertile men show considerable heterogeneity in axonemal structure. Due to the great technical difficulties and time involved in sectioning and analysing sperm ultrastructure, it is unlikely that this approach will ever be used for routine prospective appraisal. However, ultrastructural studies are of undoubted immense value for diagnostic purposes where a structural defect is suspected.

Measurement of acrosomal enzymes

The acrosome reaction is essential for normal penetration of the zona pellucida and the neutral protease acrosin is thought to be the major one responsible. Acrosin is packaged in the form of an inactive zymogen, proacrosin and there is indirect evidence that conversion of proacrosin to acrosin in human spermatozoa may precede the membrane fusion events of the acrosome reaction. Conversion of proacrosin to acrosin and then subsequent inactivation following limited proteolysis of the zona pellucida has been proposed as a mechanism of zone penetration that could explain the very limited extent of lysis that occurs in the penetration slit. The measurement of acrosin/proacrosin levels in semen may provide a valid measure of sperm competence, and this would certainly be a way of establishing total absence of acrosomes.

The gelatine substrate test is a simple way of demonstrating the presence of proteases in the acrosome. In this test, spermatozoa are washed and spread onto a thin layer of gelatin on a glass slide. Following incubation in a humid incubator, proteases leach out of the acrosome and cause a 'halo' of dissolved gelatin to appear around the sperm head. After fixation this can be seen easily using phase contrast microscopy, and the size of the halos together with the number of spermatozoa with halos can be quantitated. 'Dead' sperm that have lost their acrosomes do not develop a halo. This has the attraction of being both cheap and simple, but its relevance to fertility has not been firmly established.

Measurement of seminal ATP content

Much of sperm function depends on the production of ATP and ATP content has been proposed as a measure of fertility. However, the relationship is obscure as motility and sperm function are governed by a complex of factors including cAMP, adenosine, calcium ions and pH (Hoskins & Vijayaraghavan, 1990). Certainly the regulation of intracellular ATP levels is closely coupled with motility, as about 50% of the intracellular ATP pool is metabolized each minute (Ford & Rees, 1990). However, total seminal ATP may not necessarily reflect that available for motility or for fuelling the acrosome reaction as there is evidence (discussed again below) that high energy phosphate bonds from mitochrondrial ATP are passed to the flagellum in the intermediate form of creatine phosphate: the 'creating–creatine phosphate shuttle' (Thombes & Shapiro, 1985). Thus the measurement of total ATP is unlikely to be of more than indirect clinical interest in predicting fertility. A recent report from the World Health Organization (1992) confirms that neither ATP content nor conventional sperm parameters have any predictive value for fertility when the sperm count is 'normal' (>20 million per ml).

Other biochemical tests

Several biochemical tests have been proposed as indicators of sperm dysfunction. Thus creatine phosphokinase (CK), the major enzyme thought to be responsible for moving high energy phosphate groups from the midpiece mitochrondria to the axoneme in the 'creatine shuttle' (Tombes & Shapiro, 1985), exists in two isoforms, the 'B' (brain-type) isoform characteristic of immature cells and tissues, and the 'M' (muscle-type) isoform characteristic of mature or differentiated cells. Huszar and his co-workers have demonstrated a clear relationship between a high B:M isoform ratio and infertility (Huszar et al., 1992). It is not yet clear whether the high level of B isoform CK is directly related to sperm dysfunction (for example, by affecting the movement of high energy phosphate groups between mitochondria and the axoneme) or whether it is simply a marker for poorly differentiated cells. Other potential biochemical markers for sperm abnormalities include the sperm-specific isoenzyme for lactate dehydrogenase (LDH_x) and glutamic-oxaloacetic acid leakage; but, as Mortimer has pointed out, the clinical significance of these markers remains to be established (Mortimer, 1990).

Computer-aided semen analysis

Computer analysis falls into two broad areas. Sperm motion analysis coupled with semi-objective evaluation of concentration is commonly called CASMA (Computer aided sperm motion analysis). Automated sperm morphology analysis is also evolving, but is currently less well developed.

The development of computerized counts and motion analysis has greatly changed the way in which we can apply understanding of sperm motion to the study of fertility. The topic is the subject of exhaustive and authoritative recent reviews and a full evaluation is not strictly relevant here (Boyers et al., 1989). The instruments that are currently commercially available evolved historically from techniques such as time-exposure or multiple-exposure photography that provided an overlapping series of sperm head images that allowed tracking of sperm movement on a two-dimensional basis. In the mid-1980s the development of high speed cinematography and videomicrography coupled with digitized analysis and storage of coordinates permitted more sophisticated investigations of sperm movement. Parallel developments in image analysis in areas such as tomography and cytology allowed better analysis of sperm head shape for toxicology as well as in the investigation of infertility. Today, a number of commercial units are available and much effort is being devoted into developing suitable software and standardizing operating conditions so that results can be compared within and between laboratories. Despite these rapid developments, it

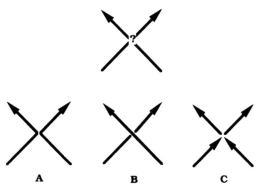

Fig. 7. This illustrates the 'bump and cross' problem in interpreting sperm tracks using computer-aided motion analysis. Intersections have a 'grey area' where the size of the overlapping heads falls outside the set defined as 'normal' for a single sperm head. Depending on the algorithms used and the definition of the 'best' fit for the available data, the computer may interpret the intersection as: A two sperm that zig-zag back on themselves; B correctly as two sperm intersecting; or C as four separate sperm tracks.

does not seem that computers can yet offer completely automated and error-free systems. Most reviewers agree that interpretation of results must be validated by expert observation. Videomicrography offers the advantage of immediate recording and multiple replaying. High-speed microcinematography, while currently capable of better resolution and higher observation frequencies, is expensive and time-consuming and therefore not suitable for routine andrological investigation.

The major inadequacies in present systems include low field rate observation frequencies, typically 30 to 60 fields per second, whereas sampling rates of at least 120 fields per second are needed to fully characterize the harmonic behaviour (oscillation frequencies) of human spermatozoa. Even higher frequencies may be needed for hyperactivated sperm or very rapidly swimming forms. Russell Davis, from the group at David, California, recommends a minimum of 200 frames per second for monkey spermatozoa (Davis *et al.*, 1992). Other problems not yet fully vanquished include the 'bump and cross' phenomenon, which occurs when sperm paths intersect and the computer is unable to resolve which sperm is emerging from the intersection. Different configurations deal with this problem in different ways. At least one system ignores all 'bump and cross' paths and does not include them in any analysis. This, however, introduces bias at higher sperm concentrations and swimming speeds when intersections are more likely to happen. Other systems look for the 'most likely' next position, but it is easy for the computer to be fooled and to identify the wrong paths. Fig. 7 demonstrates a variety of possible outcomes. In addition, problems are caused by sperm agglutination, surface effects such as 'spinning', cells entering or leaving fields, out-of-focus artefacts, and factors affected by sperm density. There is, yet, no fool-proof system, and there is no substitution for critical evaluation of all recorded paths to eliminate such artefacts.

Thus, although computer systems have been widely advertised as being suitable for routine andrology, at least one recent review recommends the user first to perform manual concentration estimations, by traditional means (haemocytometer or other counting chamber), and then adjust the concentration to <50 million per mil for motility analysis (Davis, 1992)! Despite these caveats, there is no doubt that, provided rigorous attention is paid to recommended standard procedures (Davis, 1992), good computer analysis will give more accurate results than manual equivalents. As experience accumulates in the use of these systems, advanced algorithms for evaluating sperm motion are emerging which give more accurate measures of sperm behaviour than those currently available commercially.

While most current effort is directed toward systems for tracking sperm head motion there is no doubt that future generations of computer systems will allow us to monitor the much more complex movements of the flagellum. A number of studies of flagellar beat frequency, amplitude, wavelength, rotation frequency together with progressive velocity and power output have already been accomplished for mammalian spermatozoa. Stephens and Hoskins have described a computerized semi-automatic system that evaluates flagellar form (Stephens & Hoskins, 1990). Future developments will probably also allow the three-dimensional analysis of sperm swimming free of surface effects. However, limitations in computer memory space and in the capacity to deal with the enormous volumes of data that are generated means that such systems are far from being in routine clinical use.

Turning to automated morphology assessment, several commercial systems offer fairly simple assessment of head shape based on videomicrography. These systems measure factors such as head length, width, the head perimeter and area ellipticity (defined as (length − width)/(length + width)) and form (defined as 4π area/perimeter^2). In addition, systems can report on staining characteristics such as the amount of light transmission and absorbence and overall dye staining (defined as area × absorbence). Katz (Boyers et al., 1989) has proposed a standardized set of descriptors as shown in Table 2. This can be used to produce a template defining 'normal' head shape limits (Fig. 8).

Classification systems such as these have been applied to the study of reproductive toxins and related to motility and fertility (for review see Boyers et al. (Boyers et al., 1989)). At least one commercial system ('Morphologizer' supplied by Cryo Resources, NY) will 'learn' customised classification systems, and more advanced research systems using grey-scale image processing combined with multivariate analysis have been published. No system yet appears to deal with the question of midpiece or tail abnormalities, even though these are significant for understanding impaired motility and infertility.

Table 2. *Techniques for staining the human sperm acrosome*

Technique	Target	Advantages	Disadantages
Triple-stain	Differential staining of acrosomal matrix	Uses light microscopy: incorporates live–dead stain	Inconsistent stain characteristics
FITC-Peanut (PNA) lectin	Outer acrosomal membrane	Easy to use	Small target size. Plasma membrane needs to be permeabilized: false positive results possible
Ricinus communis lectin	Acrosomal matrix	Easy to use, large target size	Extremely toxic lectin; ethanol permeabilization can give false positive results
FITC-*Pisum sativum* (PSA) lectin	Acrosomal matrix	Large target, ease of distinguishing acrosomal regions, easy to apply	Ethanol permeabilization may increase false positive results
FITC-concanavalin A lectin	Inner acrosomal membrane	Highly specific: aldehyde fixation minimises artefacts and 'false' reactions	Small target size
Indirect immuno-fluorescence using monoclonal antibodies (MABs)	Wide variety of ligands depending on MAB	Highly specific; can be used to trace movement of antigens during AR (e.g. PH20 in guinea-pig sperm	Requires access to MAB library

Direct function tests

Penetration of cervical mucus

Cervical mucus is normally the first selective barrier experienced by the spermatozoon in the female tract, and appraising the interaction between sperm and mucus should form part of every infertility investigation. Cervical mucus is a complex sialylated mucin secreted by non-ciliated epithelial cells of the cervical crypts. It is an elaborate micro-environment for the spermatozoon. It consists of

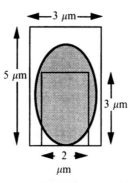

Fig. 8. This illustrates a template for judging correct head morphology. 'Normal' oval sperm head maximum width and length should lie between the two box outlines. (Adapted from Katz *et al.*, 1981.)

an aqueous phase containing serum exudates and other secretions, and an insoluble gel phase consisting of a sialoglycoprotein matrix. This complexity lends cervical mucus, like other epithelial mucins, complex physical properties such as viscosity, spinnbarkeit ('stringiness'), elasticity and the demonstration of crystalline 'ferning' patterns upon air drying. These several components show marked variation throughout the menstrual cycle in response to the changing endocrine milieu and evaluation of these physical properties gives a valuable test of the stage of the menstrual cycle at which the cervix is most (or least) receptive to sperm penetration. In addition, presence of antisperm antibodies or other 'hostile' factors can impede sperm transit and form one cause of infertility. The interaction of sperm with cervical mucus *in vitro* is complex due to the changing microstructure of mucin strands as the mucus is manipulated by stretching or shear forces.

First anticipated 60 years ago, *in vitro* tests of sperm interaction with cervical mucus either on glass slides or in capillary tubes have proven invaluable. The test was placed on a standardized practical and theoretical basis by Katz's group at Davis, California, over a decade ago (Katz, Overstreet & Hanson, 1980) and several studies have now shown that the ability of spermatozoa to penetrate cervical mucus is correlated with specific movement characteristics and with the ability of sperm to fertilize both *in vitro* and *in vivo*. To be valid, the test should be run as a cross-over trial for infertile couples: husband and fertile donor sperm should each be tested against the wife's and fertile donor mucus. However, this is logistically difficult to set up and the use of frozen mucus or mucus analogues is probably more practical (below).

Aitken has shown that the degree of lateral head displacement demonstrated by free-swimming spermatozoa is the most important single motion parameter that determines the success of penetration (Aitken, 1990). This high amplitude beat is one important characteristic of the sperm movement that increases during hyperactivation. It probably reflects the energy output of the sperm cell. There is a complex interaction between sperm mucus penetration and capacitation that is only poorly understood. Sperm that have passed through a mucus column appear to be capacitated in that they will penetrate zona-free hamster eggs very rapidly (Katz, Andrew & Overstreet, 1989) and will show increased capacity to acrosome reaction following a suitable stimulus such as exposure to the zona pellucida, or follicular fluid. However sperm recovered from the cervical mucus reservoir as long as 72 hours after coitus show no increase in the rate of spontaneous acrosome reactions. Most likely a combination of physiological interaction, physical filtering of 'good' from 'bad' sperm and suppression of the acrosome reaction is at work.

Penetration of mucus analogues

The major problem in using homologous cervical mucus as a routine test system is the difficulty of obtaining and storing mid-cycle mucus of standard physico-chemical composition. This poses severe obstacles to standardizing the test, particularly in multi-centre and cross-over trials. Alternatives to human mid-cycle mucus are now available commercially. Thus Penetrak® is a preparation of bovine mid-cycle mucus supplied frozen by Serono Diagnostics (Wellyn Garden City, UK). A purified Hyaluronate polymer gel, Sperm Select®, is also available from Pharmacia (Uppsala, Sweden). Aitken has shown (Aitken *et al.* 1992*a*) excellent correlations between penetration of the two preparations. Penetration of sperm into Sperm Select® was slightly better than Penetrak® in accounting for the results observed in an ionophore-enhanced zona-free hamster ovum penetration test (see below). The Sperm Select® test was capable of successfully identifying the group of patients in whom zero penetration occurred in the egg penetration test. Other proposed analogues for cervical mucus include egg white and serum albumen but these do not appear to have been evaluated in any systematic manner.

Hyperactivation assays

The development of computer assisted motion analysis opens the way for diagnostic tests of human sperm capacitation as manifest by the onset of hyperactivation. Burkman (1990) has defined the parameters by which hyper-activated spermatozoa may be discriminated from non-hyperactivated using computer analysis. In essence, sperm defined as hyperactivated show a simultaneous combination of high curvilinear velocity ($>100 \mu$/second), high beat amplitude ($>7.5 \mu$) and low linearity ($<65\%$). The dynamics of spontaneous onset of hyperactivation, in sperm from fertile donors cultured under capacitating conditions, show a close relationship to those of spontaneous acrosome reactions. There are no reports yet linking hyperactivation with fertility as a predictive test; however, this approach seems very likely. We have observed (unpublished observations) that metabolic enhancers such as pentoxifylline stimulate high levels of hyperactivation for normospermic samples for about 2–4 hours, and markedly enhance the rate of acrosome reactions in response to A23187. One could possibly use such techniques to determine the proportion of sperm in the population capable of undergoing hyperactivation. This may offer an attractive way of testing fertile potential, by deliberately challenging the sperm population to demonstrate its maximum capacity for hyperactivation. A hyperactivation motility assay requires only 5–10 μl of dilute sperm suspension, so that the sperm preparation that is used for IVF could be monitored simultaneously for hyperactivation status and potential. We are currently evaluating this approach as an alternative to the ARIC test described below.

Acrosomal function assays

Completion of capacitation and initiation of the acrosome reaction on or close to the zona pellucida are essential steps in fertilization. There is good evidence that failure in one of these steps is an important cause of infertility. Thus Byrd and Wolf (1986) showed that a significant subset of sperm from infertile men cultured under capacitating conditions do not respond to the calcium ionophore A23187. In oligozoospermic men, A23187 treatment does not enhance sperm penetration of zone-free hamster eggs (below), and although this can be increased by treatment with follicular fluid, there is no increase in the proportion of acrosome reacted sperm. The cause of this failure is not clear, but it is likely that the spermatozoa have either suffered damage due to free-radical-induced lipid peroxidation or are somehow incapable of completing the normal capacitation sequence.

Studying the human sperm acrosome has been difficult until fairly recently. It is relatively thin and overlies a sperm head that varies in thickness, being spatulate distally but oval in cross-section in the middle. This gives the sperm head an oval profile but a wedge-shaped sagittal section. This varying optical thickness makes the components of the human sperm head difficult to evaluate by conventional microscopical techniques such as phase contrast, that can be applied very readily to the study of acrosome reactions in species such as the hamster and guinea pig. This made study of the dynamics of the acrosome reaction difficult.

The small size of the acrosome also means that vital stains such as acridine Orange, used to differentiate the acrosomes of sperm of laboratory animals cannot be applied to human spermatozoa. The first major technical breakthrough came when Talbot and Chacon (1981) developed a triple-stain approach. This not only identified the acrosome but also included a vital stain (Trypan blue) that was incorporated by 'dead' (membrane permeable) cells. However, the technique had a number of difficulties, both in standardizing stain between-batch variations, and in applying it readily to experimental and clinical situations.

The development of fluorescently labelled lectins and specific antibodies together with other membrane stains such as chlortetracycline greatly simplified matters. We now have a variety of staining protocols that can be applied alone or in combination with vital stains such as Hoechst 33258 to distinguish 'live' from 'dead' sperm. An alternative is the combination of lectin staining with the hypoosmotic swelling test that likewise will clearly indicate whether acrosome reactions are occurring in spermatozoa with functionally competent plasma membranes. Table 2 gives a summary of the major techniques, their staining target(s) and their major advantages and disadvantages.

In studying the acrosome reaction, it is important to distinguish between spontaneous reactions and those which suitable stimuli can elicit in capacitated fertile spermatozoa. Almost certainly, the physiological reaction in human sperm accompanies the final stages of approach to the oocyte through the cumulus oophorus. Human sperm with intact acrosomes readily penetrate the cumulus *in vitro* and the reaction rate seen *in vitro* probably bears little or no relationship to fertile potential. This is very different from species such as the hamster or the guinea pig where most spermatozoa will undergo spontaneous reactions. Tesarik (Tesarik, 1989) analysed this question carefully considering other tests currently available such as the hamster ovum penetration test (qv) and concluded that, 'the only physiological acrosome reaction is that produced by an appropriate biological stimulus, while spontaneous acrosome reactions have little biological efficiancy'. He concluded that tests of sperm function based on acrosome reaction potential 'should therefore be designed to distinguish between the spontaneous and induced acrosome reactions'. Working independently, my colleagues and I had arrived at the same conclusion. We decided to use the calcium ionophore A23187 (10 μM) to induce Ca^{2+} influx in a sperm population prepared under capacitating conditions identical to those used for IVF. Besides the ionophore-treated spermatozoa we treat a control aliquot with vehicle alone (10% DMSO in protein-free culture medium). The vehicle has no significant effect on acrosome reactions. After one hour, we wash the sperm through 60% Percoll and then fix and permeabilize the sperm with 95% ethanol. The sperm are spread onto glass slides and stained with FITC-labelled *Pisum sativum* lactin. This binds to the acrosomal matrix. Sperm with an intact acrosome show complete and uniform staining over the anterior head. Sperm that have completed the acrosome reaction show a belt of staining representing the equatorial segment. Intermediate stages can also be distinguished, and sperm that were degenerate at the time of fixing generally show no staining at all. This is because the equatorial segment is relatively transient and starts to break down soon after the sperm dies or completes the acrosome reaction. The sperm are examined using fluorescence microscopy and classified according to acrosomal status.

We use the difference between the A23187-induced reaction rate and the background spontaneous (control) rate as the ARIC value (acrosome reaction following ionophore challenge) (Cummins *et al.*, 1991). We arrived at the following characteristics for the test (Table 3), based on 53 fertile and 26 sub-fertile men. The men were characterized on the grounds of their proven fertility in IVF. Sub-fertility was defined as less than 50% fertilization rate when four or more oocytes were inseminated and no other likely cause of the poor fertilization could be identified.

As can be seen, an ARIC cut-off of 5% has a high predictive value (90%) and is highly specific (98%) while giving a false-positive rate of only 2% (only one of our group of 53 controls fell in this range). We have now screened several hundred men using this test and the results are highly consistent. Men presenting with a test result of less than 5% are counselled about the likelihood of poor fertilization in IVF.

The test thus seems to be broadly comparable to the hamster ovum penetration test, described below, but is much cheaper and quicker taking at most 3–4 hours. We have been unable to compare it directly with the hamster egg penetration test as hamsters are forbidden laboratory animals in Australia. Work coming from several laboratories (Japan, Chile, UK) is now beginning to confirm that the two tests are very similar clinically. The major disadvantage of the ARIC test as currently applied is that it requires at least 2×10^5 motile sperm per ml following sperm preparation. For normospermic men this is not a problem but for severely oligoospermic men we are, occasionally, unable to recover enough motile spermatozoa for evaluation. In these cases, of course, the men will have severe difficulties in producing enough sperm for conventional IVF and may need to move to alternative approaches such as micromanipulation. We have attempted to use a micro-method for evalating acrosomal status based on preparing small sperm numbers on a filter, but without much success.

While we have found the ARIC test to be clinically useful, ionophores such as A23187 can give varied results according to protein type and concentration and the underlying metabolic state of the cell. In addition there may be batch variations and other preparative problems (e.g. photosensitivity) with ionophores. The free

Table 3. *Test characteristics for various cut-off levels of the ARIC test in distinguishing between fertile and sub-fertile men*

ARIC threshold (%)	3	5	10	15
Sensitivity (%)	23	35	54	69
Predictive value (%)	100	90	64	56
Specificity (%)	100	98	85	74
95% confidence – Intervals of specificity		95.6–100	76.9–93.5	63.2–84.0
False-positive rate (%)	0	2	15	26

From Cummins *et al.*, 1991.

acid is recommended as it shows less batch variation than the Ca^{2+}/Mg^{2+} salt, however it also shows quite strong autofluorescence that can be a disadvantage in some physiological studies (Ford *et al.*, 1991). It is essential that each laboratory using this approach titrates ionophore concentrations carefully using known fertile donor spermatozoa to ensure that only the mimimum amount of A23187 (or ionomycin) is used to stimulate a maximal acrosome reaction response. Future developments in the field may well rely on different modes of stimulating the acrosome reactions: for example, the use of fusogenic phospholipid liposomes.

Use of follicular fluid to stimulate the acrosome reaction and/or fertility ability

Various workers have proposed the use of human follicular fluid to maximize the acrosome reaction or to stimulate fertilizing ability. While follicular fluids have marked effects on sperm motility and can stimulate acrosome reactions very rapidly, within a few minutes, (Yudin, Gottlieb & Meizel, 1988) they are highly variable in this capacity. This, presumably, reflects heterogeneity in the physiological status of follicles following ovarian stimulation. This variability is due in part to the varying progesterone content of the follicular fluid. Progesterone provokes a rapid Ca^{2+} influx and will result in the acrosome reaction in competent capacitated spermatozoa, and there is some evidence from Meizel's group in California that this steroid acts through $GABA_A$ receptors in conjunction with Cl^- influx. This is an unusual pathway as normally steroids bind to nuclear receptors while GABA receptors are membrane bound. These observations are interesting given the high concentrations of progesterone and other membrane-active steroids in the cumulus following ovulation. However, until the molecular mechanisms are fully characterized it is probably inappropriate to use follicular fluids on a routine basis for sperm stimulation or enhancement of motility or fertilizing ability.

Capacitation assays

Human sperm capacitation status can be monitored by a chlortetracycline fluorescence technique originally developed for mouse spermatozoa. The assay depends on the binding of chlortetracycline and Ca^{2+} to the sperm surface during the early stages of capacitation. Chlortetracycline forms a fluorescent compound with Ca^{2+} and has been used in several physiological systems (such as blood platelets) to monitor Ca^{2+} fluxes. As sperm capacitation continues fluorescence gradually disappears, presumably as a result of Ca^{2+} influx. The technique has the advantage that small aliquots of sperm populations can be removed and the chlortetracycline-fluorescence 'frozen' with glutaraldehyde for later evaluation. The assay probably cannot distinguish between physiologically normal and spontaneous acrosome reactions, and needs controls for sperm viability. Nevertheless, it is a valuable tool and has been used to demonstrate delayed capacitation patterns, and reduced inducibility of acrosome reactions in men with abnormal semen profiles such as teratozoospermy and polyzoospermy (Kholkute, Meherji & Puri, 1992).

Bronson's group in Stony Brook, NY, have examined the expression of glucoproteins such as vitronectin and fibronectin on the surface of human sperm following capacitation, and have shown a relationship between low levels of expression and impaired capacity to undergo a progesterone-induced acrosome reaction. This is consistent with observations that the egg surface has recognition sites to the ubiquitous RGD peptide (Arg–Gly–Asp) common to a number of extracellular matrix proteins. A variety of other factors could be used to study the onset of capacitation and the acrosome reaction. One such factor is fucoidin, which inhibits human sperm–zona binding and the zona-induced acrosome reaction. A very promising approach is that of Tesarik *et al.* (Tesarik *et al.*, 1991), who studied the appearance of D-mannose binding sites on the surface of sperm cultured under capacitating conditions. As described earlier, D-mannose on the zona pellucida may interact with D-mannosidase on the sperm surface during zone binding. Tesarik observed that spermatozoa from fertile men showed a characteristic pattern of D-mannose binding over the acrosomal region. This pattern differed in infertile men. The overall proportion of motile sperm showing D-mannose binding specifically over the acrosome was less than 10%, which is consistent with observations on the background rate of spontaneous capacitation and acrosome reactions. This interesting finding, if it can be repeated, may open the way to more specific tests based on the dynamics of sperm capacitation and exposure of zone-binding factors.

Zona pellucida binding and penetration

Sperm interaction with the zona pellucida consists of a number of separate components each one of these steps requiring active sperm involvement and is a potential source of fertilization failure (Storey, 1991). Besides enabling us to understand the molecular biology of sperm–egg interaction these separate components can also serve as very specific tests of sperm fertilizing ability *in vitro* (Oehninger, 1992). The components as presently understood are as follows:

1. Loose attachment
2. Firm binding and induction of the acrosome reaction
3. Penetration of the zona matrix.

Oocytes can be prepared in bulk from surgically removed ovaries or from post-mortem material using a combination of mechanical and enzymic dissection, screening the dissociated tissue through filters of decreasing size and finally by pipetting under a dissecting microscope. Care must be taken to select mature oocytes as there is evidence that immature oocytes show reduced sperm binding compared with mature. However, even 'mature' oocytes selected from large antral follicles may differ significantly in binding and sperm penetrating characteristics despite having very similar appearance. Clearly, 'zona maturation', along with nuclear and cytoplasmic maturation of the oocytes, is another factor to consider both in designing binding assays and in understanding how differences in IVF fertilization rates are caused by inherent oocyte factors. Alternatively, tests may use surplus oocytes from IVF programmes, and even unfertilized oocytes that have been exposed to spermatozoa (this may be subject to ethical approval and legal constraints). In the latter case care must be taken to distinguish any residual spermatozoa remaining from the IVF attempt from any that are used to assess zona binding or penetration. In addition some oocytes may be activated during the IVF attempt resulting in reduced sperm binding capacity. In all cases internal controls, both positive and negative, must be used to take account of variation between oocytes and between women. This is particularly important for comparisons between centres.

As the zona material is metabolically relatively inert, it is possible to bulk-store zonae either by freezing or by the much more convenient approach of salt-storing in buffered hyperosmolar solutions. Studies have shown very similar sperm binding characteristics between oocytes pickled in this way (1.5M $MgCl_2$ with 0.1% Polyvinulpyrrolidone in HEPES buffer) and those cryopreserved in 2M DMSO: also between salt-stored and fresh oocytes (Oehninger, 1992).

Two basic approaches have been used to assess and control sperm binding and penetration. In both cases, test spermatozoa are compared with those from a fertile donor. In competitive binding assays the sperm are labelled with different fluorochromes and then mixed in approximately equal numbers. This has a twofold disadvantage: first the fluorochrome used may itself affect sperm viability or binding capacity (or both); secondly large number of oocytes must be used to account for between-oocyte variability. The hemi-zona assay pioneered by the Jones Institute in Norfolk, Virginia uses oocytes that are bisected by a micro-manipulator. One half zone is inseminated with test spermatozoa and the other control from a fertile donor. In this way each oocyte serves as its own control, and fewer oocytes are need to attain similar levels of accuracy to the competitive assay (Oehninger, 1992). The hemi-zona assay has proved very useful in assessing inherent fertilizing ability, as well as the dynamics of capacitation, hyperactivation and the acrosome reaction (Burkman, 1990). Fertile sperm cultured under capacitating conditions for a hemi-zona assay showed a peak of hyperactive movement at about 2 hours followed by a slow decline over 5 hours. There was an increase in the numbers of spontaneously acrosome reacting spermatozoa coupled with a decrease in acrosome intact spermatozoa between and 3 and $3\frac{1}{2}$ hours. Sperm–zona binding increased rapidly between 30 minutes and 2 hours and after $3\frac{1}{2}$ hours there was a steady decline in the capacity of the sperm population to initiate firm zona binding.

Penetration of heterologous oocytes

A major breakthrough in functional tests for sperm fertilizing capacity came when Yanagimachi demonstrated that the zona-free golden hamster oocyte could support the penetration of 'foreign' spermatozoa. In hamsters the major block to polyspermy lies in the zona pellucida, while the oocyte surface is remarkably non-discriminatory even after penetration and egg activation. Work from Yanagimachi's group has demonstrated that, unlike any other known species, the hamster oocyte will permit the penetration of multiple foreign spermatozoa. The capacity to fuse with spermatozoa develops in the forming oocyte at about the time the zona pellucida and the egg microvilli appear. It declines after sperm penetration and is lost by the eight-cell embryo stage. The nature of the fusogenic factor is obscure, as it resists proteinase digestion. It may be a glycolipid or a cryptic membrane protein.

Since the original observation by Yanagimachi et al. in 1976, the zona-free hamster oocyte penetration test has developed as a fundamental laboratory element in the diagnosis and treatment of male infertility. It has been applied to predicting fertility, evaluating function after contraception or medical therapy to alleviate infertility, and in assessing semen after cryopreservation. One very important clinical application of the test is in karyotyping human sperm as under careful control the penetrating spermatozoon will form a metaphase plate, and this end-point has been used to monitor possible genetic damage to sperm (Martin, 1989). The hamster egg has also been used to study the fertilizing ability of sperm from a wide range of animal species, from dolphins to birds.

In essence, the hamster egg test involves inducing superovulation in prepubertal (4–6 weeks old) female hamsters. Eggs are removed from the oviduct at a defined time after ovulation and treated with hyaluronidase to remove the cumulus. Trypsin digestion removes the zona pellucida. A standard concentration of motile spermatozoa is added to groups of eggs. Following a defined period of co-incubation (usually 3 h at 37 °C under humid 5% CO_2 in air) the eggs are removed, washed and examined for the presence of penetrating sperm heads associated with tails. The results are usually read as a penetration rate (percentage of eggs with decondensing sperm heads). However, as polyspermic penetration is common (particularly with fertile men) the penetration rate may be combined with information about the numbers of sperm heads per penetrated egg. The conditions need to be very carefully standardized with meticulous attention to media type and purity, water source and brand of tissue culture ware, as all these factors can affect the results.

While the hamster egg test has been widely applied, there are great problems in standardizing the methodology, and historically this caused unacceptable levels of false-negative results (i.e. fertile men showing failure to penetrate). Aitken (Aitken & Elton, 1984) showed that the interaction between sperm and eggs conforms to Poisson distribution theory, meaning that observed fertilization rates can be explained purely on the grounds of collision frequency between receptive oocytes and capacitated spermatozoa. This work led to a standard recommended protocol (World Health Organization, 1987), although much work still continues in attempts to reduce the variability of the test. The essential problem, which is of course common to homologous IVF, is that penetration requires collision between a capacitated spermatozoon that is ready to undergo the acrosome reaction and an oocyte. The motile sperm population in any culture consists of a heterogenous set of sperm, at different stages of capacitation, and a major subset may be incapable of completing the acrosome reaction. A variety of strategies have been advanced to maximize the number of reacting sperm and thus the penetration rate. The philosophy is that if we can induce *all* competent sperm to fertilize then we obtain the maximum amount of information about the population, thus enhancing the capacity of the test to discriminate between fertile and sub-fertile men. Strategies include pre-incubation in medium where Sr^{2+} replaces Ca^{2+}, incubation in high Ca^{2+} or hypertonic medium, and prolonged incubation at low temperature (4 °C) in TEST-egg yolk buffer. Why the latter approach works is not clear: either the stress differentially kills incompetent spermatozoa or the lipid component of the medium enhances capacitation by enhancing cholesterol efflux from the sperm membrane or otherwise affecting lipid phase transitions. Aitken's group has shown that treatment with A23187 to induce the acrosome reaction results in more consistent hamster egg test results that are better predictors of fertility after artificial insemination or IVF. In addition, the increased penetration rates allow for more economical use of hamster oocytes.

Despite these advances, the hamster ovum test remains a very expensive and labour-intensive mode of studying infertility. For many clinics the cost is prohibitive, and in Australia it is banned in several states. There are thus pressing reasons to develop alternative tests of similar predictive value.

Penetration of homologous oocytes

The definitive test of sperm function is, of course, the ability to fertilize homologous oocytes and to initiate embryonic development. However, a single episode of fertilization failure does not necessarily mean that subsequent attempts will also fail. A number of IVF units have proposed using 'spare' oocytes from IVF attempts and it is indeed possible to freeze aged oocytes and use them subsequently (following removal of the zona pellucida) in a test of fertilizing capacity. This approach depends, of course, on ethical and legal authorisation. In Western Australia it would be illegal, as both the oocyte in the process of fertilization and the resulting embryo are protected in law, and an embryo can only be created with the intention of allowing it to develop normally (paradoxically, embryos once created can be 'allowed to succumb' but cannot be used for research).

Conclusions

No single test of sperm function yet exists that will successfully predict all aspects of sperm function. Fertilization failure *in vitro* is the area of assisted reproduction that causes most distress in practice. In some cases (general biochemistry, capacitation assays and homologous zona binding or penetration assays) the cost will vary widely according to the specific test being performed, and also the degree of access to material. Some tests may well be banned in different countries due to ethical or legal constraints.

What can we predict of the future for sperm testing? There are a number of interesting possibilities. It may prove possible to separate 'good' from 'bad' sperm subsets by their surface characteristics or swimming behaviour. Monoclonal antibody-coated magnetic beads could separate acrosome-intact from acrosome reacted spermatozoa. Separation of sperm in different phases of capacitation may be possible using lectin-coated beads specific for different glycoproteins and their associated sugar moieties. Alternatively, we can start to look for the expression of exposure of specific membrane proteins as sperm capacitate. Molecular synthesis of pure human zona pellucida protein fractions such as ZP3 will give us an invaluable research tool and could serve to separate capacitated from non-capacitated sperm based on their ZP3 binding affinity. It is known that some aspects of sperm function including capacitation are modified by neurohormones and changes occur in the distribution of cholinergic binding sites during capacitation in the rabbit. If true for human spermatozoa, this could provide another route for detecting and separating capacitated from non-capacitated spermatozoa. Any of these approaches could also be used in flow cytometry. A major challenge in this approach is to develop staining and separation techniques that do not damage spermatozoa and which allow viable cells to be recovered quickly so that they can be used in assisted reproductive technology.

Acknowledgements

I wish to express my appreciation to my colleagues, Dr Anne Jequier and Dr Mary McConnell, who kindly read and commented on the manuscript.

References

Aitken RJ. Motility parameters and fertility. In: Gagnon C, ed. *Controls of Sperm Motility: Biological and Clinical Aspects.* Boca Raton: CRC Press, 1990: 285–302.

Aitken RJ, Bowie H, Buckingham D, Harkiss D, Richardson DW, West KM. Sperm penetration into a hyaluronic acid polymer as a means of monitoring functional competence. *J Androl* 1992a; **13**: 44–54.

Aitken RJ, Buckingham D, West K, Wu FC, Zikopoulos K, Richardson DW. Differential contribution of leucocytes and spermatozoa to the generation of reactive oxygen species in the ejaculates of oligozoospermic patients and fertile donors. *J Reprod Fert* 1992b; **94**: 451–62.

Aitken RJ, Elton RA. Significance of Poisson distribution theory in analysing the interaction between human spermatozoa and zona-free hamster oocytes. *J Reprod Fert* 1984; **72**: 311–21.

Boyers SP, Davis RO, Katz DF. Automated semen analysis. *Curr Probl Obstet Gynecol Fertil* 1989; **12**: 165–200.

Burkman LJ. Hyperactivated motility of human spermatozoa during *in vitro* capacitation and implications for fertility. In: Gagnon C, ed. *Controls of Sperm Motility: Biological and Clinical Aspects.* Boca Raton: CRC Press, 1990: 303–29.

Byrd W, Wolf DP. Acrosomal status in fresh and capacitated human ejaculated sperm. *Biol Reprod* 1986; **34**: 859–69.

Chan PJ, Tredway DR. Association of human sperm nuclear decondensation and *in vitro* penetration ability. *Andrologia* 1992; **24**: 77–81.

Cummins JM. Evolution of sperm form: levels of control and competition. In: Bavister BD, Cummins JM, Roldan ERS, eds. *Fertilization in Mammals*. Norwell, Massachusetts: Serono Symposia, USA, 1990: 51–64.

Cummins JM, Pember SA, Jequier AM, Yovich JL, Hartmann PE. A test of the human sperm acrosome reaction following ionophore challenge (ARIC): relationship to fertility and other seminal parameters. *J Androl* 1991; **12**: 98–103.

Davis RO. The promise and pitfalls of computer-aided sperm analysis. *Infert Reprod Med Clinics N America* 1992; **3**: 341–52.

Davis RO, Niswander PW, Katz DF. New measures of sperm motion. I. Adaptive smoothing and harmonic analysis. *J Androl* 1992; **13**: 139–52.

Eisenbach M, Ralt D. Precontact mammalian sperm–egg communication and role in fertilization. *Am J Physiol* 1992; **262**: C1095–101.

Ford WCL, Rees JM, McLaughlin EA, Goddard RJ, Hull MGR. The effect of A23187 concentration and exposure time on the outcome of the hamster egg penetration test. *Int J Androl* 1991; **14**: 127–39.

Hoskins D, Vijayaraghavan S. A new theory on the acquisition of sperm motility during epididymal transit. In: Gagnon C, ed. *Controls of Sperm Motility: Biological and Clinical Aspects*. Boca Raton: CRC Press, 1990: 53–62.

Huszar G, Vigue L, Morshedi M. Sperm creatine phosphokinase M-isoform ratios and fertilizing potential of men: a blinded study of 84 couples treated with *in vitro* fertilization. *Fert Steril* 1992; In Press.

Ivani KA, Seidel GE. At least half of capacitated, motile mouse sperm can fertilize zona-free mouse oocytes. *J Exp Zool* 1991; **412**: 406–12.

Jeyendran RR, Van der Ven HH, Perez-Pelaez M, Crabo BG, Zaneveld LJD. Development of an assay to assess the functional integrity of the human sperm membrane and its relationshiop to other semen characteristics. *J Reprod Fert* 1984; **70**: 219–28.

Johnson L, Varner DD. Effect of daily spermatozoan production but not age on transit time of spermatozoa through the human epididymis. *Biol Reprod* 1988; **39**: 812–17.

Katz DF, Andrew JB, Overstreet JW. Biological basis of *in vitro* tests of sperm function. *Prog Clin Biol Res* 1989; **302**: 95–103.

Katz DF, Overstreet JW, Hanson FW. A new quantitative test for sperm penetration into cervical mucus. *Fert Steril* 1980; **33**: 179–86.

Kessopoulou E, Tomlinson MJ, Barratt CLR, Bolton AE, Cooke ID. Origin of reactive oxygen species in human semen: spermatozoa or leucocytes? *J Reprod Fert* 1992; **94**: 451–70.

Kholkute SD, Meherji P, Puri CP. Capacitation and the acrosome reaction in sperm from men with various semen profiles monitored by a chlortetracycline fluorescence assay. *Int J Androl* 1992; **15**: 43–53.

Martin RH. Analysis of human sperm chromosome complements. In: Bavister B, Roldan E, Cummins J. eds. *Fertilization in Mammals*. Norwell, Massachusetts: Serono Symposia, USA, 1989: 365–72.

Morrell JM. Applications of flow cytometry to artificial insemination: a review. *Vet Rec* 1991; **129**: 375–8.

Mortimer D. Semen analysis and sperm washing techniques. In: Gagnon C, ed. *Controls of Sperm Motility: Biological and Clinical Aspects*. Baco Raton: CRC Press, 1990: 263–84.

Ng S-C. Micromanipulation: its relevance to human *in vitro* fertilization. *Fert Steril* 1990; **53**: 203–19.

Oehninger S. Diagnostic significance of sperm-zona pellucida interaction. *Reprod Med Reviews* 1992; **1**: 57–81.

Palermo G, Joris H, Derde M-P, Camus M, Devroey P van Steirteghem A. Sperm characteristics and outcome of human assisted fertilization by sub-zonal insemination and intracytoplasmic sperm injection. *Fertil Steril* 1993; **59**: 826–35.

Serres C, Feneux D, Jouannet P. Abnormal distribution of the periaxonemal structures in a human sperm flagellar dyskinesia. *Cell Motil Cytoskel* 1986; **6**: 68–76.

Stephens DT, Hoskins DD. Computerized quantitation of flagellar motion in mammalian sperm. In: Gagnon C, ed. *Controls of Sperm Motility: Biological and Clinical Aspects.* Boca Raton: CRC Press, 1990: 251–60.

Storey BT. Sperm capacitation and the acrosome reaction. In: Robaire B, ed. *The Male Germ Cell: Spermatogonium to Fertilization.* 637. New York: NY Academy of Sciences, 1991: 459–73.

Suarez SS, Katz DF, Owen DH, Andrew JB, Powell RL. Evidence for the function of hyperactivated motility in sperm. *Biol Reprod* 1991; **44**: 375–81.

Talbot P, Chacon R. A triple-stain technique for evaluating normal acrosome reactions in human sperm. *J Exp Zool* 1981; **215**: 201–8.

Tesarik J. Appropriate timing of the acrosome reaction is a major requirement for the fertilizing spermatozoon. *Human Reprod* 1989; **4**: 957–61.

Tesarik J, Mendoza C, Carreras A. Expression of D-mannose binding sites on human spermatozoa: comparison of fertile donors and infertile patients. *Fert Steril* 1991; **56**: 113–18.

Tombes RM, Shapiro BM, Metabolite channelling. A phosphorylcreatine shuttle to mediate high energy phosphate transport between sperm mitochondrion and tail. *Cell* 1985; **41**: 325–34.

Wassarman PM. Fertilization in the mouse. 1. The egg. In: Dunbar BS, O'Rand MG, eds. *A Comparative Overview of Mammalian Fertilization.* NY: Plenum Press, 1991: 151–65.

World Health Organization. WHO laboratory manual for the examination of human semen and semen – cervical mucus interaction. In: eds. *WHO Laboratory Manual for the Examination of Human Semen and Semen – Cervical Mucus Interaction.* Cambridge: Cambrdge University Press, 1987.

World Health Organization Task Force on the Prevention and Management of Infertility. Adenosine triphosphate in semen and other sperm characteristics: their relevance for fertility prediction in men with normal sperm concentration. *Fert Steril* 1992; **57**: 877–81.

Yanagimachi R. Mechanisms of fertilization in mammals. In: Mastroianni L, Biggers JD, eds. *Fertilization and Embryonic Development In Vitro.* New York: Plenum Press, 1981; 81–182.

Yanagimachi R. Mammalian fertilization. In: Knobil E, Neill JD, eds. *The Physiology of Reproduction.* New York: Raven Press, 1988*a*: 135–85.

Yanagimachi R. Sperm-egg fusion. In: Duzgunes N, Bronner F, eds. *Current Topics in Membrane and Transport.* 32. NY: Academic Press, 1988*b*: 3–43.

Yanagimachi R, Yanagimachi H, Roger BJ. The use of zona-free animal ova as a test-system for the assessment of the fertilizing capacity of human spermatozoa. *Biol Reprod* 1976; **15**: 471–6.

Yudin AI, Gottlieb W, Meizel S. Ultrastructural studies of the early events of the human sperm acrosome reaction as initiated by human follicular fluid. *Gamete Res* 1988; **20**: 11–24.

5

The sperm cell: genetic aspects

R. H. MARTIN

Introduction

The ability to karyotype human sperm has made a tremendous impact in the field of reproductive genetics. Prior to the first published technique which used hamster ova to reactivate human sperm (Rudak, Jacobs & Yanagimachi, 1978), information about the frequency, type and aetiology of chromosomal abnormalities had to be inferred from indirect studies of spontaneous abortions and livebirths. Since the majority of chromosomal abnormalities result in early pregnancy loss, these studies were confounded by extreme ascertainment bias.

The analysis of human sperm chromosome complements has provided the first information available on the frequency and type of chromosomal abnormalities in human gametes. The majority of studies have been on normal males to obtain baseline data (Martin *et al.*, 1983; Martin, 1991*a*; Brandriff, Gordon & Watchmaker, 1985; Brandriff *et al.*, 1990; Sele *et al.*, 1985; Kamiguchi & Makamo, 1986; Jenderny & Röhrborn, 1987; Pellestor & Sele, 1989; Navarro *et al.*, 1990; Mikamo, Kanaguchi & Tateno, 1990). There have also been studies on the effect of donor age on the frequency of chromosomal abnormalities in human sperm (Martin & Rademaker, 1987*b*), evaluation of sperm sex preselection techniques (Brandriff *et al.*, 1986; Ueda & Yanagimachi, 1987; Beckett, Martin & Hoar, 1989); the effect of microinjection of human sperm into hamster oocytes (Martin, Ko & Rademaker, 1988) the effect of cryopreservation (Chernos & Martin, 1989; Martin, Chernos & Rademaker, 1991), and the effect of culture media (Martin *et al.*, 1990*c*; Benet *et al.*, 1991; Martin *et al.*, 1992). Men at increased risk of sperm chromosomal abnormalities have also been studied, such as men exposed to radiotherapy (Martin *et al.*, 1986*a*, 1989; Jenderny & Röhrborn, 1987; Genesca *et al.*,1990) and men carrying constitutional chromosomal rearrangements such as translocations and inversions (Balkan & Martin, 1983*a,b*; Balkan, Burns & Martin, 1983; Martin, 1984; Brandriff *et al.*, 1986; Martin, 1986*a,b*; Martin *et al.*,

1986b; Burns et al., 1986; Pellester, Sele & Jalbert, 1987; Benet & Martin, 1988; Martin, 1988a,b; Templado et al., 1988; Pellestor et al., 1989; Pellestor, 1990; Martin et al., 1990a,b; Templado et al., 1990; Estop et al., 1992; Martin, 1991b; Spriggs, Martin & Hulten, 1992; Martin, 1992; Martin et al., 1992; Jenderny, 1992; Jenderny et al., 1992; Martin & Hulten, 1993; Syme & Martin, 1992; Martin, 1993; Martin et al., 1994b; Spriggs & Martin, 1994; Martin, 1994a,b; Martin & Spriggs, 1994).

In this report, I will summarize the information on sperm chromosomal abnormalities in normal men, discuss the effect of donor age on the frequency and type of chromosomal abnormalities in sperm, analyse the distribution of aneuploidy in the various chromosome groups and demonstrate how these data provide clues to the aetiology of numerical chromosomal abrnormalities and review results of sperm chromosome studies in 42 men with constitutional chromosomal abnormalities.

Materials and methods

Technique

I have previously published a detailed technique for obtaining pronuclear human sperm chromosome complements after sperm penetration of golden hamster eggs that have had the zona pellucida removed (Martin, 1983). The methods reported here are similar with alterations in the preparation of sperm, manipulation of eggs, and the culture of eggs in colcemid.

Media

Biggers-Whitten-Whittingham medium (BWW: Biggers, Whitten & Whittingham, 1971) with some modifications (Martin, 1983) was used for sperm and egg preparation. This medium was filtered through a cellulose acetate membrane (pore size 0.22 μm) to sterilize it. The pH was adjusted to 7.4–7.5 with a small amount (0.1 ml) of acid or base Hepes solution. TEST-yolk buffer (Bolanos, Overstreet & Katz, 1983; Brandriff et al., 1985) was used for sperm capacitation and preservation. The medium used for egg culture was Ham's F10 (Flow Laboratories, McLean, Va) supplemented with 15% fetal bovine serum (Flow Laboratories, heat inactivated at 60 °C for 1 h, 100 IU penicillin G/ml and 50 μg streptomycin sulphate/ml). Just before use, the pH was adjusted to 7.2 with 1 M HCl.

Human sperm preparation

The semen sample was collected in a sterile container, was liquefied for 30 min at 37 °C, at which time volume was measured and an equal volume of TEST-yolk buffer added. The sample was well mixed with the buffer and sealed in a tube, which was immersed in a jar of room-temperature water. This jar, in turn, was sealed and plunged into a styrofoam box of crushed ice, which was closed and refrigerated at 4 °C for 18–24 hours. On the experiment day, the sperm in TEST-yolk buffer were removed from refrigeration and room temperature BWW was added to a total volume of 10 ml, the components were mixed, the suspension was centrifuged at 600 g for 6 min, the supernatant was decanted, and the pellet resuspended in 10 ml BWW. The sperm were washed two more times to remove seminal fluids, TEST-yolk buffer, and debris. Sperm were assessed for forward progression and motility and the final sperm pellet was resuspended in BWW to a final concentration of approximately 0.5×10^6 to 20×10^6/ml, depending on sperm quality. Using an Eppendorf pipette, four 20 μl drops of sperm suspension were made per 60×15 mm petri dish and 10–15 ml of light mineral oil (Fisher 0-121 Edmonton, Alberta) were added to cover the drops. Dishes of sperm drops were kept at 37 °C, 5% CO_2, 95% relative humidity.

Hamster egg preparation

The hamsters (*Microcetus auratus*) were superovulated with an intraperitoneal injection of 25 to 30 IU of pregnant mare's serum gonadoptropin (Sigma, G-4877, St. Louis M.) 69–73 h before egg retrieval followed by an intraperitoneal injection of 25 IU of human chorionic gondatropic (hCG: A.P.L., Ayerst Laboratories, New York, NY) 16–17 h before egg retrieval.

Each hamster yielded approximately 40–60 eggs. The hamsters were stunned with ether and killed by cervical dislocation approximately 16–17 h after hCG injection. The oviducts were punctured, the cumulus cell mass was removed and 0.1% hyaluronidase (Type 1-S, Sigma) in BWW was added. The hyaluronidase dispersed the cumulus cells in 2–3 min, freeing the eggs, which were then washed two times in BWW, treated with 0.1% trypsin until the zonae pellucidae were removed, washed three times in BWW and put into the prepared sperm drops in groups of 20–30 eggs.

Gamete coincubation

Fertilization checks (Martin, 1983) were performed every 15 min during the gamete coincubation time. At the first appearance of swollen sperm heads, the eggs were washed briefly in F10 to remove excess sperm, then were transferred to prepared 100 μl drops of F10 under oil in 60×15 mm petri dishes. After incubation in F10 for 13.0–15.5 h, colcemid (Gibco/BRL, Burlington, Ontario) was added to the drops to a concentration of 0.4 μg/ml and the eggs were incubated for approximately 5 h.

Chromosome preparation

The eggs were transferred to a hypotonic solution (1% sodium citrate) for 3–6 min. A maximum of ten eggs were transferred in a small drop of hypotonic solution (2 mm diameter) to the centre of a glass slide pre-cleaned with alcohol. Four drops of fixative (3:1 96% ethanol:glacial acetic acid), each 20 μl, were dropped over the eggs (Tarkowski, 1966). After 2 weeks, the chromosomes were stained with 0.5% quinacrine dihydrochloride (pH 4.5) for 25 min followed by three rinses in distilled H_2O (pH 4.5) for a total of 10 min. The slides were mounted in distilled H_2O at pH 4.5 and examined and photographed with a Zeiss fluorescence microscope with a DC-powered HBO W2 mercury lamp. The barrier filter was set at No. 47 and the excitation filter at BG3. The slides were subsequently stained with 3 ml Giemsa (Harleco, Sibbstown, NJ) in 47 ml Gurr buffer (pH 6.8) for 5 min. An example of a Q-banded sperm chromosome complement with a structural abnormality is presented in Fig. 1.

Sperm chromosome complements from normal men

Our laboratory has analysed a total of 6524 sperm chromosome complements from 84 normal healthy men. The mean frequency of abnormalities in this population was 12.8%. Structural chromosomal abnormalities accounted for 8.6% and numerical for 3.7%. Of the numerical abnormalities, 0.5% were hyperhaploid and 3.2% were hypophaploid. If all of these numerical abnormalities were produced by meiotic non-disjunction, we would expect an equal frequency of hyperhaploid and hypohaploid complements. Since we observed a significant excess of hypohaploid complements, some of these complements must have arisen by other mechanisms such as anaphase lag or by artefactual loss of chromosomes during slide preparation. Since we used Tarkowski's technique (1966) for fixation of the fertilized eggs on slides and this technique is known to be associated with an excess of hypohaploidy, it is likely that our elevated frequency of hypohaploidy is a technical artefact. A conservative estimate of aneuploidy can be obtained by doubling the frequency of hyperhaploidy which yields an aneuploidy frequency of 1.0%. Using this conservative estimate of aneuploidy, the total mean of sperm chromosomal abnormalities was 9.6%. These results are summarized in Table 1.

Table 1. *Cytogenetics of sperm in 84 normal men*

Abnormalities	Observed	Conservative estimate[a]
Structural	8.6%	8.6%
Numerical	3.7%	1.0%
Hyperhaploid	0.5%	
Hypohaploid	3.2%	
Total abnormal	12.8%	9.6%

Total sperm 6524
[a]See text for explanation of conservative estimate of chromosomal abnormalities.

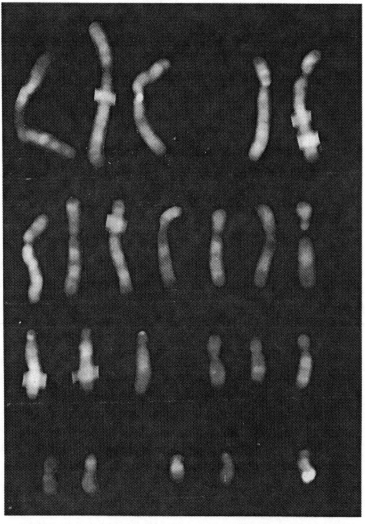

Fig. 1. Q-banded human sperm chromosome complement with a chromosome break in the long arm of chromosome 12, 23, Y, csb 12 q15.

Table 2. *Sperm chromosomal abnormalities observed in 129 normal men from three large studies*

Laboratory	Number of donors	Number of karyotypes	% Abnormalities	
			Numerical (2 × hyperhaploid)	Structural
Bandriff *et al.* (1990)	20	5126	1.4	6.9
Martin (this report)	84	6524	1.0	8.6
Mikamo *et al.* (1990)	26	9820	1.4	13.9

Eight other laboratories in five different countries have also reported on chromosomal abnormalities in sperm of normal men (Rudak *et al.*, 1978; Brandriff, Gordon & Carrano, 1990; Jenderny *et al.*, 1987; Pellester & Sele, 1989; Navarro *et al.*, 1990; Mikamo, Kanaguchi & Tateno, 1990; Estop *et al.*, 1991; Rosenbusch, Strehler & Sterzik, 1992) for a total of more than 20 000 sperm chromosome complements analysed. The majority of the reports are on very small sample sizes, with no actual karyotypes. However, three large studies have reported on 5000 or more sperm karyotypes in three different countries. Brandriff *et al.* (1990), in the United States, have analysed 5000 Q-banded sperm chromosome complements from 20 men. We have studied 6524 Q-banded sperm complements from 84 normal Canadian men (as above). Mikamo *et al.* (1990), in Japan, have reported on 9280 unbanded sperm karyotypes from 26 donors. Results from these three laboratories represent over 90% of the worldwide data and these are summarized in Table 2. A conservative estimate of the mean frequency of aneuploidy is very similar in all three studies (1.0–1.4%). For the study by Mikamo *et al.*, this is the actual value of hyperhaploid and hypohaploid complements combined. Both of the other studies had significantly more hypohaploid than hyperhaploid complements, thus the numerical frequency is a conservative estimate based on a doubling of the hyperhaploid frequency. The mean frequency of structural abnormalities showed more variability in the three studies but all three were in the general vicinity of 9–10%. However, there was considerable inter-donor variability in the frequency of structural abnormalities with large ranges reported in all three studies. Brandriff *et al.* (1990) found a range in the frequency of structural abnormalities of 2–15% in 20 donors, Martin (1991*a*) found 0–22% in 83 donors and Mikamo *et al.* (1990) reported 4–22% in 26 donors. Nevertheless, both Brandriff's group and Mikamo's group have shown that the frequency of chromosomal abnormalities in human sperm is donor-specific and stable over time. In summary, these studies suggest that an estimate of the frequency of chromosomal abnormalties in human sperm is 1–2% numerical and 9–10% structural.

The effect of age on the frequency of sperm chromosomal abnormalities

We have studied the effect of age on the frequency of sperm chromosomal abnormalities because it has been suggested that advanced paternal age (independent of maternal age) is associated with an increased incidence of trisomy. We studied *sperm chromosome complements from 30 normal men to proven* fertility stratified by age with five males in each of six age categories (20–24, 25–29, 30–34, 35–39, 40–44, 45 +). A minimum of 30 complements was analysed for each male. The analysis was performed 'blindly', without knowledge of the donor's age (Martin & Rademaker, 1987*b*).

There was a significant negative relationship between the proportion of hyperhaploid sperm and age. Thus young men had the highest frequency of hyperhaploid sperm, this finding was certainly unexpected but has, in fact, been reported previously. Hook & Regal (1984) studied cases of trisomy 21 in which the extra chromosome was of paternal origin and found a negative trend of Down syndrome with paternal age. Also, Carothers & Fillippi (1988) found that 47,XXY of paternal original had a significant decrease in paternal age.

We found a highly significant increase in the frequency of structural chromosomal abnormalities with age from 2.8% in the youngest age group of 13.6% in men older than 44 years. A number of studies have determined that over 80% of *de novo* structural aberration are of paternal origin (Olson & Magenis, 1988). An increasing frequency of structural chromosomal abnormalities with age could be explained by the continued cell divisions of spermatogenesis and the long time exposure to elastogens which could gradually increase the frequency of chromosome breaks with age.

In summary, this study did not find evidence for an increased risk of trisomy with paternal age. In contrast, the frequency of hyperhaploid sperm decreased while the frequency of sperm with structural abnormalities increased with age. This age effect must be taken into account with any future studies on human sperm chromosomes.

Distribution of aneuploidy among the different chromosomes

We have recently looked at the distribution and frequency of aneuploidy among the different chromosomes in sperm to determine whether all chromosomes are equally likely to be involved in aneuploid events or if some chromosomes are particularly susceptible to non-disjunction. It is important to determine the incidence of non-disjunction for different chromosomes because this information will give us clues about the mechanisms of non-disjunction and survival of chromosomally abnormal embryos. If all chromosome groups have the same frequency of non-disjunction, then the mechanism that causes non-disjunction must be common to all chromosomes, e.g. errors of spindle formation or attachment. If specific chromsomes have an increased frequency of non-disjunction, then we would focus on the specific characteristics of the chromosomes (e.g. small size, presence of heterochromatin, nucleolar organizing regions) to elucidate some of the factors which influence the rate of non-disjunction.

Results on the distribution of aneuploidy were pooled from a number of studies encompassing 8356 sperm chromosome complements from normal men and 3259 sperm complements from men carrying a constitutional chromosomal abnormality (Martin, Ko & Rademaker, 1991). For the latter group, aneuploid complements unrelated to the constitutional chromosomal rearrangement were only included if no interchromosomal effect had been ascertained. The analysis was based on hyperhaploid complements since hypohaploid complements might be caused by technical artefact (as discussed above). The data were analysed separately for the two groups of men and then pooled after statistical analysis demonstrated no difference in the two groups (chi square analysis). For statistical analysis, it was assumed that all chromosomes had an equal probability of non-disjunction and two-tailed binomial tests using exact binomial probabilities were performed (Rosner, 1986) to determine if each chromosome (or chromosome group) had a frequency of hyperhaploidy that differed significantly from the expected frequency.

All chromosome groups were represented among the hyperhaploid sperm demonstrating that all groups are susceptible to non-disjunction, not just those commonly observed in studies of newborns and spontaneous abortions. There was a significantly increased frequency of hyperhaploidy for chromosome 1 ($p = 0.02$), 21 ($p = 0.002$) and the sex chromosomes ($p = 0.0001$). The increased frequency of hyperhaploidy for chromosome 1 is surprising since this is the only chromosome which has not been observed as a trisomy in spontaneous abortions. However, trisomy 1 has been observed in an eight-cell human pre-embryo (Watt *et al.*, 1987) and it is possible that trisomy 1 is common in human conceptuses but is always lost in an early preimplantation stage.

The highly significant increase in the frequency of hyperhaploidy for the sex chromosomes in human sperm is interesting since, in many studies of meiosis I in human males, the X and Y chromosomes are often unpaired (Laurie & Hulten, 1985). It is possible that these univalents might predipose to non-disjunction of the sex chromosomes in males. There are four common aneuploidies for the sex chromosomes in humans: 45,X; 47,XYY; 47,XXY and 47,XXX. Recent evidence has demonstrated that the majority of these originate from a paternal error, unlike autosomal aneuploidies, in which maternal errors predominate (Hassold, Benham & Leppert, 1988; Jacobs *et al.*, 1988).

These results suggest heterogeneity in the aetiology of non-disjunction: a common mechanism affecting all chromosomes and mechanisms targeting specific chromosomes such as sex chromosome pairing in the male.

Studies in men heterozygous for translocations and inversions

Men with a constitutional chromosomal abnormality have an increased risk of chromosomally abnormal children and spontaneous abortions. The ability to karyotype sperm has allowed detailed analysis of the segregation of chromosomes in men carrying a translocation or inversion. Forty-two men have been analysed from six different laboratories and this has provided our first glimpse of how these rearrangements affect meiosis. Of these 42 men, 30 carried different reciprocal translocations, six were heterozygous for Robertsonian translocations and six were heterozygous for inversions. A summary of the translocations and inversions and the frequency of chromosomally unablanced sperm in each case is presented in Table 3.

The majority of the information available is on reciprocal translocations. Alternate and adjacent 1 segregations were present in all of the translocations with means of 46% and 38%, respectively. Adjacent 2 and 3:1 segregations were rare with means of 11% and 5%, respectively. Adjacent 1 segregation was the most common segregation leading to chromosomal imbalance, even in those translocations known to have abnormal livebirths exclusively from another segregation, such as the common t(11; 12) translocation for which only 3:1 segregations have been reported in livebirths (Martin, 1984). Thus it appears that the adjacent 1 segregation occurs preferentially during spermatogenesis. This is not surprising, since both adjacent 2 and 3:1 segregations require nonseparation of homologues and are thus akin to non-disjunction.

Alternate segregation yields normal offspring: theoretically 1/2 should have normal chromosomes and 1/2, the two balanced translocated chromosomes. This expectation was met in 28 of the reciprocal translocations studied by sperm chromosomal analysis. This adherence to the theoretical 1:1 ratio of normal to balanced complements corroborates the validity of the system demonstrating no selective advantage of chromosomally normal sperm compared to sperm carrying

Table 3. *Segregation of sperm chromosomes in translocation and inversion heterozygotes*

Type of rearrangement	Laboratory (reference)	% unbalanced sperm
Reciprocal		
t(5; 18)	Balkan & Martin (1983*a*)	19
t(5; 13)	Pellestor *et al.* (1989)	23
t(5; 11)	Burns *et al.* (1986)	30
(t; 14)	Balkan & Martin (1983*a*)	32
t(4; 17)	Pellestor *et al.* (1989)	44
t(2; 17)	Jenderny (1992)	44
t(2; 3)	Martin (1994*b*)	45

Table 3. *Continued*

Type of rearrangement	Laboratory (reference)	% unbalanced sperm
t(7; 14)	Martin et al. (1990a)	48
t(6; 7)	Pellestor et al. (1989)	49
t(3; 11)	Martin & Hulten (1993)	53
t(9; 13)	Martin & Spriggs (1994)	53
t(1; 4)*	Estop et al. (1992)	54
t(12; 20)	Martin et al. (1990b)	54
t(1; 9)	Martin (1992)	55
t(4; 6)	Martin et al. (1990a)	55
t(2; 9)	Martin et al. (1990a)	56
t(1; 2)	Templado et al. (1990)	59
t(9; 10)	Martin (1988a)	59
t(16; 19)	Martin (1992)	60
t(1; 4)*	Estop et al. (1992)	61
t(7; 20)	Martin & Hulten (1993)	61
t(11; 27)	Spriggs et al. (1992)	62
t(3; 16)	Brandriff et al. (1986)	62
t(8; 15)	Brandriff et al. (1986)	63
t(2; 5)	Templado et al. (1988)	64.5†
t(7; 14)	Burns et al. (1986)	65
t(9; 18)	Pellestor et al. (1989)	65
t(3; 8)	Jenderny (1992)	66
t(15; 22)	Martin & Hulten (1993)	66
t(1; 11)	Spriggs et al. (1992)	67
t(11; 22)	Martin (1984)	77
Robertsonian		
t(21; 22)	Syme & Martin (1992)	3
t(13; 14)	Pellestor et al. (1987)	8
t(13; 15)	Pellestor (1990)	10
t(15; 22)	Martin et al. (1992)	10
t(14; 21)	Balkan & Martin (1983b)	13
t(13; 14)	Martin (1988b)	27
Inversions		
1. peri(3)	Balkan et al. (1983)	0
2. para(7)	Martin 1986a)	0
3. peri(1)	Martin et al. (1994a,b)	0
4. peri(20)	Jenderny et al. (1992)	0
5. peri(8)	Martin (1993)	11
6. peri(3)	Martin (1991b)	31

*Two cousins carried the same translocation.
†Some alternate and adjacent segregations could not be distinguished, so the 64.5% unbalanced frequency assumes that each segregation comprised 50% of the unidentified karyotypes.

the translocation. The only exception in the reciprocal translocations studied was one translocation in the male carrying two different reciprocal translocations and this was probably caused by the small sample size, since only 23 sperm karyotypes were studied.

The frequency of chromosomally unbalanced sperm varied from 19–77% with a mean of 54%. In fact, most of the translocations have had approximately half of the sperm chromosomally unbalanced. This frequency of imbalance observed in sperm is much higher than seen in studies of human fetuses from translocation heterozygotes. The most likely explanation for this difference is that many chromosomally unbalanced embryos are lost early in embryological development. It is also possible that sperm selection *in vivo* might account for the lower frequency of unbalanced fetuses. However, this is unlikely since paternal reciprocal translocations carriers have been found to have the same frequency of chromosomally unbalanced fetuses as maternal carriers (11.4%) in the European Collaborative Study of Prenatal Diagnosis (Boué & Gallano, 1984).

Six men with Robertsonian translocation have been studied to date: three DD translocations, two DG and one GG. The frequency of chromosomal imbalance in sperm is much lower in Robertsonian translocation carriers than reciprocal translocation heterozygotes. In Robertsonian translocation carriers the mean is 12%, with a range of 3–27%. The decrease in the frequency of abnormalities in Robertsonian translocations compared to reciprocal translocations is interesting, since males and females carrying a reciprocal translocation have an equivalent risk of producing chromosomally abnormal offspring, whereas males carrying a Robertsonian translocation have a lower risk of producing an unbalanced child compared to female carriers (Boué & Gallano, 1984). Results from sperm chromosome studies suggest that this lower risk for male Robertsonian translocation carriers comes about by a meiotic mechanism which produces a low frequency of unbalanced sperm. It is possible that *cis* pairing of Robertsonian translocations is more common during male meiosis, as this type of pairing is more conducive to alternate segregation which yields chromosomally normal and balanced gametes.

A total of six inversion heterozygotes have been studied by sperm chromosomal analysis: five pericentric inversions and one paracentric inversion. Four of the inversions had no recombinant chromosomes and two inversions had 11% and 31% recombinant sperm. In order to produce recombinant chromosomes, a cross-over must occur within the inversion loop. Three of the inversions which did not produce recombinant sperm [(3)(p11q11); (7)(q11q22); (1)(p31q12)] were relatively small (less than 30% of the chromosome length) and it is likely that either crossing-over did not occur within the small inversion loop or that pairing was accomplished by heterosynapsis. The other three pericentric inversions are all larger than 50% of the chromosome length and could produce recombinant chromosomes if pairing was accomplished via an inversion loop or by pairing of homologues only within the inverted segment and an uneven number of chiasmata within the inverted region. The two large pericentric inversions studied by this laboratory fulfilled these expectations with 30.8% [inv(3); 25q21); Martin 1991a,b] and 11.4% [inv(8)(p23q22); Martin, 1993] recombinant sperm. The inversion (20)(p13q11.2) studied by Jenderny et al. (1992) failed to produce recombination sperm. This may simply be a matter of sample size as only 26 sperm were analysed. Alternatively, the inversion (20) chromosome may not pair as an invertion loop, despite the proportionately large size of the inverted segment.

Cases of trisomy 21 and sex chromosomal aneuploidy have been reported in association with translocations (Aurias et al., 1978). A number of researchers have suggested that there is an increased frequency of chromosomal abnormalities unrelated to the specific translocation or inversion and have termed this an 'interchromosomal effect'. The frequency of numerical chromosomal abnormalities unrelated to the translocation was not significantly increased for any of the translocations with the exception of the man who is heterozygous for two reciprocal translocations (Burns et al., 1986). This man had an extremely high frequency of numerical chromosomal abnormalities, unrelated to the translocation. It is possible that the presence of two reciprocal translocations greatly disrupted pairing and crossing-over at meiosis, causing the anomalous segregations that were observed. The evidence to date does not support the concept of large inter-chromosomal effect for carriers of a single translocation. However, studies on sperm chromosomal analysis have been based on small numbers and have not had the statistical power to rule out an interchromosomal effect. For example, I have calculated that, for the frequency of aneuploidy observed from sperm of normal men in my laboratory, approximately 160 sperm complements would need to be analysed to detect a tripling in the aneuploidy frequency and that approximately 500 would need to be analysed to detect a doubling (Rosner 1986; pp. 225). To date, we have studied a sufficient number of sperm complements in 11 translocation heterozygoes to detect a tripling of the aneuploidy frequency and in only one translocation to detect a doubling. It is not trivial to attempt to study 160–500 sperm karyotypes in each translocation heterozygote, since the technique is still extremely labour intensive. However, this sample size is required to assess the possibility of an interchromosomal effect adequately.

It would be very interesting to compare meiotic pairing data in an inversion heterozygote with the outcome in sperm. Similarly, it would be valuable to determine if predominantly *cis* pairing in Robertsonian translocation carriers is followed by a low frequency of chromosomally unbalanced sperm. Sequential analysis of meiotic chromosomes and the gametic outcome in sperm would also provide some insight into the question of an interchromosomal effect. For example, chromosomes unrelated to structural abnormalities have been observed to associate with structurally rearranged chromosomes at meiosis I and this association could lead to non-disjunction of the chromosomes involved. This could be analysed by studying chromsomes and sperm, as well as meiosis. These studies are currently in progress.

New developments

A wealth of new information has been amassed on human sperm from the cross-species fertilization technique. However, the technique is limited because it is time consuming, labour intensive and difficult to learn. Thus progress has been slow. A rapid simple inexpensive technique is required to provide an alternate method of obtaining information on the genetic content of human sperm. Fluorescence *in situ* hybridization (FISH) may provide a rapid screen for aneuploidy detection in human sperm. Several laboratories have reported preliminary data with *in situ* hybridization in interphase sperm nuclei (Joseph, Gosden & Chandley, 1984; Burns et al., 1985; Guttenbach & Schmid, 1990, 1991; Wyrobek et al., 1990; Pieters et al., 1990; Coonen et al., 1991; Han et al., 1992, 1993; Goldman et al., 1993; Robbins et al., 1993; Williams et al., 1993). In our laboratory we have studied more than 300 000 interphase sperm nuclei using multicolour FISH to analyse DNA probes specific for chromosomes 1, 12, 15, 16, X and Y. The technique appears reliable and reproducible and generates data much faster than the cross-species fertilization technique (Holmes & Martin, 1993; Martin, Ko & Chan, 1993; Martin et al.. 1994a,b; Martin, 1994a,b & unpublished data). Also the frequency of aneuploidy detected is very similar to the frequency observed in sperm chromosome complements. However, there is still the disadvantage that it is an indirect test and that a fluorescent spot does not necessarily correspond to the presence of a chromosome. Nevertheless, fluorescence *in situ* hybridization does have the potential of providing a screen for aneuploidy detection in large numbers of men exposed to occupational or environmental hazards.

Acknowledgements

Sincere thanks go to Leona Barclay, Evelyn Ko and Kathy Hildebrand for expert technical assistance. Renée Martin is an Alberta Heritage Foundation for Medical Research Scientist, whose research is funded by the Medical Research Council of Canada and the Alberta Children's Hospital Foundation.

References

Aurias A, Prieur M, Dutrillaux B, Lejeune J. Systematic analysis of 95 reciprocal translocations of autosomes. *Hum Genet* 1978; **45**: 259–82.

Balkan W, Burns K, Martin RH. Sperm chromosome analysis of a man heterozygous for a pericentric inversion of chromosome number 3. *Cytogenet Cell Genet* 1983; **35**: 295–7.

Balkan W, Martin RH. Chromosome segregation into the spermatozoa of two men heterozygous for different reciprocal translocations. *Hum Genet* 1983a; **63**: 345–8.

Balkan W, Martin RH. Segregation of chromosomes into the spermatozoa of a man heterozygous for a 14;21 Robertsonian translocation. *Am J Med Genet* 1983b; **16**: 169–72.

Beckett TA, Martin RH, Hoar DI. Assessment of Sephadex technique for selection of X chromosome-bearing human sperm by analysis of sperm chromosomes, deoxyribonucleic acid and Y-bodies. *Fertil Steril* 1989; **52**: 829–35.

Benet J, Martin RH. Sperm chromosome complements in a 47,XXY man. *Hum Genet* 1988; **78**: 313–15.

Benet J, Navarro J, Genesca A, Egozcue J, Templado C. Chromosome abnormalities in human spermatozoa after albumin or TEST-yolk capacitation. *Hum Repro* 1991; **6**: 369–75.

Biggers JD, Whitten WK, Whittingham DG. The culture of mouse embryos *in vitro*. In: Daniel JC, ed. *Methods in Mammalian Embryology*. San Francisco: Freeman, 1971: 86–116.

Bolanos JR, Overstreet JW, Katz DF. Human sperm penetration of zona-free hamster eggs after storage of semen for 48 hours at 2 °C to 5 °C. *Fertil Steril* 1983; **39**: 536–41.

Boué A, Gallano P. A collaborative study of the segregation of inherited chromosome structural rearrangements in 1356 prenatal diagnosis. *Prenat Diagn* 1984; **4**: 45–67.

Brandriff B, Gordon L, Ashworth LK, Littman V, Watchmaker G, Carrano AV. Cytogenetics of human sperm: meiotic segregation in two translocation carriers. *Am J Hum Genet* 1986; **38**: 197–208.

Brandriff B, Gordon L, Ashworth L, Watchmaker G, Moore D, Wyrobek AJ, Carrano AV. Chromosomes of human sperm: variability among normal individuals. *Hum Genet* 1985; **70**: 18–24.

Brandriff BF, Gordon LA, Carrano AV. Cytogenetics of human sperm: structural aberrations and DNA replication. In: Mendelsohn ML, Albertini RJ, eds. *Mutation and the Environment Part B: Metabolism Testing Methods and Chromosomes*. New York: John Wiley, 1990: 435–46.

Brandriff BF, Gordon LA, Haendel S, Singer, Moore DHII, Gledhill BL. Sex chromosome ratios determined by karyotypic analysis in albumin-isolated human sperm. *Fertil Steril* 1986; **46**: 678–85.

Brandriff B, Gordon L, Watchmaker G. Human sperm chromosomes obtained from hamster eggs after sperm capacitation in TEST-yolk buffer. *Gamete Res* 1985; **11**: 253–9.

Burns JP, Chan VTW, Jonasson JA, Fleming KA, Taylor S, McGee JOD. Sensitive system for visualization biotinylated DNA probes hybridized *in situ*: rapid sex determination of intact cells. *J Clin Pathol* 1985; **38**: 1085–92.

Burns JP, Koduru PRK, Alonso ML, Chaganti RSK. Analysis of meiotic segregation in a man heterozygous for two reciprocal translocation using hamster *in vitro* penetration system. *Am J Hum Genet* 1986; **38**: 467–78.

Carothers AD, Filippi G. Klinefelter's syndrome in Sardinia and Scotland. *Hum Genet* 1988; **81**: 71–5.

Chernos JE, Martin RH. A cytogenetic investigation of the effects of cryopreservation on human sperm. *Am J Hum Genet* 1989; **45**: 766–77.

Coonen E, Pieters MHEC, Dumoulin JCM, Meyer H, Evers JLH, Ramaekers FCS, Geraedts JPM. Nonisotopic *in situ* hybridization as a method for nondisjunction studies in human spermatozoa. *Molecular Repro Develop* 1991; **28**: 18–22.

Estop AM, Cieply K, Vankirk V, Mune S, Garver K. Cytogenic studies in human sperm. *Hum Genet* 1991; **87**: 447–51.

Estop AM, Levinson F, Cieply K, Van Kirk V. The segregation of a t(1;4) in two male carriers heterozygous for the translocation. *Hum Genet* 1992; **89**: 425–9.

Genesca A, Miro R, Caballin MR, Benet J, Germa JR, Egozcue J. Sperm chromosome studies in individuals treated for testicular cancer. *Hum Repro* 1990; **5**: 286–90.

Goldman ASH, Fomina A, Knights PA, Hill CJ, Walker AP, Hulten MA. Analysis of the primary sex ratio, sex chromosome aneuploidy and diploidy in human sperm using dual-colour fluorescence *in situ* hybridization. *Eur J Hum Genet* 1993; **1**: 325–34.

Guttenbach M, Schmid M. Determination of Y chromosome aneuploidy in human sperm nuclei by non-radioactive *in situ* hybridization. *Am J Hum Genet* 1990; **46**: 553–8.

Guttenbach M, Schmid M. Non-isotopic detection of chromosome 1 in human meiosis and demonstration of disomic sperm nuclei. *Hum Genet* 1991; **87**: 261–5.

Han TL, Ford JH, Webb GC, Flaherty SP, Corell A, Matthews CD. Simultaneous detection of X- and Y-bearing human sperm by double fluorescence *in situ* hybridization. *Mol Rep Devel* 1993; **34**: 308–13.

Han TL, Webb GC, Flaherty SP, Correll A, Matthews CD, Ford JH. Detection of chromosome 17- and X-bearing human spermatozoa using fluorescence *in situ* hybridization. *Mol Rep Devel* 1992; **33**: 189–94.

Hassold T, Benham F, Leppert M. Cytogenetics and molecular analysis of sex chromosome monosomy. *Am J Hum Genet* 1988; **42**: 534–41.

Holmes JM, Martin RH. Aneuploidy detection in human sperm. *Am J Hum Genet* Suppl 1991; **49**(4): 218.

Holmes JM, Martin RH. Aneuploidy detection in human sperm nuclei using fluorescence *in situ* hybridization. *Hum Genet* 1993; **91**: 20–4.

Hook EB, Regal RR. A search for a paternal age effect upon cases of 47, + 21 in which the extra chromosome is of paternal origin. *Am J Hum Genet* 1984; **36**: 413–21.

Jacobs P. Hassold T, Whittington E, Butler G, Collier S, Keston M, Lee M. Klinefelter's syndrome: an analysis of the origin of the additional sex chromosome using molecular probes. *Ann Hum Genet* 1988; **52**: 93–109.

Jenderny J. Sperm chromosome analysis of two males heterozygous for a t(2;17)q35;p13) and t(3;8)(p13;p21) reciprocal translocation. *Hum Genet* 1992; **90**: 171–3.

Jenderny J, Gebauer J, Röhborn G, Ruger A. Sperm chromosome analysis of a man heterozygous for a pericentric inversion of chromosome 20. *Hum Genet* 1992; **89**: 117–19.

Jenderny J, Röhrborn G. Chromosome analysis of human sperm. 1. First results with a modified method. *Hum Genet* 1987; **76**: 385–8.

Joseph AM, Gosden JR, Chandley AC. Estimation of aneuploidy levels in human spermatozoa using chromosome specific probes and *in situ* hybridization. *Hum Genet* 1984; **66**: 234–8.

Kamiguchi Y, Mikamo K. An improved, efficient method for analysing human sperm chromsomes using zona-free hamster ova. *Am J Hum Genet* 1986; **38**: 724.

Laurie DA, Hulten MA. Further studies on bivalent chiasma frequency in human males with normal karyotypes. *Ann Hum Genet* 1985; **49**: 189–201.

Martin RH. A detailed method for obtaining preparations of human sperm chromosomes. *Cytogenet Cell Genet* 1983; **35**: 253–6.

Martin RH. Analysis of human sperm chromosome complements from a male heterozygous for a reciprocal translocation t(11;22)(q23q11). *Clin Genet* 1984; **25**: 257–61.

Martin RH. Sperm chromosome analysis in a man heterozygous for a paracentric inversion of chromosome 7 (q11q22). *Hum Genet* 1986a; **73**: 97–100.

Martin RH. A fragile site 10q25 in human sperm chromosomes. *J Med Genet* 1986b; **23**: 279.

Martin RH. Meiotic segregation of human sperm chromosomes in translocation heterozygotes. Report of a t(9;10)(q34;q11) and a review of the literature. *Cytogenet Cell Genet* 1988a; **47**: 48–51.

Martin RH. Cytogenic analysis of sperm from a male heterozygous for a 13;14 Robertsonian translocation. *Hum Genet* 1988b; **80**: 357–61.

Martin RH. Chromosomal analysis of human spermatozoa. In: Verlinsky Y and Kuliev A, ed. *Preimplantation Genetics*. New York: Plenum Press, 1991a: 91–102.

Martin RH. Cytogenetic analysis of sperm from a man heterozygous for a pericentric inversion inv (3)(p25q21). *Am J Hum Genet* 1991b; **48**: 856–61.

Martin RH. Sperm chromosome analysis of two men heterozygous for reciprocal translocations t(1;9)(q22;q31) and t(16;19)(q11.1;q13.3). *Cytogenet Cell Genet* 1992; **60**: 18–21.

Martin RH. Analysis of sperm chromosome complements from a man heterozygous for a pericentric inversion, inv (8)(p23q22). *Cytogenet Cell Genet* 1993; **62**: 199–202.

Martin RH. Detection of aneuploidy for chromosomes 1,12,X and Y in human sperm using multicolour fluorescence *in situ* hybridization (FISH). *Human Reproduction* 1994a 'in press'.

Martin RH. Sperm chromosome complements in a man heterozygous for a reciprocal translocation t(2;3)(q24;p26). *Human Reproduction* 1994b 'in press'.

Martin RH, Balkan W, Burns K, Rademaker AW, Lin CC, Rudd NL. The chromosome constitution of 1000 human spermatozoa. *Hum Genet* 1983; **63**: 305–9.

Martin RH, Barclay L, Hildebrand K, Ko E, Fowlow SB. Cytogenetic analysis of 400 sperm from three translocation heterozygotes. *Human Genet* 1990a; **86**: 33–9.

Martin RH, Chan K, Ko E, Rademaker AW. Detection of aneuploidy in human sperm by fluorescence *in situ* hybridization (FISH): different frequencies in fresh and stored sperm nuclei. *Cytogenet Cell Genet* 1994a; **65**: 95–6.

Martin RH, Chernos JE, Lowry RB, Pattinson AA, Barclay L, Ko E. Analysis of sperm chromosome complements from a man hetetozygous for a pericentric inversion of chromosome 1. *Hum Genet* 1994b; **93**: 135–8.

Martin RH, Chernos JE, Rademaker AW. The effect of cryopreservation on the frequency of chromosomal abnormalities and sex ratio in human sperm. *Molecular Reproduction and Development* 1991; **30**: 159–63.

Martin RH, Hildebrand KA, Yamamoto J, Peterson D, Rademaker AW, Taylor P, Lin CC. The meiotic segregation of human sperm chromosomes in two men with accessory marker chromosomes. *Am J Med Genet* 1986b; **25**: 381–8.

Martin RH, Hildebrand K, Yamamoto J, Rademaker A, Barnes M, Douglas G, Arthur K, Ringrose T, Brown IS. An increased frequency of human sperm chromosomal abnormalities after radiotherapy. *Mut Res* 1986a; **174**: 219–25.

Martin RH, Hulten M. Chromosome complements in 695 sperm from three men heterozygous for reciprocal translocations and a review of the literature. *Hereditas* 1993; **118**: 165–76.

Martin RH, Ko E, Chan K. Detection of aneuploidy in human interphase spermatozoa by fluorescence *in situ* hybridization (FISH). *Cytogenet Cell Genet* 1993; **64**: 23–6.

Martin RH, Ko E, Hildebrand K. Analysis of sperm chromosome complements from a man heterozygous for a Robertsonian translocation, 45,XY,t(15q22q). *Am J Med Genet* 1992; **43**: 855–7.

Martin RH, Ko E, Rademaker A. Human sperm chromosome complements after microinjection of hamster eggs. *J Repro Fertil* 1988; **84**: 179–86.

Martin RH, Ko E, Rademaker A. The distribution of aneuploidy in human gametes: comparison between human sperm and oocytes. *Am J Med Genet* 1991; **39**: 321–31.

Martin RH, McGillivray B, Barclay L, Hildebrand K, Ko E, Fowlow SB. Sperm chromosome analysis in a man heterozygous for a reciprocal translocation 46,XY,t(12;20)(q24.3;q11). *Hum Repro* 1990b; **5**: 606–9.

Martin RH, Rademaker AW. The effect of age on the frequency of sperm chromosomal abnormalities in normal men. *Am J Hum Genet* 1987b; **41**: 484–92.

Martin RH, Rademaker A, Hildebrand K, Barnes M, Arthur K, Ringrose T, Brown IS, Douglas G. A comparison of chromosomal aberrations induced by *in vivo* radiotherapy in human sperm and lymphocutes. *Mut Res* 1989; **226**: 21–30.

Martin RH, Rademaker AW, Hildebrand K, Long-Simpson L, Peterson D, Yamamoto J. Variation in the frequency and type of sperm chromosomal abnormalities among normal men. *Hum Genet* 1987a; **77**: 108–14.

Martin RH, Rademaker AW, Ko E, Barclay L, Hildebrand K. A comparison of the frequency and type of chromosomal abnormalities in human sperm after different sperm capacitation conditions. *Biology of Reproduction* 1992; **47**: 268–70.

Martin RH, Spriggs EL. Sperm chromosome complements in a man heterozygous for a reciprocal translocation 46,XY,t(9;13)(q21.1;q21.2) and a review of the literature. *Clin Genet* 1994 'in press'.

Martin RH, Templado C, Ko E, Rademaker A. Effect of culture conditions and media on the frequency of chromosomal abnormalities in human sperm chromosome complements. *Molecular Repro Develop* 1990c; **26**: 101–4.

Mikamo K, Kanuguchi Y, Tateno H. Spontaneous and *in vitro* radiation-induced chromosome aberrations in human spermatozoa: application of a new method. In: Mendelsohn ML, Albertini RJ, eds. *Mutation and the Environment Part B: Metabolism Testing Methods and Chromosomes*. New York: John Wiley, 1990: 447–56.

Navarro J, Templado C, Benet J, Lange K, Rajmil O, Egozcue J. Sperm chromosome studies in an infertile man with partial complete asynapsis of meiotic bivalents. *Hum Repro* 1990; **5**: 227–9.

Olson SB, Magenis RE. Preferential paternal origin of de novo structural chromosome rearrangements. In: Daniel A, ed. *The Cytogenetics of Mammalian Autosomal Rearrangements*. New York: Alan R. Liss Inc., 1988: 583–99.

Pellestor F. Analysis of meiotic segregation in a man heterozygous for a 13;14 Robertsonian translocation and a review of the literature. *Hum Genet* 1990; **85**: 49–54.

Pellestor F, Sele B, Jalberg H. Chromosome analysis of spermatozoa from a man heterozygous for a 13;14 Robertsonian translocation. *Hum Genet* 1987; **76**: 116–20.

Pellestor F, Sele B. Etude cytogénétique du sperme humain. *Méd Sci* 1989; **5**: 244–51.

Pellestor F, Sele B, Jalbert H. Chromosome analysis of spermatozoa from a male heterozygous for a 13:14 Robertsonian translocation. *Hum Genet* 1987; **76**: 116–20.

Pellester F, Sele B, Jalbert H, Jalbert P. Direct segregation analysis of reciprocal translocations: a study of 283 sperm karyotypes from four carriers. *Am J Hum Genet* 1989; **44**: 464–73.

Pieters MHEC, Geraedts JPM, Meyer H, Dumoulin JCM, Evers JLH, Jongblood RJE, Nederlof PM, van der Flier. Human gametes and zygotes studied by non-radioactive *in situ* hybridization. *Cytogenet Cell Genet* 1990; **53**: 15–19.

Robbins WA, Segraves R, Pinkel D, Wyrobek A. Detection of aneuploid human sperm by fluorescence in situ hybridization: evidence for a donor difference in frequency of sperm disomic for chromosomes 1 and Y. *Am J Hum Genet* 1993; **52**: 799–807.

Rosenbusch B, Strehler E, Sterzik K. Cytogenetics of human spermatozoa: correlations with sperm morphology and age of fertile men. *Fertility and Sterility* 1992; **58**: 1071–2.

Rosner B. *Fundamentals of Biostatistics.* 2nd edn. Boston: Duxbury Press, 1986: 225.

Rudak E, Jacobs PA, Yanagimachi R. Direct analysis of the chromosome constitution of human spermatozoa. *Nature* 1978; **274**: 911–13.

Sele B, Pellestor F, Jalbert P, Estrade C. Analyse cytogenetique des pronucleus a partir due moldele de fecondation interspectifique homme hamster. *Ann Genet* 1985; **28**: 81.

Spriggs EL, Martin RH. Analysis of segregation in a human male reciprocal translocation carrier, t(1;11)(p36.3;q13.1), by 2-colour fluorescence *in situ* hybridization. *Molecular Reproduction and Development* 1994 'in press'.

Spriggs EL, Martin RH, Hulten M. Sperm chromosome complements from two human reciprocal translocation heterozygotes. *Hum Genet* 1992; **88**: 447–52.

Syme RH, Martin RH. Meiotic segregation of a 21;22 Robertsonian translocation. *Human Reproduction* 1992; **7**: 825–9.

Tarkowski AK. An air-drying method for chromosome preparation from mouse eggs. *Cytogenetics* 1966; **5**: 34–400.

Templado C, Navarro J, Benet J, Genesca A, Mar Penez M, Egozcue J. Human sperm chromosome studies in a reciprocal translocation t(2;5). *Hum Genet* 1988; **79**: 24–8.

Templado C, Navarro J, Requena K, Bene J. Ballesta F, Egozare J. Meiotic and sperm chromosome studies in a reciprocal translocation t(1;2)(q32;q36). *Hum Genet* 1990; **84**: 159–62.

Ueda KU. Yanagimachi R. Sperm chromosome analysis as a new system to test human X- and Y-sperm separation. *Gamete Res* 1987; **17**: 221–8.

Watt JL, Templeton AA, Messinis I, Bell L, Cunningham P, Duncan RO. Trisomy 1 in an eight cell human preembryo. *J Med Genet* 1987; **24**: 60–4.

Williams BJ, Ballenger C, Malter H, Bishop F, Tucker M, Zwingman TA, Hassold TJ. Nondisjunction in human sperm: results of fluorescence *in situ* hybridization studies using two and three probes. *Human Molecular Genetics* 1993; **2**: 1929–36.

Wyrobek AJ, Alhborn T, Balhorn R, Stanleer L, Pinkel D. Fluorescence in situ hybridization to Y chromosomes in decondensed human sperm nuclei. *Molec Reprod Develop* 1990; **27**: 200–8.

6

The motility of human spermatozoa before and after capacitation

L. J. BURKMAN

Introduction

For many years, the detailed study of human sperm motility was considered a nonessential topic in the field of fertility. This viewpoint was a natural consequence of the paucity of information about relationships between the quality of sperm motility and fertilizing capacity. However, the earliest investigators into animal and human *in vitro* fertilization (IVF) soon learned that *in vitro* success required specific sperm preparation for fertilization, that is 'capacitation'. Even now, when human IVF is no longer considered experimental, clinicians and scientists are vigorously pursuing a better understanding of sperm capacitation and practical methods for altering sperm function. While sperm capacitation and function can be approached from numerous angles, the focus of this chapter is on sperm movement as a critical parameter and a tangible marker of capacitation.

At the microscope, a patient observer can readily detect differences in the movements of individual human spermatozoa as they progress through three states: (1) motility within semen; (2) enhanced vigour of motion as capacitation is just completed; and (3) the declining movement of ageing, capacitated sperm. In this chapter, the reader will receive practical guidance for carrying out initial observations at the microscope. In addition to briefly reviewing sperm movement within semen and cervical mucus or during clinical preparation, the author will focus principally on the physiology of capacitation, hyperactivated motility, computer-assisted evaluation, human IVF and clinical correlations.

Motility of spermatozoa within seminal plasma

Although mammalian spermatozoa typically acquire forward progression within the mid and distal portions of the epididymis, ejaculated sperm are not immediately capable of fertilization. *In vivo* fertilizing capacity is not achieved until sperm have proceeded through a number of functional changes called capacitation (see below) and subsequent events. The patterns of motility seen with semen are influenced by the viscous structure of seminal plasma, as well as the presence of 'decapacitation' factors, which prevent sperm from initiating capacitation.

Motility assessment of seminal sperm can be carried out immediately after the ejaculated seminal gel has liquified (liquefaction requires 10 to 30 minutes). In addition to the most common subjective methods for motility evaluation (e.g. grading the vigour of forward movement as 0 to 4), there also exist a number of preferred objective protocols. These include: 1) a timed-exposure photographic approach as shown in Fig. 1 (Overstreet *et al.*, 1979); 2) videorecordings made at high speed and assessed either frame-by-frame (Katz & Overstreet, 1979) or by slow-motion analysis (Burkman, 1984); and most recently, 3) computer software programs linked to digitized video tracking (Katz & Davis, 1987; Robertson, Wolf & Tash, 1988; Burkman, 1991). For seminal sperm (as well as sperm in artificial media), the movement patterns, velocity and other characteristics are dependent on: 1) temperature (controlled warming induces higher velocities; Milligan, Harris & Dennis, 1978); 2) chamber depth (greater depth accommodates greater flagellar amplitude and more vigorous patterns); 3) rate of data acquisition (higher video framing rates capture more points on the sperm path, resulting in a higher relative velocity; Mortimer, 1990); and 4) elapsed time (as ejaculated sperm age within semen, percentage motility and vigour will steadily decrease).

The typical movement characteristics within semen (Burkman, 1986*b*) include a relatively straight path and rolling of the sperm. The flagellum shows minimal bending, hence small side-to-side movements of the sperm head (minimal amplitude of head movement) and a lower velocity. The reader can gain familiarity with such motility by loading a drop of fresh semen into a chamber and visually following sperm at the microscope under high magnification ($\times 40$ objective, phase contrast). For semen having a low count, utilize a deep chamber (e.g. haemacrytometer, flat capillary tube, etc.); however, if the sperm count is about 50 million/ml, visualization will be best in a shallow chamber having a depth of 20–30 microns (e.g. slide mount, Micro-cell, Cell-Vu, etc.). One should note the change in sperm vigour when the observations are made first at room temperature then repeated after warming the semen for 10 minutes at 37 °C.

Whether determined by the older subjective methods or the newest computerized analyses, the data on sperm movement within semen can provide some indication of the probable fertilizing capacity of the sample. Computer-assisted analysis (CASA) of sperm movement typically represents averaged values across the whole sperm population. Currently, no specific CASA values have been accepted which reliably predict fertilization potential. The overall seminal data are most

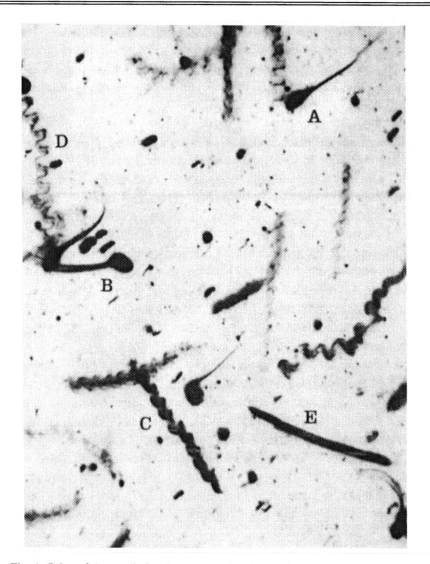

Fig. 1. Print of 1-second timed exposure showing various movement patterns within semen. A, nonmotile sperm. B, sperm with no forward progression but showing slight flagellar movement. C, active sperm with rolling pattern. D, vigorous sperm with pronounced side-to-side head motion (yaw). E, sperm with straight trajectory but no roll or yaw (× 666; from Overstreet *et al.*, 1979).

diagnostic only when these values are well below normal. In this instance, repeated low values for sperm density and percentage motility, or mean velocity and amplitude of head movement, are generally indicative of compromised fertilization function (see also chapter by Cummins in this volume). At the other end of the scale, the presence of large numbers of moving sperm in the semen cannot ensure that fertility is normal. In contrast, demonstrating that some of the sperm can complete capacitation is an objective indicator that fertilizing capacity is likely (refer also to the sections below on sperm capacitation and sperm/egg testing).

Sperm motility within cervical mucus

If coitus occurs at midcycle (periovulatory), a limited number of sperm will quickly leave the vaginal pool of seminal plasma and penetrate the cervical mucus. Sperm which have relatively normal morphology and good flagellar vigour will show effective progression through the glycoprotein mesh which comprises the backbone of cervical mucus (Katz, Drobnis & Overstreet, 1989). Compared to sperm movement within seminal plasma, sperm motility in cervical mucus is marked by higher flagellar beat frequencies, less axial rolling of the sperm, a decrease in the amplitude of flagellar beating, and an altered beat shape (Katz *et al.*, 1989; Chapter 8).

Sperm capacitation

Capacitation of mammalian spermatozoa denotes numerous changes in sperm membrane structure, metabolism and ionic fluxes, the sum of which confers the 'capacity' to fertilize an intact oocyte/ovum (Yanagimachi, 1988). The entire process of capacitation is not yet fully understood; even the definition for completion of capacitation has produced debate (Bedford, 1983; Chang, 1984). Capacitation is often defined (Yanagimachi, 1988) as the membrane changes which prepare sperm for *initiating* a functional acrosome reaction and (stated with increasing frequency) acquiring a more vigorous motility pattern (hyperactivation). Once freshly ejaculated sperm are removed from the seminal plasma and transferred to a suitable medium, capacitation can begin. Practically speaking, therefore, capacitation is initiated as sperm swim through the cervical mucus (Yanagimachi, 1988) or during the dilution and washing steps which are often performed during *in vitro* handling (Chapter 14). At the microscope ($\times 40$ magnification), the reader can observe the altered, more vigorous sperm movement which appears after removing the seminal fluid and incubating sperm with a known IVF fertilization medium. Such observations can be made immediately after washing the sperm and again after 2–3 hour of sperm incubation (37 °C).

Hyperactivated motility

As introduced earlier, the completion of capacitation will lead to a change in sperm movement, namely, the acquisition of a distinctive, vigorous motility called hyperactivation (Yanagimachi, 1988). Hyperactivation, first detected in 1969 by

Yanagimachi and also by Gwatkin & Anderson, is a physiological event closely associated with ovulation and fertilization in those animals studied. In the past 40 years, examination of reproductive tract fluids from many species and the successful development of *in vitro* fertilization systems were the necessary prelude to detection of hyperactivated swimming. In later studies, Katz & Yanagimachi (1980) were able to make direct observations of hyperactivated (HA) sperm within the oviduct of golden hamsters near the time of ovulation. By all current evidence, sperm HA is required for zona pellucida penetration (Fraser, 1981; Fleming & Yanagimachi, 1982) and may be required for effective oviductal sperm transport and penetration of the cumulus oophorus (Katz, Drobnis & Overstreet, 1989; Tesarik, Mendoza & Testart, 1990). Between 1969 and 1984, HA swimming was described for about a dozen mammalian species, including the primate (Yanagimachi, 1981; Cummins, 1982; Boatman & Bavister, 1984).

The relatively recent success of *in vitro* therapy for human fertilization has provided the critical milieu for observing sperm movements in the context of proven fertilization. Before the advent of human IVF, there existed only scant information on sperm within the female reproductive tract. Without the link to actual fertilization, no conclusions could be drawn about the physiology of human sperm capacitation and the phenomenon of hyperactivation.

Early observations on human sperm capacitation

The earliest reports describing human sperm HA were published six years after the world's first IVF birth and three years following the United State's initial IVF success. In 1984, Burkman, and separately, Mortimer *et al.*, reported that intact sperm prepared for human IVF inseminations demonstrated classical hyperactivation. More specifically, these human spermatozoa displayed extreme bending of the flagellum (high-amplitude, high-curvature), resulting in large side-to-side movements of the sperm head (great lateral displacement of the head). Although these HA sperm moved with very high velocities along the swimming path (high curvilinear velocity), their total path (trajectory) was always quite non-linear (i.e. linearity was *low* – where linearity of 100 is defined as a 'straight' trajectory). In contrast to seminal sperm, which swim with a high 'straight-line' velocity, these hyperactivated sperm have limited 'forward progression'. Lastly, HA spermatozoa often show an erratic behaviour, switching from one swimming pattern to another (biphasic, multiphasic). In contrast to other mammals, hyperactivation in the human is not a well-synchronized event; that is, among all of the sperm which will eventually exhibit HA, one subpopulation will show HA early in capacitation, while other subpopulations will demonstrate HA at intermediate or very late periods in capacitation. Some evidence suggests that

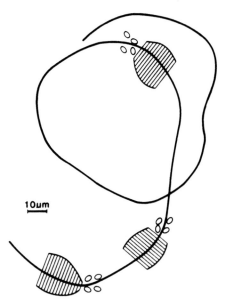

10um

Fig. 2. Representation of a hyperactivated human spermatozoon (circling, high-curvature pattern) observed by eye through a phase contrast microscope. The large amplitude head movements appear 'double'.

those sperm with early HA are not the same sperm which exhibit HA after 24 hours of capacitation (Burkman, 1986*b*).

Direct observation of these vigorous HA patterns is possible by returning to the microscope. Fresh human sperm from a fertile donor should be washed twice with any common IVF medium (e.g. Ham's F10, Human Tubal Fluid, Menezo's B2 medium) which has first been supplemented with crystallized human serum albumin or heat-inactivated human serum. This washed sperm suspension should be incubated at 37 °C for 1–3 hours before loading a drop in a deep chamber. Using a typical fertile specimen, sperm with the most common HA pattern will be swimming in a roughly circular path (50 to 200 microns in diameter). At the microscope, such sperm are easily identified (see Fig. 2) owing to the vigorous side-to-side head movements (they may appear 'double-headed') and the broad 'blur' of the lashing flagellum. As described below, the other principal HA patterns are easily detected by eye due to their erratic, very rapid and nonlinear movement.

The first illustrations of human HA patterns were published in 1984 by Mortimer *et al.* and by Burkman. The human patterns were similar to hyperactivated modes previously detailed for capacitated rabbit sperm (Johnson, Katz & Overstreet, 1981) and for other species. Initial work (Burkman, 1984, 1986*a*) described four general HA patterns in the human: 1) circling, high-curvature (the predominant pattern already mentioned above); 2) thrashing (an extremely erratic trajectory); 3) star-spin (spinning in place, sometimes stuck to glass); and 4) helical. Figs. 3–6 provide examples of each of the four patterns, along with the values of their movement characteristics as derived from computerized assessment. The biphasic nature of human HA can also produce complex paths such as the series shown in Fig. 7, where the extended trajectory of a single spermatozoon is captured in six serial segments covering a total of four seconds (Burkman, 1990a). In 1988, Robertson et al. reported on a different strategy for identifying HA motility, describing three patterns (star, transitional and HA). Hoshi et al. (1988) attempted to define the orderly transition of motility patterns as capacitation time elapsed. It is possible that their Type C and Type D motion represent the two modes of a biphasic pattern. For a more detailed discussion of the early HA literature, please refer to the chapter by Burkman (1990b).

The author has shown that reliable and quantitative evaluations of the percentage of sperm swimming with HA patterns can be obtained by three methods (Burkman, 1990b). The oldest approach utilized a high-speed video camera and recordings made at 30 frames/s which were played back in slow-motion (15 frames/s) as a trained technicial evaluated each sperm for the

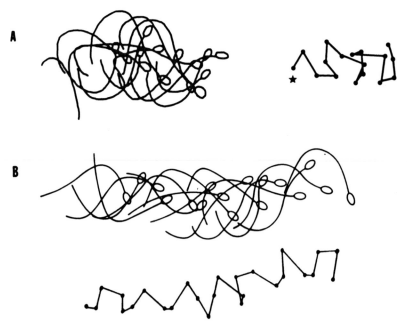

Fig. 3. Hyperactivated human spermatozoon (circling, high-curvature). High-speed videorecorded images were first traced frame-by-frame and also tracked by CASA analysis (30 Hz; from Burkman, 1990a).

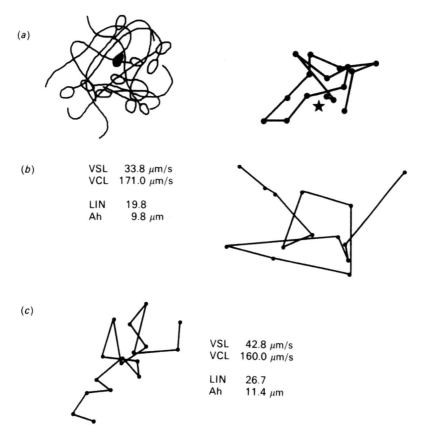

(a)

(b)   VSL   33.8 μm/s
       VCL   171.0 μm/s

       LIN   19.8
       Ah   9.8 μm

(c)   VSL   42.8 μm/s
       VCL   160.0 μm/s

       LIN   26.7
       Ah   11.4 μm

Fig. 4. Hyperactivated human spermatozoon (thrashing). Manual frame-by-frame tracing in (A). Tracks also analysed by CASA (30 Hz) with individual velocities (VSL, VCL), linearity (LIN) and amplitude (Ah). (From Burkman, 1990a.)

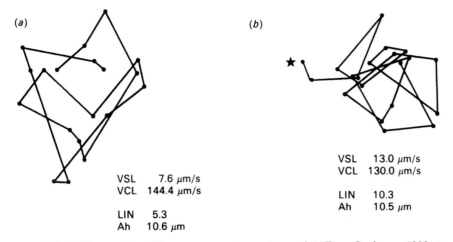

(a)

VSL   7.6 μm/s
VCL   144.4 μm/s

LIN   5.3
Ah   10.6 μm

(b)

VSL   13.0 μm/s
VCL   130.0 μm/s

LIN   10.3
Ah   10.5 μm

Fig. 5. Hyperactivated human spermatozoon (star-spin). (From Burkman, 1990a.)

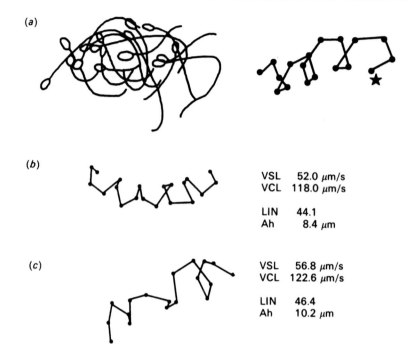

(a)

(b)

VSL   52.0 μm/s
VCL   118.0 μm/s

LIN   44.1
Ah   8.4 μm

(c)

VSL   56.8 μm/s
VCL   122.6 μm/s

LIN   46.4
Ah   10.2 μm

Fig. 6. Hyperactivated human spermatozoon (helical). (From Burkman, 1990*a*.)

presence or absence of HA motility ('semi-objective' method). In this manner, individual spermatozoa could be observed continuously for approximately five seconds. Alternatively, a trained technician can follow the sperm movement directly at the microscope (× 40 objective, deep chamber, 37 °C), where each sperm is also visually tracked for about five sectonds. For these two methods, each motile sperm is classified (Yes/No) for the presence of HA (≥ 200 motile sperm evaluated). For twelve sperm samples evaluated in the 1990 methodological study, the semi-objective method and the simple microscope protocol gave indistinguishable results.

The most technical method is that of computer-automated identification of hyperactivation (e.g. in the 1990 study, a Hamilton–Thorne Motility Analyzer with automatic track sorting was used). For such CASA analyses, the author has reported on a triple criterion for identifying hyperactivated sperm prepared in Ham's F10 medium and fetal cord serum (curvilinear velocity ≥ 100 microns/s *and* linearity ≤ 65 *and* amplitude of head movement ≥ 7.5 microns; Burkman, 1991). Mortimer & Mortimer (1990) arrived at very similar HA criteria using a different culture medium and female serum. Although very objective, most CASA software packages will track each sperm for approximately one second only. Therefore, compared to the other two methods which rely on 5-second readings,

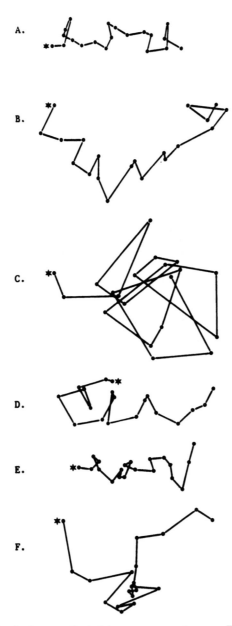

Fig. 7. A multiphasic, hyperactivated human spermatozoon. These consecutive patterns represent 4 seconds of movement. Tracks analysed by CASA (30 Hz).

the computerized assessment detected about one-fourth of the HA seen visually (Burkman, 1990*b*). This issue of duration of observation time is relevant in view of the biphasic (on/off) nature of hyperactivation: short observation periods miss HA sperm which are momentarily in the 'off' mode (see Burkman, 1990*a*).

Clinical correlates of human sperm hyperactivation

During 1982–1983, the author was able to document the movement characteristics of sperm from subfertile patients participating in the IVF program at Norfolk, Virginia. There were clear differences in the vigour and quality of movement when comparing washed, capacitating sperm from men with primary infertility problems versus men who had normal semen characteristics. After two to four hours of incubation in Ham's F10 medium and 7.5% human fetal cord serum, only 8% of the motile subfertile sperm exhibited HA, whereas a mean of 20% of motile sperm from proven fertile men displayed hyperactivation patterns (Burkman, 1984). Individual men also differed with respect to the duration of incubation required to support peak levels of HA (Burkman, 1986b). Most commonly, the peak occurred after three hours, whereas percentage HA fell to statistically lower levels after 6 and 24 hours of incubation. Since these ageing sperm exhibited much less HA, this observation may provide one physiological rationale behind a specific IVF laboratory practice. When human oocytes were inseminated the day after aspiration (either reinsemination of older eggs or initial insemination for newly matured oocytes), the use of sperm prepared the previous day usually required a two- to five-fold increase in the motile concentration. This manoeuvre actually compensated for the steady decline in hyperactivated motility within the original sperm suspension.

In 1987, Jinno, Burkman & Coddington reported that sperm populations having high levels of HA penetrated hamster ova at a high rate; conversely, sperm exhibiting low HA showed significantly less egg penetration (see also Burkman, 1990a). When performed optimally, the zona-free hamster ovum penetration assay (see Rogers, 1985) can provide significant information about the fertilizing potential of a specific sperm preparation. Results from the hamster assay also give indirect evidence concerning the completion of the acrosome reaction (Zaneveld & Jeyendran, 1988). Therefore, the data from Jinno et al. imply that sperm samples showing high levels of HA are also undergoing the acrosome reaction at a relatively high rate. Thus, the peak incidence of HA may be indicative of the potential for completing the functional acrosomal reaction below.

Before fertilization can occur, capacitated sperm must bind tightly to the zona pellucida (Fig. 8). Data from the hemizona sperm binding assay (Burkman et al., 1988; Burkman, 1990a) have been predictive of eventual IVF success (Coddington et al., 1991). The hemizona assay has also contributed valuable information on the relationships between HA, zona binding and normal sperm morphology (Coddington et al., 1991). In that study, the sperm from fertile men exhibited a mean incidence of 30% HA (direct microscopic evaluation) and a mean of 37 sperm bound to the hemizona, where an average of 16% of the semen population

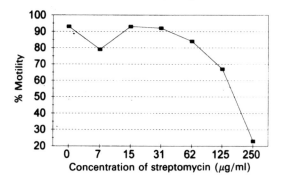

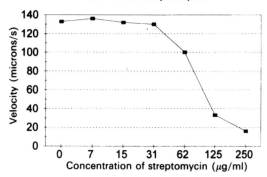

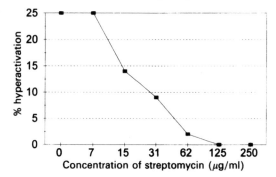

Fig. 8. Representative results from a dose–response study of human sperm behaviour when exposed to increasing concentrations of a toxic factor (% motility, curvilinear velocity and % hyperactivation). Each data point represents a single reading.

had perfectly normal morphology (strict method; Kruger, 1988). In contrast, all mean values for the group of subfertile men were significantly less (15% HA, 7 sperm bound, 1.4% normal morphology). Here, the incidence of HA was positively and statistically correlated with morphology and zona binding capacity. These data suggested that HA analysis might also give indirect information on membrane-related functions required for fertilization, that is, a normally shaped acrosome (included in morphology) which recognizes the zona receptor, and completion of the acrosome reaction, a requirement for tight zona binding.

It remained to be shown whether critical assessment of hyperactivation might be predictive of fertilization success. Karande, Burkman and colleagues (1990, 1995) reported that 89% of the IVF cases with excellent fertilization could be predicted based on two new criteria. At two hours and four hours after the initial sperm wash (Ham's F10 medium and cord serum) HA assessment was performed using a Hamilton–Thorne Motility Analyzer (37 °C, chamber depth of 200 microns). Automatic identification of hyperactivation was carried out using the triple-criterion presented above (curvilinear velocity, linearity and amplitude). Analysis of the data indicated two significant endpoints: the relative *change* in HA between the two timepoints, and the *lowest* HA percentage for that patient. Cases which had a poor fertilization rate (<75%) were characterized by a lower HA which was ≤14%, and/or no change in percentage HA between the two timepoints. For laboratories using a different capacitation medium or a different protein, it should be noted that these specific numerical thresholds will probably change somewhat.

The development of a hyperactivation assay (diagnostic and quality control)

The IVF study detailed in the previous section and other work to evaluate HA as a quality control endpoint (Burkman et al., 1991) have both accelerated the development of a hyperactivation assay. Experience of the past several years has indicated that human sperm HA is significantly affected by altered culture conditions. The peak incidence of HA is suppressed: 1) in a simple salts solution versus a complex medium (e.g. BWW versus Ham's F10); 2) in samples held at room temperature versus 37 °C; and 3) in medium containing bovine serum albumin compared to human fetal cord serum or human serum albumin (unpublished observations). These facts suggested that sperm HA might also be sensitive to contaminants in the medium or other deleterious conditions.

Our 1991 study (Burkman et al.) compared three reproductive assays for quality control purposes: human sperm hyperactivation and percentage motility (CASA), the zona-free hamster penetration (SPA), and the one-cell mouse zygote (embryo) growth assay. Twenty-four product samples (liquids and powders) used commonly by infertility clinics were initially tested. For the ten samples evaluated by all three assays, nine of ten had the same Pass/Fail result for the three assays (rate of assay agreement was 90%). Continued testing which utilized this mouse assay and the sperm HA/motility protocol still revealed >90% agreement for a total of 50 products.

This combined diagnostic and quality control experience with HA has suggested the following guidelines in carrying out a hyperactivation assay. Since the medium and supplement will influence the peak value of HA and the time required to attain that peak, we have recommended a common culture medium and a common protein (Ham's F10 medium and human serum albumin, at 3 mg/ml). After a swim-up procedure, either from a washed pellet or from semen, a resulting high concentration of supernatant sperm should be diluted with the medium in order to optimize sperm tracking during computer-assisted analysis (CASA). Our experience suggests that no more than 30 motile sperm should be present in the field of data acquisition for optimal CASA analysis. After sperm loading, the chamber should be warmed for ten minutes at 37 °C before collecting data; this temperature should be maintained throughout data collection. When utilizing the assay to gain some assessment of sperm fertilizing potential, HA and motility assessment at one timepoint is not very adequate. Due to patient-to-patient variation in the time to peak HA (Burkman, 1986b), these diagnostic observations should be made at both two and four hours after initiating the first wash. For quality control/toxicity purposes the assay results can be read after six hours, with an optimal reading at 24 hours of capacitation.

A recent effort to further delineate this quality control (QC) assay examined dose response relationships when human sperm were exposed to a model toxin (Burkman, 1994). Donor sperm were incubated in Ham's F10 medium which was supplemented with increasing concentrations of a toxic batch of streptomycin sulphate. Data were recorded by CASA methods for %HA, ALH, VSL and % motility after 2, 4, 6 and 24 hours of exposure. Analysis for ED_{50} (the dose required to suppress each endpoint by 50%) versus time revealed that %HA was the most sensitive movement parameter (50% loss in less than 6 hours) and that % motility was the least sensitive parameter (50% loss required 24 hours), while ALH and VCl fell in-between. Using the streptomycin model as well as other deleterious supplements, a QC analysis carried out for just six hours appeared sufficient for detecting a problematic supplement or agent. As illustrated in Fig. 8, the dose–response decline in % motility, VCL and %HA is quite marked for individual donors and single readings.

Further studies on a hyperactivation assay might focus on comparing the diagnostic accuracy of the protocol given above against the HA identification schemes proposed by Tash, Wolf and colleagues (Robertson, 1988) and by

Mortimer & Mortimer (1990). With time, it is certainly expected that the protocols, the critical parameters, as well as the specific threshold values will be modified and improved.

Summary of additional studies on the physiology of human hyperactivation

Preliminary observations requiring considerably more study from a number of reports serve to define a basic framework for understanding hyperactivation in the human. The biphasic nature of human sperm HA complicates any discussion of the optimal duration of CASA motility analysis. After continuously video-recording sperm movement for > 60 seconds (Burkman & Coddington, 1986), only 55% of the HA sperm were correctly classified as hyperactivated based on their movement during the first *two* seconds. Only 20% of these HA sperm showed continuous hyperactivation when tracked for 20 to 60 seconds. The protocols for HA analysis must eventually wrestle with this fact (learn to live with the curtailed data, or extrapolate back to the 'actual' %HA, or extend the duration of automated HA analysis).

The relationship of hyperactivation to zona binding was also investigated in a preliminary study by Burkman and Coddington (1986). Using videomicrography, the behaviour of HA sperm was examined as they approached and attached to a human intact zona (frozen–thawed and non-viable). The HA spermatozoa tended to have longer periods of zona interaction. Specifically, about two-thirds of the arriving non-hyperactivated sperm had a brushing contact with the zona (less than one second), while two-thirds of the HA sperm actually attached to the zona pellucida for 1 to 60 seconds or longer. It is plausible that this enhanced zona interaction reflected concomitant acrosomal changes in HA sperm.

To date, there is only meager information available on the control of mammalian sperm hyperactivation, both at the membrane level and intracellularly. Lindemann and Kanous (1989) have modelled a pathway thought to control hyperactivation. Depending on fluctuating intracellular calcium concentrations, HA might be turned on (high calcium) then turned off (low calcium). Suarez & Osman (1989) has shown that exposure to calcium ionophore will directly stimulate the appearance of HA. Incubation of sperm with dibutyryl cyclic AMP will increase intracellular cAMP levels and act to accelerate capacitation, including the induction of HA (Fraser, 1981). Coincubation with human follicular fluid can enhance hyperactivation, most likely due to the progesterone content (Mbizvo, Burkman & Alexander, 1990). A rise in superoxide anion levels could also provide one mechanism for controlling HA (De Lamirande & Gagnon, 1993).

Lastly, there has been some investigation of hyperactivation's physiological role and its relationship to other fertilization events. Two studies have examined

HA motion in connection with sperm penetration of viscous fluids, with particular focus on the cumulus oophorous matrix. Both laboratories concluded that the subpopulation of sperm with hyperactivated movement more readily penetrated the viscous solutions (Tesarik *et al.*, 1990; Suarez *et al.*, 1991). Simultaneous evaluation of human sperm acrosomal reactions, tight binding to the zona pellucida and hyperactivation was carried out by Burkman *et al.* (1988). These strictly timed experiments revealed that rapid induction of the acrosome reaction occurred just slightly after the peak in HA for each donor. The peak in zona binding occurred at essentially the same time as the hyperactivation maximum. These data also suggested that some HA sperm never lose their acrosome. This particular study was the first to suggest that hyperactivation, completion of the acrosome reaction, and tight zona binding may be temporally (and perhaps functionally) linked events for an individual sperm.

Future investigation

Although the information from animal species relating to hyperactivated motility is still minimal, it substantially exceeds our knowledge of human sperm motion. Effective diagnostic and therapeutic help for subfertile males will require concerted investigation of the physiology and control mechanisms for typical motility as well as hyperactivation. Although some have heralded assisted reproduction by micromanipulation as the panacea for any man with primary or secondary infertility, the future treatment for male infertility cannot be viewed so narrowly. Our sights are often limited by the short span of time since laboratories proved that human sperm could fertilize *in vitro* – a mere 15 or so years – and much is yet to be learned. Today's challenge is to accelerate data acquisition on human sperm function and control, so that male therapy will commonly include oral medications, or highly effective protocols for intra-uterine insemination, or new proven surgical interventions.

References

Bedford JM. Significance of the need for sperm capacitation before fertilization in eutherian mammals. *Biology of Reproduction* 1983; **28**: 108–20.

Boatman DE, Bavister BD. Stimulation of rhesus monkey sperm capacitation by cyclic nucleotide mediators. *J Reprod Fertil* 1984; **71**: 357–66.

Burkman LJ. Characterization of hyperactivated motility by human spermatozoa during capacitation: comparison of fertile and oligozoospermic sperm populations. *Arch Androl* 1984; **13**: 153–65.

Burkman, LJ. Experimental approaches to the evaluation and enhancement of sperm function. In: Jones HW, ed. In vitro *fertilization at Norfolk*. Baltimore: Williams & Wilkins, Co., 1986*a*: 201–14.

Burkman LJ. Temporal pattern of hyperactivation-like motility in human spermatozoa. *Biol Reprod* 1986b; Supplement (1) **34**: 226.

Burkman LJ, Coddington CC. Interaction of hyperactivated-like human spermatozoa with the human zona pellucida. 1986; program supplement: 129.

Burkman L, Coddington C, Franken C, Kruger T, Rosenwaks Z. Hodgen G. The hemizona assay (HZA): development of a diagnostic test for the binding of human spermatozoa to human hemizona pellucida to predict fertilization potential. *Fertil Steril* 1988; **49**: 688–97.

Burkman LJ. Hyperactivated motility of human spermatozoa during *in vitro* capacitation. In: Gagnon C, ed. *Controls of sperm motility*. Boca Raton: CRC Press, 1990a: 303–29.

Burkman LJ. Computer-automated versus visual analysis of human sperm hyperactivation (HA). Program supplement 1990b; S32.

Burkman LJ. Discrimination between nonhyperactivated and classical hyperactivated motility patterns in human spermatozoa using computerized analysis. *Fertil Steril* 1991; **55**: 363–71.

Burkman L, Rogers B, Kiessling A, Epstein D. Comparing three reproductive assays for their quality control (QC) potential. 1991; program supplement, p. S145.

Burkman LJ. Human sperm hyperactivation (HA) and CASA analysis as a rapid QC/toxicity assay. *Fertil Steril* 1994; program supplement; S174.

Chang, MC. The meaning of sperm capacitation; a historical perspective. *J Andrology* 1984; **5**: 45–50.

Coddington C, Franken D, Burkman L, Oosthuizen W, Kruger T, Hodgen G. Functional aspects of human sperm binding to the zona pellucida using the hemizona assay. *J Andrology* 1991; **12**: 1–8.

Cummins JM. Hyperactivated motility patterns of ram spermatozoa recovered from the oviducts of mated ewes. *Gamete Res* 1982; **6**: 53–63.

Fleming AD, Yanagimachi R. Fertile life of acrosome-reacted guinea pig spermatozoa. *J Exp Zool* 1982; **220**: 109–15.

Fraser LR. Dibutyrul cyclic AMP decreases capacitance time *in vitro* in mouse spermatozoa. *J Reprod Fertil* 1981; **62**: 63–72.

Gwatkin RBL, Anderson OF. Capacitation of hamster spermatozoa by bovine follicular fluid. *Nature* 1969; **221**: 1111–12.

Hoshi K, Yanagida K, Aita T, Yoshimatsu N, Sato A. Changes in the motility pattern of human spermatozoa during *in vitro* incubation. *Tohoku J Exp Med* 1988; **154**: 47.

Jinno B, Burkman LJ, Coddington CC. Human sperm hyperactivated motility (HA) and egg penetration. *Biol Reprod* 1987; **36**: 53.

Johnson LL, Katz DF, Overstreet JW. The movement characteristics of rabbit spermatozoa before and after activation. *Gamete Res* 1981; **4**: 275–82.

Karande V, Mbizvo M, Burkman L, Veeck L, Alexander N. Hyperactivation (HA) of human sperm is a prognostic indicator of fertilization during IVF. (abstract). *J Andrology* 1990; Program supplement: 28-P.

Karande V, Burkman L, Mbizvo M, Veeck L, Alexander N. Hyperactivated motility (HA) of human spermatozoa may be a prognostic indicator of fertilization during IVF. *Fertil Steril* 1995; manuscript submitted.

Katz DF, Overstreet JW. Biophysical aspects of human sperm movement. In: Fawcett DW, Bedford JM, eds. *The spermatozoon*. Baltimore: Urban & Schwarzenberg, 1979: 413–23.

Katz DF, Yanagimachi R. Movement charcateristics of hamster spermatozoa within the oviduct. *Biol Reprod* 1980; **22**: 749–64.

Katz DF, Overstreet JW. Sperm motility assessment by videomicrography. *Fertil Steril* 1981; **35**: 188–93.

Katz DF, Davis RO. Automatic analysis of human sperm motion. *J Androl* 1987; **8**: 170–81.

Katz DF, Drobnis EZ, Overstreet JW. Factors regulating mammalian sperm migration through the female reproductive tract and oocyte vestments. *Gamete Res* 1989; **22**: 443–69.

Kruger TF, Acosta A, Simmons KF, Swanson RJ, Matta JF, Oehninger S. Predictive value of abnormal sperm morphology in *in vitro* fertilization. *Fertil Steril* 1988; **49**: 112–17.

Lindemann CD, Goltz JS, Kanous KS, Gardner TK, Olds-Clarke P. Evidence for an increased sensitivity to calcium in the flagella of sperm from two 32± mice. *Mol Reprod Dev* 1990; **26**: 69–77.

Mbizvo MT, Burkman LJ, Alexander NJ. Follicular fluid stimulates human sperm hyperactivation. *J Andrology* 1990; program supplement: 28-P.

Milligan MP, Harris SJ, Dennis KJ. The effect of temperature on the velocity of human spermatozoa as measured by time-lapse photography. *Fertil Steril* 1978; **30**: 592.

Mortimer D, Courtot AM, Giovangrandi Y, Jeulin C, David G. Human sperm motility after migration into, and incubation in, synthetic media. *Gamete Res* 1984; **9**: 131.

Mortimer D. Objective analysis of sperm motility and kinematics. In: Keel BA, Webster BW, eds. *Handbook of the laboratory diagnosis and treatment of infertility*. Boca Raton: CRC Press, 1990: 97–133.

Mortimer ST, Mortimer D, Kinematics of human spermatozoa incubated under capacitating conditions. *J Androl* 1990; **11**: 195–203.

Oehninger S. Diagnostic significance of sperm–zona pellucida interaction. *Reprod Med Rev* 1992; **1**: 57–81.

Overstreet JW, Katz DF, Hanson FW, Fonseca J. A simple inexpensive method for objective assessment of human sperm movement characteristics. *Fertil Steril* 1979; **31**: 162–72.

Robertson L, Wolf DP, Tash JS. Temporal changes in motility parameters related to acrosomal status: identification and characterization of populations of hyperactivated human sperm. *Biol Reprod* 1988; **39**: 797–805.

Rogers BJ. The sperm penetration assay: its usefulness reevaluated. *Fertil Steril* 1985; **43**: 821–9.

Saurez S, Osman R. Initiation of hyperactivated flagellar bending in mouse sperm within the female reproductive tract. *Biol Reprod* 1989; **131**: 475–82.

Suarez SS, Latz DF, Owen DH, Andrew JB, Powell RL. Evidence for the function of hyperactivated motility in sperm. *Biol Reprod* 1991; **44**: 375–81.

Tesarik J, Mendoza C, Testart J. Effect of human cumulus oophorus on movement characteristics of human capacitated spermatozoa. *J Reprod Fertil* 1990; **88**: 665–75.

Yanagimachi R. *In vitro* capacitation of hamster spermatozoa by follicular fluid. *J. Reprod Fertil* 1969; **18**: 275–86.

Yanagimachi R. Mechanisms of fertilization in mammals. In: Mastroianni L, Biggers JB, eds. *Fertilization and embryonic development* in vitro. New York: Plenum, 1981; 81–182.

Yanagimachi R. Mammalian fertilization. In: Knobil E, Neill JD, Euing LL, Markert CI, Greenwald GS, Pfaff DN, eds. *The physiology of reproduction*. New York, Raven Press, 1988: 135–55.

Zaneveld LJD, Jenendran RS. Modern assessment of semen for diagnostic purposes. *Semin Reprod Endrocinol* 1988; **4**: 323–37.

7

Post-testicular sperm maturation and transport in the excurrent ducts

H. D. M. MOORE

Introduction

On release from the seminiferous epithelium of the testis, the spermatozoon has completed a striking and unique morphological transformation from a round undifferentiated germ cell (Bellve & O'Brien, 1983; De Kretser & Kerr, 1988). Nearing the end of a developmental process which has taken already about 64 days, the spermatozoon makes a final journey out of the testis and along the highly convoluted, epithelial-lined tubules of the vasa efferentia, epididymis and vas deferens before eventually passing out of the body (via the urethra) at ejaculation (Figs. 1 and 2). But the excurrent duct system is much more than a passive conduit between the testis and the outside. Not only does it maintain the viability of spermatozoa for a sojourn which might last several weeks but it also promotes the development of their fertilizing capacity, culminating in the acquisition of full motility and the ability to bind to and penetrate the ovum. This sperm maturation, as it is termed, appears to be a feature of all mammalian species and has been extensively studied in laboratory animals (for reviews see Cooper, 1986; Moore 1990a). Although we know less about the details of human sperm maturation, techniques such as microsurgical aspiration, or re-anastomosis of the epididymis, along with *in vitro* fertilization and cell culture are now providing important new information about the process in men (Cooper, 1990).

The passage of spermatozoa along the excurrent duct is associated with a number of distinct functional processes. Rather than a description based on the various anatomical regions it is more appropriate to consider the physiological and biochemical interactions undergone by spermatozoa and the tract. These include (in order from the testis), resorption of fluid secreted by the testis, the development of sperm fertilizing capacity and finally sperm storage and ejaculation. Many of these processes are mediated by the secretory and absorptive activity of the epithelial lining of the excurrent duct which in turn is under the control of androgens (Moore, 1990b).

140

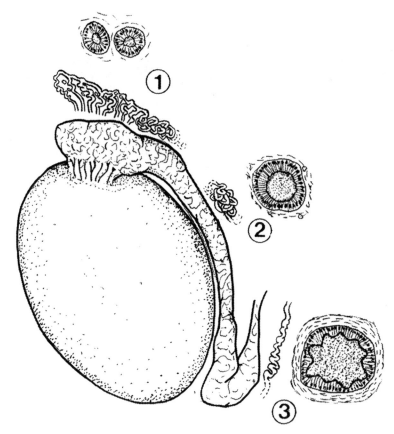

Fig. 1. A diagram of a human testis and epididymis displaying tubule anatomy and histology. (1) From the Rete testis a number of narrow efferent ducts allow passage of spermatozoa to the proximal caput region. (2) The diameter of the convoluted tubule widens in the corpus region while there is a decrease in the thickness of the epithelium. (3) The tubule of the cauda region and the vas deferens is less convoluted and is surrounded by smooth muscle and connective tissue. The tubule diameter is at its widest for sperm storage.

Sperm transport to the epididymis and function of the vasa efferentia and initial segment

Spermatozoa within the testis and male tract are quiescent and therefore play no active role in their own transport along the tract. Passage out of the seminiferous tubules and through the main testicular collecting duct, the Rete canal, is due to the flow of secretion from Sertoli cells and Rete epithelium (testicular fluid) and intrinsic smooth muscle contractions of the tubules and entire testicular capsule. The secretory output from the testis is considerable and in laboratory or domestic animals can be collected over extended periods by

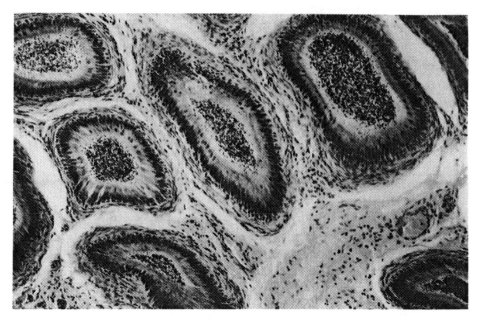

Fig. 2. Light micrograph of human corpus epididymidis. Epithelial-lined sections of the convoluted tubule, packed with spermatozoa are shown. Note the thick connective tissue surrounding sections of tubule.

cannulation of the Rete (4–20 μl/g testis/h); in man, the secretory rate is in the order of 15 μl/g testis/h (Howards, Lechene & Vigersky, 1979; Setchell & Brookes, 1988). On leaving the testis, spermatozoa must pass through one of an array of tubules (10–15), or vasa efferentia (ductuli efferenti), that splay out from the Rete and connect with a broad area of the proximal epididymidis (Baumgarten, Holstein & Rosengren, 1971). This anatomy is somewhat different from that seen in laboratory or domestic species where just a few efferent ducts (usually less than five) make a narrow connection with the most proximal end of the epididymis. Such a difference may be important when comparing epididymal function in different species. Ciliated epithelial cells are present in the vasa efferentia, but not elsewhere in the excurrent ducts, and presumably serve to aid the movement of spermatozoa at this juncture and prevent any cellular aggregation that could block testis outflow and lead to a hazardous increase of pressure in the seminiferous tubules (Fig. 3). At this point the concentration of spermatozoa is relatively low, however, it rises rapidly as luminal fluid is actively resorbed by the epithelial cells of both the efferent ducts and the first portion of the epididymis, called the initial segment. The main epithelial cells of this region, the principal cell type, are particularly tall and have many long microvilli on their apical surface which increase the membrane surface area in contact with the luminal

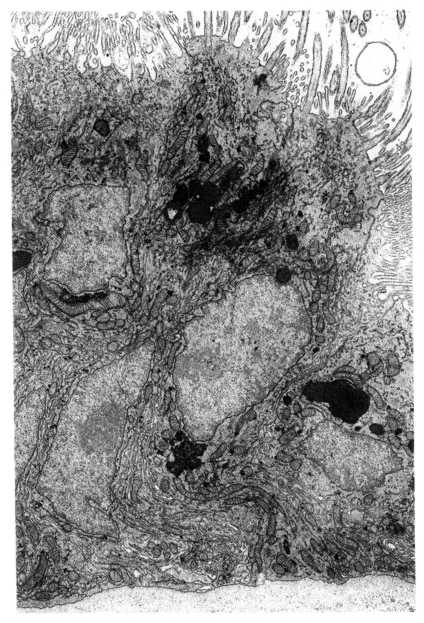

Fig. 3. An electron micrograph of the epithelim of a human efferent duct. Mitochondria-rich ciliated cells (*) interspersed between principal cells facilitate transport of spermatozoa to the epididymis.

microenvironment (Fig. 4). Passive fluid resorption driven by active ionic exchange (sodium and chloride) takes place across this apical membrane with water being pumped into the lateral intercellular spaces in a process similar to that occurring in the distal tubules of the kidney with which it shares a common embryological

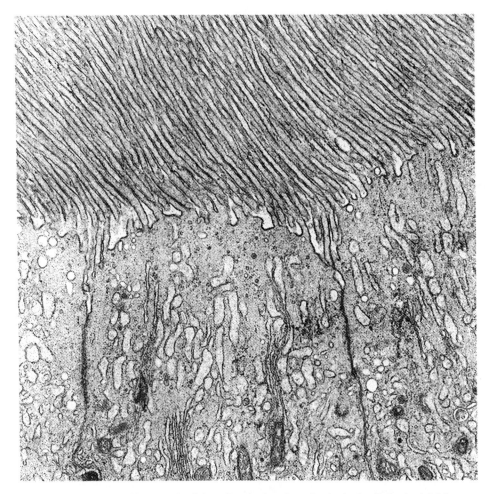

Fig. 4. Electron micrograph of the adluminal region of principal cells in the initial caput epididymidis. Long microvilli are present on the apical cell surface increasing the membrane area for fluid resorption. Note the tight junctions between adjacent epithelial cells.

origin. In keeping with this function the most dense capillary network for the excurrent ducts surrounds the vasa efferentia and initial segment and results in a higher blood flow than for the rest of the tract (Kormano & Reijonen, 1976).

The initial segment of the epididymis has been shown in laboratory rodents, at least, to be dependent on high levels of androgen (testosterone and dihydro-testosterone), derived directly from Rete testis fluid as well as from the peripheral circulation, to maintain function. Ligation of the vasa efferentia in rats, for example, leads to regression of the initial segment within a few days because androgens bound to androgen binding protein (ABP), a carrier protein secreted by Sertoli cells, are prevented from reaching receptors on and in principal cells

(Fawcett & Hoffer, 1979). In this case, the androgen concentration in the peripheral circulation is insufficient to compensate for the loss of hormone in the luminal fluid. Whether the human epididymis would react in such a rapid manner is not known, as the clinical investigation of blocked ducts is usually undertaken at a relatively late stage after the initial lesion. Interestingly, compared with that of the rodent, the human epididymis does not exhibit such a distinctive morphological differentiation of the epithelium in the proximal part of the duct. Indeed, this poor regional epithelial differentiation may be one consequence of the lack of a marked androgen gradient along the duct in man (Moore & Pryor, 1981).

Changes to spermatozoa during epididymal passage

Perhaps the most conspicuous change to spermatozoa passing along the epididymal lumen, is the potential for flagellum movement such that a sustained progressive sperm motility is induced by the appropriate culture medium. For men of proven fertility, the best assessment of this aspect of sperm maturation has been made by examining samples of luminal contents recovered from various regions of epididymis of volunteers undergoing vasectomy under general anaesthetic (Moore, Hartman & Pryor, 1983). In these cases, most of the spermatozoa recovered from the caput region remained immotile or show weak tail twitching in a modified Tyrode's medium with just 3% displaying forward motility (Fig. 5(i)). By contrast, more than 60% of spermatozoa from the cauda region were progressively motile. Since it is known that the fertilizing potential of an ejaculate is correlated with the proportion of spermatozoa with a velocity above 25 μm/s, this induction of forward motility is clearly crucial for the development of sperm fertilizing ability (Holt, Hillier & Moore, 1985).

Equally important as changes in motility, epididymal spermatozoa also acquire the ability to recognize and bind to oocytes. Because of practical and ethical difficulties of experimenting with human oocytes, the first *in vitro* studies were undertaken using zona-free hamster eggs. With these preparations, fertile human spermatozoa will bind and fuse to the oolemma and their nuclei decondense in the egg cytoplasm. Although indirect, this technique provides a partial but convenient assessment of sperm fertilizing capacity. Spermatozoa retrieved from the initial segment or caput region of proven fertile men failed to bind to these oocytes while spermatozoa from the cauda epididymidis attached and penetrated them (Hinrichsen & Balquier, 1980; Fig. 5(ii), Moore, Hartman & Pryor, 1983). Recently, experiments with human oocytes have confirmed the conclusion that, in the normal fertile man, spermatozoa obtain the capacity to bind and penetrate oocytes during epididymal passage (Moore *et al.*, 1992). As discussed later, in exceptional circumstances the natural process may occasionally be circumvented.

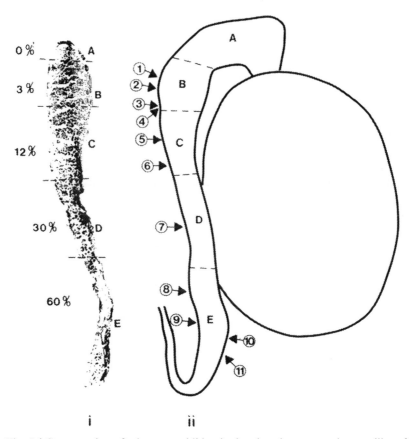

Fig. 5. **i** Cross-section of a human epididymis showing the progressive motility of spermatozoa in different regions **A**, efferent ducts; **B**, proximal caput; **C**, distal caput; **D**, corpus; **E**, cauda. **ii** Diagram showing where sperm samples were obtained from men undergoing vasectomy in order to assess sperm fertilising capacity (from Moore *et al.*, 1983).

These critical functional alterations to spermatozoa during epididymal transit are accompanied by numerous physiological and biochemical modifications. Some of these maturation changes are probably 'housekeeping' to ensure that the cell remains viable during its stay in the excurrent ducts. For example, alterations in the lipid composition of the sperm membranes may help to stabilise them for prolonged storage. Likewise, the movement of the cytoplasmic droplet along the flagellum during maturation does not impart an obvious benefit on human spermatozoa in terms of fertility, but the sequestering of redundant enzymes in such vesicles may help to protect the cell. On the other hand, a number of biochemical changes may be directly associated with the development of full sperm fertility. Structural stabilization of the dense fibres of the tail with disulphide bonds probably leads to the more rigid tail movement that enables the mature spermatozoon to be progressively motile. A similar stabilization occurs in sperm chromatin thereby hardening the nucleus for penetration through the zona pellucida and perhaps in preparation for pro-nucleus formation in the zygote. Interestingly, unlike those of almost any other mammals (with the exception of the gorilla), human spermatozoa are extremely heterogeneous with regard to nuclear stability as detected by the swelling reaction in detergents (Bedford, Calvin & Cooper, 1973). This poses the intriguing question as to whether spermatozoa lacking adequate disulphide cross-linking of their chromatin are as fertile in terms of fertilization and/or sustaining embryonic development as those with normal disulphide content. In laboratory animals, inseminations carried out with immature spermatozoa not only lead to lower conception rates but also to increased early embryonic loss (Orgebin-Crist, 1967) suggesting that sperm chromatin may require epididymal maturation to be fully functional.

Modification of determinants on the plasmalemma undoubtedly enable spermatozoa to recognise and bind to the zona surface of the egg as a prelude to fertilization. It is now believed that during the final stages of epididymal maturation, spermatozoa acquire specific receptors on the plasma membrane overlying the acrosome. These sperm receptors engage with complementary ligands on the zona surface to initiate binding and probably the acrosome reaction of the fertilizing spermatozoon (Moore, 1990*b*). At present the nature of the sperm receptor molecules is not known (for any mammal) although possible candidates have been identified. Certainly, human spermatozoa display a changing distribution and density of moieties over their surface during maturation which is reflected grossly in an increase in the negative charge brought about in part by an increase in sialic acid residues. Significantly, ejaculated spermatozoa focussed in a pH/density gradient form more than one band, possibly indicating populations of cells at different stages of maturation. In one set of experiments, selected motile spermatozoa formed a discrete homogeneous band which was consistently lower (more negative) than motile sperm samples from infertile men with apparently normal semen parameters. Such results favour the notion that infertility may result from inadequate maturation of the sperm surface (Moore, 1979).

Does the epididymis play an active or passive role during sperm maturation?

As spermatozoa pass down the epididymis, they are bathed in a continuously changing milieu of the luminal fluid, derived from Rete testis fluid and modified by the secretory and absorptive activity of the epididymal epithelium. This environment maintains the viability of spermatozoa in the tract until their expulsion at ejaculation. A crucial issue is whether the epididymal epithelium and the fluid it creates is directly responsible for promoting the acquisition of

Table 1. *The proportion of hamster oocytes fertilized in vitro with immature spermatozoa from the corpus epididymidis pre-incubated in the presence or absence of epithelial cultures. Epithelial vesicles cultured for 3 days with androgen promoted sperm maturation*

Distal corpus spermatozoa			Cauda spermatozoa
Epithelial culture with androgen	Epithelial culture without androgen	Without culture	Without culture
93*/240 (39%)	21/226 (9%)	5/124 (4%)	69/78 (88%)

*Significantly different from control P ⩽ 0.005.

sperm fertilizing capacity, or acts passively during an inherent sperm 'ageing' process? To answer this question it is important to consider studies carried out in laboratory and domestic animals as well as reviewing the rather scant information in man. Certainly in all non-human mammals there is compelling evidence that the epididymal epithelium does provides essential factors for sperm maturation. In the rabbit, for example, ligation experiments that retain spermatozoa in various regions of the epididymis indicate that spermatozoa must pass through at least the initial segment and caput region to acquire fertilizing capacity (Bedford, 1967; Orgebin-Crist, 1967). Similar conclusions are reached from 'bypass' experiments involving the surgical removal of regions of the rabbit epididymis and the rejoining of the tract by re-anastomosis (epididymovasostomy). Even after two years, end-to-end anastomosis of the vas deferens to the proximal or distal caput region severely compromised buck fertility (Temple-Smith, Southwich, Herrera Casteneda, Hamer & McClatchey, 1989). Further evidence for epithelial involvement comes from the incubation of immature rabbit or hamster spermatozoa in the presence of homologous epididymal epithelial cell cultures (Moore & Hartman, 1986). Only spermatozoa incubated with functional epithelium (cultured with androgen) acquire the ability to bind to, and fertilize, oocytes *in vitro* (Table 1).

In contrast to the consistent findings in animals, the involvement of the epididymis in human sperm maturation would, at first sight at least, seem to be more equivocal. In part, this is due to the fact that most information has been obtained from the treatment of pathological cases rather than from normal fertile men. However, species differences between the commonly used animal models (rabbit and rodents) and man may also exist. Evidence supporting a direct role for the epididymis comes from results of epididymovasostomy bypass operations in men to relieve epididymal obstruction. In these case, anastomosis of the vas deferens to the proximal 10 mm of duct results in significantly reduced fertility compared to anastomosis to the more distal regions of the tract (Schoysman & Bedford, 1986). But, exceptions have been reported and anastomosis of the vas deferens to even the efferent ducts has subsequently resulted in pregnancies with paternity confirmed (Silber, 1988). Perhaps most surprisingly, spermatozoa have been retrieved from the efferent ducts and proximal caput region of men with congenital absence of the vas and used for successful *in vitro* fertilization and pregnancy (Silber *et al.*, 1988). Unfortunately, such results are difficult to interpret as pathological rather than normal tissue is involved and therefore local conditions for limited sperm maturation may have been created. On the other hand, there does seem to be more individual variation as to when sperm fertility commences in the epididymis of men compared with the situation in laboratory animals, and a small population of spermatozoa ($<3\%$) may be progressively motile in the proximal caput epididymidis. Since *in vitro* fertilization techniques require relatively small numbers of motile spermatozoa (about 25 000), this small proportion of motile sperm can sometimes be utilised. However, perhaps the best evidence for epididymal involvement has come recently from studies in my own laboratory where immature epididymal spermatozoa recovered from proven fertile men have been incubated with human epithelial cell cultures (Fig. 6). In the presence of epithelium, spermatozoa improved their motility and showed a significant increase in their capacity to attach to human zona *in vitro* (Moore *et al.*, 1992).

Morphology of the epididymal epithelium and function during sperm maturation

Given that the epididymal epithelium is actively involved in sperm maturation this begs the question as to what function it plays. The majority of cells (85%) that constitute the pseudostratified epithelium are tall columnar principal cells that are present throughout the length of the duct. Each principal cell possesses long microvilli on its luminal border, has an elaborate Golgi apparatus and numerous vesicles, dense bodies and mitochondria consistent with an absorptive and secretory function. Human principal cells are somewhat unusual in containing many more inclusions, such as dense bodies and lysosomes, than seen in equivalent cells in other species (Fig. 7). These often distort the organization of the cell but whether function is affected is not known. In the proximal epididymis a small (10%) population of apical cells also reside. These and a related type in the corpus and cauda region called the clear cell are mitochondrial rich with many multivesicular vesicles in their apical cytoplasm. The remaining cell types are basal cells (stem epithelial cells?) and wandering intra-epithelial lymphocytes (Fig.

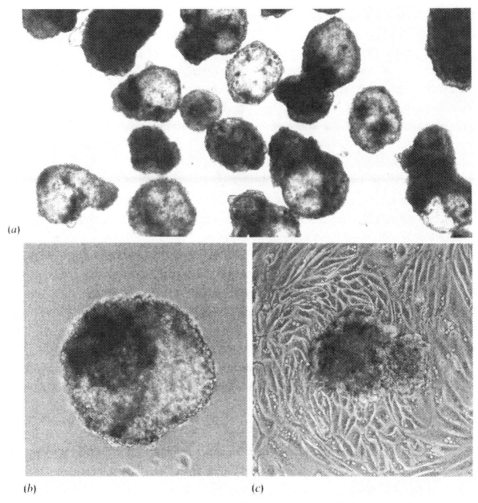

Fig. 6. (a) Micrograph of everted vesicles of human epididymal epithelium. Prepared from fragmented epididymal tubule, these vesicles (b) have epithelium facing outwards and in the presence of androgen continue to produce secretion. (c) With prolonged culture, epithelium plates out onto the bottom of culture dishes.

8). Beneath the basal lamina of the epithelium lies connective tissue containing fibroblasts, smooth muscle cells, a capillary bed and nerve fibres (Moore, 1990a).

Overall, this epithelium is involved in an array of secretory and absorptive functions including the transport of ions, small organic molecules and proteins and glycoprotein as summarized in Fig. 8. Most of these processes appear to be dependent on androgens. As demonstrated with specific antisera or monoclonal antibodies, particular polypeptides are secreted by principal cells in different segments of the duct suggesting that the changing profile in the protein composition of the luminal fluid along the epididymis is directly mediated by the

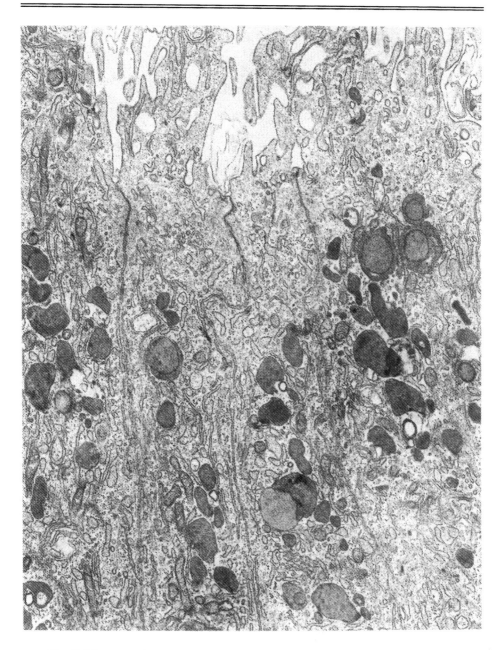

Fig. 7. Electron micrograph of human epididymal epithelium from the corpus region. The disorganized cytoplasm of principal cells with many dense bodies is a feature of human epididymis not seen in laboratory animal models.

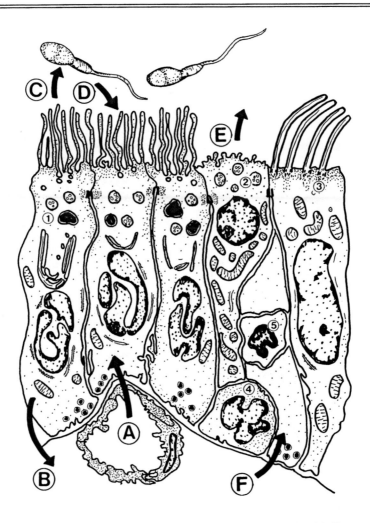

Fig. 8. A schematic diagram of the cell types of the epididymal epithelium and their various functions. (1) Principal cell; (2) Apical (caput region) or Clear cell (cauda region); (3) Ciliated cell (efferent duct); (4) Basal cell; (5) Intra-epithelial lymphocyte. (A) Androgens from the systemic blood supply via the capillary bed (and from Rete testis fluid) control secretory and absorptive activity of the epithelium. (B) Passive fluid resorption driven by active ionic exchange (sodium and chloride) takes place across the apical membrane with water being pumped into the lateral intercellular spaces. (C) Macromolecule secretions from principal cells modify the sperm surface and promote acquisition of fertilizing capacity. (D) Resorption of ions (Na^+, Cl^-) maintain osmolarity of luminal fluid. (E) Apical cells secrete H^+ ions helping to maintain the correct acidity of the luminal fluid. Particulate matter from degenerating spermatozoa is also actively endocytosed by these cells. (F) Active transport mechanisms across the epithelium (carnitine, inositol, glycerol) result in a changing luminal environment as spermatozoa pass along the duct.

epithelium activity. Immunocytochemical studies have shown that epitopes synthesised and secreted by principal cells are expressed on the surface of spermatozoa either through direct covalent binding or possibly via enzymes such as transferases (Eddy *et al.*, 1985). Hence, discrete sequential modifications to the sperm surface may occur during epididymis passage, rather like a production line. Such secretory factors may induce forward motility and provide sperm receptors for zona recognition. Due to the difficulty of obtaining normal human epididymis, the nature of these glycoproteins is still unclear although the molecular weights of a number of proteins secreted by the epithelium have now been identified (Tezon, Ramella, Cameo, Vasquez & Blaquier, 1985; Moore *et al.*, 1992).

Usually, the secretory and absorptive activity of the epididymal epithelium is finely tuned so that the viscosity of the luminal fluid remains within normal limits. However, under certain pathological conditions this balance may be disrupted with catastrophic results. In genetic diseases such as cystic fibrosis or Young's syndrome, mucoprotein secretion occurs without the correct water content (owing to defective chloride transport) and a thick viscous plug may develop causing obstructive azoospermia (Wong *et al.*, 1992).

Sperm storage in the epididymis and transport along the distal excurrent ducts

In laboratory animals it has been shown that spermatozoa retain fertility for several weeks in the cauda epididymidis which acts as a sperm reservoir prior to ejaculation. This storage process is affected by scrotal temperature and is under the control of androgens. In the rat, castration leads to a loss of sperm viability within 3–4 days (Orgebin-Crist, Danzo & Davies, 1975). Compared with the rodent or rabbit, the human cauda epididymidis has a relatively poor storage capacity and due to the secretory flow of epididymal fluid, spermatozoa are continually voided in urine when not ejaculated. Considerable mixing of spermatozoa in the cauda epididymidis and vas deferens probably occurs leading to variations in the quality of the ejaculate. The capacity for sperm storage decreases distally and spermatozoa in the distal vas deferens may only be fertile for a few days. Ejaculated spermatozoa from men who had previously undergone vasectomy (i.e. distal to a scrotal ligature) retained fertilizing capacity for just a few days.

Although occasionally spermatozoa are endocytosed by the epithelium of the epididymis or vas deferens, under normal conditions the duct's capacity for sperm resorption or spermiophagy is believed to be small. Particulate protein matter is, however, readily endocytosed by apical/clear cells and to a lesser extent by principal cells (Moore & Bedford, 1979). After vasectomy, an increase in spermiophagy by the epithelium often occurs but in this situation the majority of spermatozoa are disposed of by macrophages which invade the tract at rupture sites and form focal granuloma (Bedford, 1976). Rupture or damage to the excurrent duct such as that caused by vasectomy may provoke the formation of autoantibodies against spermatozoa which may subsequently lead to infertility. A proportion of men who have had vasovasostomy operations to reverse their vasectomy remain infertile even though spermatozoa are present in the ejaculate. High titres of sperm agglutinating antibodies are often found in the seminal plasma of these individuals (Linnet, Hjort & Fogh-Andersen, 1981). The epithelium of the intact excurrent duct may therefore act as an immunological barrier in the same way as the blood–testis barrier. In this respect, the tight junctions near the apical surface of principal cells have been shown to prevent lanthanum, an electron dense marker, from reaching the epididymal lumen.

Ejaculation results from a coordinated contraction of the smooth muscle surrounding the cauda epididymis and vas deferens mediated by sympathetic and parasympathetic nerves. A bolus of luminal fluid is ejected along the urethra resulting in a 'sperm-rich' fraction with little mixing with accessory gland secretions until spermatozoa leave the tract. Misappropriate stimulation of the tract or disease may cause retrograde ejaculation into the bladder (Benson, 1988). Patients with spinal injury and damage to motor nerves serving the genital tract can be helped by electroejaculation techniques carried out under anaesthesia. Using electrodes placed in the rectum, a small electrical stimulation across the rectal mucosa induces erection and ejaculation.

References

Baumgarten HG, Holstein AF, Rosengren E. Arrangement, ultrastructure and adrenergic innvervation of smooth musculature of the ductuli efferentes, ductus epididymidis and ductus deferens in man. *Z Zellforsch Mikrosk Anat* 1971; **120**: 39–71.

Bedford JM. Effect of duct ligation on the fertilising capacity of spermatozoa in the epididymis. *J Exp. Zool* 1967; **166**: 271–81.

Bedford JM. Adaptions of the male reproductive tract and fate of spermatozoa following vasectomy in the rabbit, rhesus monkey, hamster and rat. *Biol Reprod* 1976; **14**: 118–42.

Bedford JM, Calvin HI, Cooper GW. The maturation of spermatozoa in the human epididymis. *J Reprod Fert* 1973; **18** (suppl): 199–213.

Bellve AR, O'Brien DA. The mammalian spermatozoon: structure and temporal assembly. In: Hartmann JF, ed. *Mechanism and Control of Animal Fertilisation*. New York: Academic Press, 1983: 55–137.

Benson GS. Male sexual function: erection, emission and ejaculation. In: Knobil E, Neill J, eds. *The Physiology of Reproduction*. New York: Raven Press, 1988: 1121–39.

Cooper TG. *The Epididymis: Sperm Maturation and Fertilisation*. Heidelberg: Springer Verlag, 1986.

Cooper TG. In defense of a function for the human epididymis. *Fertil Steril* 1990; **54**: 965–75.

De Kretser DM, Kerr JB. The cytology of the testis. In: Knobil E, Neill J, eds. *The Physiology of Reproduction*. New York: Raven Press, 1988: 837–932.

Eddy EM, Vernon RB, Muller CH, Hahnel AC, Fenderson BA. Immunodissection of sperm surface modifications during epididymal maturation. *Am J Anat* 1985; **174**: 225–37.

Fawcett DW, Hoffer AP. Failure of exogenous androgen to prevent regression of the initial segments of the rat epididymis after efferent duct ligation or castration. *Biol Reprod* 1979; **20**: 162.

Hinrichsen MJ, Balquier JA. Evidence supporting the existence of sperm maturation in the human epididymis. *J Reprod Fert* 1980; **60**: 291–5.

Holt WV, Hillier SG, Moore HDM. Computer assisted measurements of sperm swimming speed in human semen: correlation of results with *in vitro* fertilization assays. *Fertil Steril* 1985; **44**: 112–19.

Howards S, Lechene C, Vigersky R. The fluid environment of the maturing spermatozoon. In: Fawcett DW, Bedford JM, eds. *The Spermatozoon*. Urban & Schwarzenburg: Baltimore, 1979: 35–41.

Kormano M, Reijonen K. Microvascular structure of the human epididymis. *Am J Anat* 1976; **143**: 23–38.

Linnet L, Hjort T, Fogh-Andersen P. Association between failure to impregnate after vasovasostomy and sperm agglutinins in semen. *Lancet*, 1981: 117–19.

Moore HDM. The net surface charge of mammalian spermatozoa as determined by isoelectric focusing, changes following sperm maturation, ejaculation, incubation in the female tract and after enzyme treatment. *Int J Androl* 1979; **2**: 449–62.

Moore HDM. The epididymis. In: Chisholm GD, Fair WD. eds. *Scientific Foundation of Urology*. Oxford: Heinemann Medical, 1990a: 399–410.

Moore HDM. The development of sperm–egg recognition processes in mammals. *J Reprod Fert* 1990b; 42 (suppl): 71–8.

Moore HDM, Bedford JM. The differential absorptive activity of epithelial cells in the rat epididymis. *Anat Rec* 1979; **193**: 313–21.

Moore HDM, Hartman TD, *In vitro* development of the fertilising ability of hamster epididymal spermatozoa after co-culture with epithelium from the proximal cauda epididymidis. *J Reprod Fert* 1986; **78**: 347–52.

Moore HDM, Pryor JP. The comparative ultrastructure of the epididymis in monkeys and man: a search for a suitable animal model for studying primate epididymal physiology. *Am J Primatol* 1981; **1**: 241–50.

Moore HDM, Hartman TD, Pryor JP. Development of the oocyte penetrating capacity of spermatozoa in the human epididymis. *Int J Androl* 1983; **6**: 310–18.

Moore HDM, Curry MR, Penfold LM, Pryor JP. The culture of human epididymal epithelium and *in vitro* maturation of epididymal spermatozoa. *Fertil Steril* 1992; **58**: 776–83.

Orgebin-Crist M-C. Maturation of spermatozoa in the rabbit epididymis: fertilising ability and embryonic mortality in does inseminated with epididymal spermatozoa. *Ann Biol Anim Biochim Biophys* 1967; **7**: 373–9.

Orgebin-Crist M-C, Danzo BJ, Davies J. Endrocrine control of the development and maintenance of sperm fertilising ability in the epididymis. In: Hamilton D, Greep R. eds. *Handbook of Endocrinology V, section 7, Male Reproductive System*. Washington: American Physiological Society, 1975: 319–37.

Schoysman RJ, Bedford JM. The role of the human epididymis in sperm maturation and sperm storage as reflected in the consequences of epididymovasostomy. *Fertil Steril* 1986; **46**: 293–9.

Setchell BP, Brookes DE. Anatomy, vasculature, innervation and fluids of the male reproductive tract. In: Knobil E, Neill J, eds. *The Physiology of Reproduction*. New York: Raven Press, 1988: 753–836.

Silber SJ. Pregnancy caused by sperm from vasa efferentia. *Fertil Steril* 1988; **49**: 373–5.

Silber SJ, Balmaceda J, Borrerco C, Ord T, Asch R. Pregnancy with sperm aspiration from the proximal head of the epididymis: a new treatment for congential absence of the vas deferens. *Fertil Steril* 1988; **50**: 525–8.

Temple-Smith PD, Southwich GJ, Herrera Casteneda E, Hamer J, McClatchey M. Surgical manipulation of the epididymis: an experimental approach to sperm maturation. In: Serio M, ed. *Perspectives in Andrology*. New York: Raven Press, 1989: 281.

Tezon JG, Ramella E, Cameo MS, Vasquez MH, Blaquier, JA. Identification of androgen induced proteins in human epididymis. *Biol Reprod* 1985; **32**: 584–90.

Wong PYD, Huang SJ, Leung AYH, Fu WO, Chung YW, Zhou TS, Yip WWK, Chan WKL. Physiology and pathophysiology of electrolyte transport in the epididymis. In: Nieschlag E, Habenicht U-F, eds. *Spermatogenesis, Fertilization, Contraception*. Berlin, Springer-Verlag, 1992: 319–44.

8

Sperm transport in the female genital tract

D. MORTIMER

Introduction

Sperm transport is the process whereby spermatozoa traverse the female genital tract from the site of insemination around the external cervical os in the vagina to the site of fertilization in the ampulla of the Fallopian tube or oviduct. Since the first report of an experimental study on mammalian sperm transport in rabbits by van Leeuwenhoek in 1685, this has been a fascinating area of reproductive biology that has attracted the interest of numerous workers anxious to understand how the male gamete traverses the expanse of the female genital tract to reach the oocyte. More recently, attention has focussed on how sperm fertilizing ability might be regulated in the dynamic series of environments through which they must pass: vagina, cervical mucus, uterine cavity, uterotubal junction (UTJ), tubal isthmus, ampullo-isthmic junction (AIJ) and, finally, the tubal ampulla. Certainly the female genital tract is rather inaccessible for simple experimentation beyond the level of the cervical mucus and many studies have suffered criticisms of artefact and lack of physiological relevance.

Great differences exist not only in the quantity and composition of the inseminate, but also in the site of its deposition (primarily vagina *versus* uterine cavity), between mammalian species. Furthermore, although the site of fertilization is usually the lower region of the tubal ampulla, just above the AIJ, the anatomy of the female tract is another source of interspecies variation. Taken together, those aspects which confound our study of the mammalian sperm transport process also make the extrapolation from other species to our own fraught with questions of relevance. Consequently, this chapter will focus upon what information we have concerning human sperm transport, review it in a critical, but constructive, manner, and only augment these data with information drawn from other eutherian species (i.e. placental mammals) where they themselves are reliable and may genuinely help resolve difficulties in interpreting data on human sperm transport.

Several specific aspects of human sperm transport will be considered: (i) the evidence for the basic concept of sperm transport as a series of reservoirs separated by selective barriers; (ii) sperm selection by the cervix and the existence and location of the so-called 'cervical sperm reservoir'; (iii) the occurrence and physiological role of 'rapid' sperm transport in the reproductive tract of women; (iv) possible mechanisms of sperm transport through the higher levels of the human female tract and the likely existence of an 'isthmic sperm reservoir'; and (v) possible mechanisms whereby sperm function might be regulated during transport through, and storage within, the female reproductive tract.

Although many studies and reviews of human sperm transport were published in the 1970s (see Mortimer, 1983), this was a rather quiet area of research during the 1980s (although many studies were performed in other eutheria). Recent reviews of sperm transport have been published by Barratt & Cooke (1991); Hunter (1987, 1989); Katz. Drobnis & Overstreet (1989); and Overstreet & Katz (1990).

The 'barriers amd reservoirs' concept of sperm transport

This concept evolved from the writings of Hafez during the 1970s in an attempt to rationalize and understand the many and varied observations on eutherian sperm transport to a unified hypothesis (Hafez, 1980). However, in the absence of substantial contradictory evidence for many years, this 'preferred' hypothesis has almost achieved the status of dogma. While it is certainly true that the cervical mucus at the external os (at least in species with vaginal insemination, which includes man), and also the UTJ, do function as selective barriers, there is no evidence that the internal cervical os or the AIJ have any such function. Furthermore, since spermatozoa are rapidly immobilized in the vagina after ejaculation, the vaginal seminal pool cannot be considered as a functional sperm reservoir (see below).

As will be seen later in this chapter, our understanding of sperm transport through the female tract is now rather more advanced, allowing the construction of a more physiological hypothesis.

Spermatozoa in the cervix

At the moment of ejaculation some 100 to 300 million spermatozoa from the caudae epididymides are mixed with the secretions of the various accessory glands in a specific sequence and deposited around the external cervical os and in the posterior fornix of the vagina. It is well established that the first portion of the human ejaculate contains the majority of the spermatozoa, suspended in primarily prostatic secretion. Consequently these are the spermatozoa most probably deposited actually at the external os, from which at midcycle there is a 'cascade' of cervical mucus.

Spermatozoa in this first fraction of the ejaculate not only have significantly better motility and survival than those in later fractions, but their motility is markedly stimulated by the prostatic secretion which also acts to protect them from the deleterious factor(s) present in the seminal vesicular fluid (Eliasson & Lindholmer, 1984). Certainly spermatozoa can be found in cervical mucus samples taken within $1\frac{1}{2}$ minutes of intercourse, at which time semen in the vagina was still visibly coagulated (the 'immediate post-coital test': Sobrero & MacLeod, 1962). Liquefaction of coagulated human semen takes some 5 to 20 minutes and is caused by a protease of prostatic origin (Tauber *et al.*, 1980).

Much debate has surrounded the physiological role of the immediate coagulation of human semen upon ejaculation, although a viable proposition is that it is merely an evolutionary vestige of the copulation plugs seen in many groups of eutheria, including primates. Seminal vesicular fluid coagulates upon emission and contact with other accessory gland secretions (e.g. prostatic fluid) or spermatozoa is not essential for coagulum formation (Tauber *et al.*, 1980). The finding of a motility inhibitor in seminal plasma, originating from the seminal vesicles (for review see Iwamoto *et al.*, 1990), has been suggested to be related to the need to keep spermatozoa quiescent within the coagulum until after liquefaction. However, the results of immediate post-coital tests argue against this as a physiological process as do observations that the majority of spermatozoa which are to penetrate cervical mucus do so within 15 to 20 minutes of ejaculation (Tredway *et al.*, 1975; Tredway, Buchanan & Drake, 1978).

An important point to remember is that just because the whole ejaculate coagulates when a semen specimen is collected by mastubation into a jar, this does not necessarily mean the same happens *in vivo*. It may well be that the first, sperm-rich fraction remains fluid and only the vesicular fraction coagulates, as is usual in the formation of copulation plugs in many other eutheria.

The pH of the vagina around midcycle is strongly acid, a highly detrimental environment for sperm survival. However, although seminal plasma has a strong buffering capacity, and is able to protect spermatozoa from the hostile vaginal environment, the vaginal pool of liquefied semen is unlikely to play any significant part in sperm transport since (i) the spermatozoa rapidly (within 35 minutes) lose their ability to penetrate cervical mucus (Kremer, 1968) and are quickly inactivated (Wallace-Haagens, Duffy & Holtrop, 1975), (ii) most of the ejaculate flow out of the vagina soon after coitus (Wallace-Haagens *et al.*, 1975), and (iii) later re-colonization of the cervix from the vagina is apparently minimal (Tredway *et al.*, 1975, 1978; Insler *et al.*, 1980).

Sperm penetration of cervical mucus

When liquefied semen and cervical mucus come into contact (at least *in vitro*) the rheological phenomenon of phalanges formation occurs. Finger-like projections of seminal material protrude into the mucus phase and motile spermatozoa migrate along them before finally crossing the semen–mucus interface at their tip. This process may serve to entrap large numbers of spermatozoa within the mucus at the external os so that they are able to migrate into the mucus column gradually, protected from detrimental influences acting upon the residual semen. Some component(s) of seminal plasma is/are important for the efficient entry of human spermatozoa into cervical mucus (Katz *et al.*, 1990), and it is known that the ability to migrate across the semen–mucus interface is highly dependent upon specific movement patterns of the motile spermatozoa (for review see Mortimer, 1990). There is also a well-established selection of morphologically normal spermatozoa at the level of sperm penetration into the cervical mucus, a selection based upon the differential motility of normal vs abnormal spermatozoa (Mortimer, 1978; 1983; Katz *et al.*, 1990). Once within the cervical mucus, spermmotility is modified dramatically and the physical penetration of the mucus by spermatozoa causes some alteration in its microstructure so that the motility of 'following' spermatozoa is different to that of 'vanguard' spermatozoa (for review see Katz *et al.*, 1989).

Sperm presence in the cervix induces a massive leukocytosis, the function of which remains unclear, but may serve to eliminate dead spermatozoa from the mucus column – although suggestions of immunological sperm selection have also been made (Pandya & Cohen, 1985). Recent evidence has also confirmed that the leukocytosis phenomenon also extends into the uterine lumen (Williams *et al.*, 1993b).

The receptivity of cervical mucus to penetration by spermatozoa is cyclic, increasing over a period of about four days before, and decreasing rapidly (within two days) after, ovulation. Receptivity is maximal on the day before and the day of the LH peak, although *in vitro* studies of sperm penetration into samples of cervical mucus collected daily have revealed that the optimum penetrability may occur on unpredictable days so that tests performed on predetermined 'ideal' days can often be poor, resulting in misleading clinical results (for review see Mortimer, 1983). Sperm penetrability of cervical mucus is dependent upon the carbohydrate composition of the mucus glycoproteins (Morales, Roco & Vigil, 1993).

Spermatozoa probably enter the uterine cavity from the internal cervical os by virtue of their own motility. This is in accordance with the reported 90-minute delay between insemination and the appearance of spermatozoa in the uterine cavity (Settlage, Motoshima & Tredway, 1974).

The concept of a cervical sperm reservoir

The concept of a cervical sperm reservoir originates primarily from work in the sheep (Mattner, 1973) and, being an attractive hypothesis, has been widely adopted for all species with vaginal insemination. Even though there is only minimal real evidence for any such mechanism in the human female tract, the concept still receives wide support (Overstreet & Katz, 1990). Human spermatozoa certainly populate the crypts of the cervical epithelium, but a shift from the lower to the upper levels of the cervix has not been demonstrated (Insler *et al.*, 1980). Indeed, the number of spermatozoa within the mucus column at the two hours post-insemination studies by Insler *et al.* (1980) is at least equal to, and often greater than, the number in the cervical crypts (Tredway *et al.*, 1975). Since a continuous migration from the vaginal pool into the lower crypts, which could mask such an upward transfer of spermatozoa, is known not to occur (see above), we are forced to accept that spermatozoa 'stored' in any particular crypt remain there until being either transferred directly to the uterus or disposed of, most probably by phagocytosis since there is a pronounced leukocytosis from the cervical epithelium after insemination (for review see Barratt, Bolton & Cooke, 1990).

In the continued absence of any definite evidence that any spermatozoa actually leave a crypt after entering it, there is no sound basis for considering the crypts of the cervical mucosa to be organs of sperm storage in the human. Indeed, a more plausible hypothesis is that, because spermatozoa swimming in cervical mucus are constrained to follow lines to the mucin structure, it may be that spermatozoa which follow this orientation all the way back to its secretory origin, the crypts, are those that are later found there; only those spermatozoa which continue to swim within the mucus column to the internal os eventually reach the uterine cavity. This population of spermatozoa within the mucus column, each swimming at its own speed, may well be the real 'cervical reservoir'. a concept that is supported by various observations in the dynamics of sperm distributions within the cervical mucus *post coitum* (Drake, Tredway & Buchanan, 1979; Inlser *et al.*, 1980).

The post-coital test

The post-coital test (PCT) has been in common use since the work of Hühner in the 1920s. It involves sampling the cervical mucus at an appropriate time after intercourse and examining it for the presence of spermatozoa. Astonishingly, despite this very simple basis, the test has proven impossible to standardize in clinical practice, even though rigorously standardized, objective methods have been established for its laboratory assessment (for review see Mortimer, 1994).

Nevertheless, the PCT is still very widely used in infertility evaluations, and has many strong proponents, even in the face of a recent clinical review which concluded that 'the PCT lacks validity and should be used more selectively and interpreted with greater caution' (Griffith & Grimes, 1990).

Also, the value of the 'fractional PDT', where mucus is sampled as a column from the external os to the internal os of the cervical canal for studying the dynamics of sperm migration through the mucus, has been discounted. No one level of the cervical canal, as sampled for a fractional PCT, can be distinguished from any other level, and so mucus from any level of the cervical canal may be used for a clinical PCT (Drake *et al.*, 1979).

Rapid sperm transport

The occurrence of a phase of 'rapid' sperm transport, whereby spermatozoa are transported by the actions of the female tract from the site of insemination to the oviducts within a very few minutes after insemination, has been based upon studies in other species (which are probably of minimal relevance to the human situation) and a few, poorly controlled studies in women. This literature has been extensively and critically reviewed elsewhere (Mortimer, 1983; Hunter, 1987) and the existence of such a physiological process cannot be substantiated in the human. Nevertheless, the rapid transport theory, which has only been conclusively demonstrated in the rabbit, still has some strong proponents (Overstreet & Katz, 1990), although this may be considered in the light of recent evidence in domesticated species (Hunter, 1989) and an ideal primate model (Wehner *et al.*, 1985).

The only study which reports the rapid transfer of spermatozoa to the Fallopian tubes in women (Settlage *et al.*, 1974) has several intrinsic inconsistencies. While no spermatozoa were found in oviducts excised before, or two minutes after, insemination (although no data were presented to substantiate these statements), there were spermatozoa in oviducts excised at later times (minimum of five minutes), with maximum numbers being present during the period 15 to 45 minutes post-insemination, and very much reduced numbers at two hours and later. However, no spermatozoa were found in the uterus until 90 minutes: so we must conclude that immediate post-insemination rapid sperm transport occurs in the absence of any sexual stimulation of the female tract (since all patients were artificially inseminated), *and* that such a process deposits spermatozoa in the tubal isthmus, ampulla and fimbriae but not in the uterus. In view of the established sperm storage capacity of the oviduct (Hunter, 1987), perhaps a more realistic interpretation of these data might be that the early oviductal spermatozoa had remained there, probably associated with the tubal mucosa (see below), from a previous insemination.

An important finding is that, even in the rabbit where rapid sperm transport has been unequivocally demonstrated, the rapidly transported spermatozoa are non-functional, indeed mostly dead and therefore cannot participate in fertilization (for review see Overstreet & Katz, 1990). Their biological significance, if any, remains unknown.

Spermatozoa in the uterus

In the adult nulliparous state the uterine cavity is merely a slit, more of a potential rather than an actual lumen, although in parous women it does remain somewhat larger. Spermatozoa entering the uterine cavity are probably suspended in the small volume of uterine fluid bathing the endometrium. Their intrinsic motility may help maintain them in suspension while the fluid is mixed throughout the uterus by segmental pattern myometrial contractions. More or less uniform distribution of spermatozoa throughout the uterine cavity would therefore be established. This hypothesis awaits confirmation or disproof.

The leukocytosis phenomenon seen when spermatozoa are present in the cervix (see above) has also recently been reported to extend into the uterine cavity (Williams *et al.*, 1993*b*).

Likewise, only theories exist as to how spermatozoa traverse the UTJ to reach the tubal isthmus. The UTJ is clearly at least a physical barrier since pressure has to be exerted to force fluid through it. Sperm motility is probably also important, and general evidence from studies on sperm selection *in vivo* suggests that the UTJ constitutes a barrier to spermatozoa with impaired motility (for review see Mortimer, 1978).

Spermatozoa in the oviduct

There is a progressive reduction in the numbers of spermatozoa along the length of the female tract (Croxatto *et al.*, 1974; Settlage *et al.*, 1974). Although there may be several hundreds or even thousands of spermatozoa in hydrosalpinges, in normal oviducts there are normally only a maximum of 200 spermatozoa at any time (Ahlgren, Boström & Malqvist, 1974). Fewer spermatozoa are transported during the luteal phase of the cycle than during the follicular phase (Croxatto *et al.*, 1974). However, recent evidence has suggested that the sperm:egg ratio at the site of fertilization may actually be closer to unity, at least in experimental models (for review see Barratt & Cooke, 1991). The only recent studies (Williams *et al.*, 1992, 1993*a*), which conclude that the isthmus does not appear to act specifically as a sperm reservoir are only very small numbers of cases, all but two of which were examined after the proposed peri-ovulatory redistribution of spermatozoa (and in one of these cases only 23 spermatozoa were recovered in total). Clearly additional, very carefully timed, studies on human oviductal sperm populations are still required to extend Ahlgren's preliminary data obtained more than 20 years ago.

In addition to its function as a sperm reservoir (see below), the oviductal isthmus also regulates the number of spermatozoa at the site of fertilization to minimize the incidence of polyspermic fertilization (for review see Hunter, 1977).

The isthmic sperm reservoir

Critical review of all careful studies to date on the dynamics of sperm transport in the eutherian female tract have supported the common existence of a sperm reservoir in the lower isthmus in every species studied carefully (Hunter, 1987). These isthmic reservoir spermatozoa apparently show reduced motility and switch to the hyperactivated pattern upon transfer into ampullary fluid or culture medium (for review see Katz *et al.*, 1989). This quiescence seems to be regulated by a high extracellular potassium ion concentration (see below), although an elevated viscosity of their environment due to the presence of oviductal mucus (Jansen, 1980) may also play a role. Recent studies on human oviducts have provided conflicting evidence (Williams *et al.*, 1992, 1993a), while another reported finding spermatozoa embedded deeply within the oviductal microvilli (Mansour *et al.*, 1993).

Close associations between spermatozoa and the oviductal mucosa have been described in several non-human eutherian species (for reviews see Katz *et al.*, 1989; Suarez *et al.*, 1990). These interactions variously involve either sequestration within the folds of the epithelium itself, in close association with the mucosal surface, or attachment of spermatozoa by their heads to the mucosal surface, and the epithelial cilia. However, spermatozoa do not seem to associate with the ampullary epithelium, perhaps due to capacitation-induced changes in the sperm surface but more likely due to differences between the isthmic and ampullary epithelia (Suarez *et al.*, 1990).

Although our understanding of the physiological interactions between the oviduct lumen and gametes (and also embryos) is still far from complete, we are becoming aware of its complexity and subtlety. We now recognize the existence of a series of microenvironments within the female tract, especially within the oviduct. Interaction of components of the pre-ovulatory isthmic environment with spermatozoa are probably responsible for the capacitation, quiescent storage, and subsequent reactivation. Evidence exists for a temperature gradient along the pig oviduct with the caudal isthmus being 0.7 °C cooler than the ampulla before ovulation in mated animals (Hunter, 1989). This difference may also cause reduced oxygen tension in the isthmus. There are also differences in the chemical compositions of isthmic and oviductal fluid, most notably that isthmic fluid has a higher concentration of potassium ions: probably of the order of 25 to 30 meq/l compared to the 5 to 10 meq/l in ampullary fluid (for review see Mortimer, 1986).

Spermatozoa from this isthmic reservoir are redistributed in the immediate periovulatory phase, so that they appear in the ampulla of the oviduct synchronously with the oocyte. This system is regulated by local hormonal messengers, probably including steroids, protein hormones and prostaglandins, from the ovarian follicles via a counter-current mechanism (Hunter, Cook & Poyser, 1983; Hunter, 1989).

Evidence for an isthmic sperm reservoir in women

To date, only anecdotal evidence is available as to the existence of an isthmic sperm reservoir in the human female tract (A.A. Templeton & D. Mortimer, unpublished observations). While laparoscopic sperm recovery in couples with idiopathic infertility was positive in 55.3% of cases (Templeton & Mortimer, 1982), spermatozoa were recovered in only one-third of bilateral salpingectomy cases studied at comparable times after insemination, contrary to an expected higher rate of sperm recovery in these normal fertile couples. It is probably significant that, at salpingectomy, the distal part of the oviductal isthmus, being located within the wall of the uterus, was not removed. The intra-mural part of the oviduct is considered the most likely location for an isthmic sperm reservoir in man. Further support comes from the recovery of large numbers of spermatozoa in two normal fertile couples where the intact uterus and oviducts were removed at hysterectomy (again at equivalent times post-insemination), thereby allowing the oviducts to be flushed from the UTJ.

While such limited observations clearly cannot constitute anything more than circumstantial evidence for the existence of an isthmic reservoir in the intra-mural, caudal portion of the human oviductal isthmus, they are the only data presently available.

Spermatozoa in the peritoneal cavity

It has now been known for 30 years that spermatozoa may be recovered in peritoneal fluid and/or fimbrial rinses at laparotomy (Horne & Thibault, 1962). With the establishment of the laparoscope as a primary tool in the investigation of suspectedly infertile women, this became the basis of several studies on 'laparoscopic sperm recovery' (LSR: for review see Mortimer, 1983; also see below).

The more or less free communication between the Fallopian tubes and the peritoneal cavity has also been employed in the opposite sense with the use of direct intra-peritoneal injection (DIPI) as a treatment for infertility in some centres.

Regulation of sperm fertilizing ability *in vivo*

Capacitation

Human spermatozoa, like those of all other eutheria, are incapable of fertilizing oocytes immediately after ejaculation. A final stage of maturation, which has been termed capacitation (defined as the process by which spermatozoa acquire the capacity to undergo the acrosome reaction to fertilize oocytes) is required (Yanagimachi, 1988). Capacitation is essential for fertilization both *in vivo* and *in vitro*, and commences upon release of the spermatozoa from the inhibitory environment of the seminal plasma. Recent studies suggest that acquisition of the capacitated state *in vivo* involves a close communication between the spermatozoa and the female tract. Consequently, capacitation may proceed rather faster *in vivo* than has been believed from experimental studied *in vitro*, and capacitated spermatozoa may be held (perhaps in a quiescent state) for prolonged periods perhaps protected from undergoing spontaneous acrosome reactions as is typically seen during their incubation *in vitro*. Capacitation is more or less completed before sperm reach the site of fertilization in the oviductal ampulla, and it may be hypothesized that spermatozoa reach a late, or even terminal, stage of capacitation during their stay in the isthmic reservoir.

In evolutionary terms, capacitation has been viewed as a mechanism for regulating sperm fertilizing ability necessitated by the emergence of internal fertilization coupled with reproductive (oestrus) cycles, changes in the oocyte and the concomitant appearance of more formidable egg vestments that must be penetrated (for reviews see Bedford, 1983*a,b*).

The charactistic highly active, but non-progressive, pattern of motility that is associated with capacitation ('hyperactivated motility': see below) has been described in most species not to occur *in vivo* until the spermatozoa enter the oviductal ampulla. *In vitro*, human spermatozoa seem to show hyperactivated motility quite early in capacitation (Burkman, 1990; Mortimer & Mortimer, 1990), perhaps suggesting that hyperactivation may be an early concomitant of the capacitation process as opposed to an expression of the acquisition of the capacitated state. It might also be a reflection of heterogeneity of human sperm populations in that the time required for the capacitation of some spermatozoa could be far shorter than previously thought. Regulation of the expression of hyperactivation by human spermatozoa, at both the cellular and physiological levels, remains unknown.

The acrosome reaction

By definition, capacitated spermatozoa are in a state ready to undergo the acrosome reaction. While it has been generally accepted that the acrosome reaction occurs prior to a fertilizing spermatozoon's penetration of a cumulus, there is increasing support for a 'modern' hypothesis that the acrosome reaction is induced by some component(s) of the zona pellucida (Kopf, 1990; Kopf & Gerton, 1990). Consequently the occurrence of spontaneous acrosome reactions are most probably related to sperm senescence and are not associated with fertilization. Totally capacitated spermatozoa are highly labile and it may be that some spermatozoa respond to non-specific stimuli such as follicular fluid, and perhaps other constituents of the cumulus matrix, before reaching the zona pellucida (Mortimer, 1991).

At least part of the acrosome reaction-inducing ability of follicular fluid is attributable to its high glycoaminoglycan content (Yanagimachi, 1988), although progesterone is also able to induce calcium influx into human spermatozoa, thereby initiating not only hyperactivated motility (Mbizvo, Burkman & Alexander, 1990) but also acrosome reactions (Meizel *et al.*, 1990).

Chemotaxis of spermatozoa

A recent report suggested that follicular fluid contains a chemotactic factor for human spermatozoa (Ralt *et al.*, 1991). However, the study failed to disprove the alternative mechanism of chemokinesis, and therefore cannot be taken as sufficient evidence for the existence of chemotaxis. Whereas chemotaxis is a modulation in the direction of travel (for review see Cosson, 1990), chemokinesis involves an alteration in the speed of travel, for example by a switch in sperm motility between progressive and non-progressive patterns. Obviously if fillicular fluid induces hyperactivation, which is defined as a non-progressive pattern of movement (Burkman, 1990; Mortimer & Mortimer, 1990), there would be an accumulation of spermatozoa within the observation chamber which might be misinterpreted as chemotaxis.

Further recent reports from the same group have extended their observations describing a partial purification of the chemotactic factor and purporting to demonstate a chemotactic response in a small, but changing sub-population of spermatozoa (2 to 12%), but a response only elicited by about half the follicular fluid samples tested (Ralt *et al.*, 1994; Cohen-Dayag *et al.*, 1994). However, the evidence for changes in sperm directionality was not provided in quantitative terms, and the data were extensively reported using 'representative' results only. Furthermore, these authors' arguments for physiological relevance of chemotaxis in human spermatozoa do not account for much of the published data on the dynamics of sperm transport.

In conclusion, the existence of chemotaxis remains unproven in objective terms and physiologically unfounded, whereas chemokinesis is well established and can be used to explain almost all the effects described to date. Objective, quantitative data testing the fundamental hypothesis as to whether chemotaxis exists, against a substantial background of chemokinesis, from experiments based upon changes in sperm directionality (c.f. Cosson, 1990), must be provided before any real credence can be given to the existence of chemotaxis in human spermatozoa.

The fertile life of spermatozoa

Sperm survival in the vagina has already been considered (see above) and, although it may be of forensic interest, the prolonged survival of spermatozoa at this level of the female tract is of little relevance to the physiological process whereby spermatozoa attain the site of fertilization.

A maximum number of spermatozoa is already present in the cervix by 15 to 20 minutes post-insemination, and the number of cervical spermatozoa remains constant for at least 24 hours, although a rapid decline has commenced by 48 hours. It is probably only during the first day *post coitum* that the continued existence of motile spermatozoa in the cervix is important, although motile spermatozoa can be found at $2\frac{1}{2}$ days, and even up to seven days *post-coitum* (for review see Mortimer, 1983). Potentially fertile spermatozoa have been recovered from cervical mucus for up to three days (Zinaman *et al.*, 1989).

Unfortunately, the methods used to recover human spermatozoa from higher regions of the female tract have not permitted assessment of their motility or functional state. It has been concluded from older observational studies that some human spermatozoa may remain motile at the site of fertilization for up to $3\frac{1}{2}$ days, although the figures for those eutherians with demonstrated long-term storage (e.g. bats) are much longer (for review see Mortimer, 1983). Reliable values for human spermatozoa are really unavailable since no studies have yet been published investigating the recovery of spermatozoa from the isthmic reservoir and their functional competence. However, a recent case report described the recovery of motile spermatozoa from the oviduct after 25 days (Mansour *et al.*, 1993), and furthermore these spermatozoa remained alive in co-culture for another 9 days.

Clinical assessment of sperm transport

The cervical level

The problems of using the PCT to assess sperm transport have already been mentioned briefly. Of great clinical significance for infertility diagnosis is the well-established poor correlation between PCT results and the presence/absence of spermatozoa in the higher levels of the female tract or peritoneal cavity (for review see Mortimer, 1983). Comparison of the clinical significance of PCT results and *in vitro* sperm–mucus interaction tests (SMITs) revealed that while PCT results were not predictive of pregnancy, good SMITs had a higher prognosis for pregnancy (30.5% *cf* 8.5% with poor SMITs: Eggert-Kruse *et al.*, 1989*a*). Consequently, the PCT is now viewed with increasing skepticism as a clinical test.

The diagnostic evaluation of the interaction between a man's spermatozoa and his partner's cervical mucus *in vitro* does, however, have substantial physiological and clinical relevance since penetration of cervical mucus is the first obstacle that spermatozoa must face if conception is to be achieved *in vivo*. These tests are derived from two basic techniques: 'slide tests' using apposed drops of semen and mucus under coverslips; and 'tube' (or 'Kremer') tests where mucus-filled capillary tubes are placed with one end in contact with liquefied semen. Penetration in either system is assessed by counting motile spermatozoa at various distances from the semen–mucus interface at certain times after establishment of this contact (for review see Mortimer, 1994).

The outcome of *in-vitro* SMITs is dependent upon semen analysis assessments of both percentage sperm motility and morphology, and is impaired by the presence of certain types of antisperm antibodies either on the sperm surface or locally secreted by the cervical epithelium (for review see Mortimer, 1994). Furthermore, several laboratories have demonstrated an influence of sperm movement characteristics upon the success of sperm penetration of cervical mucus, particularly the progression velocity of the spermatozoa and the amplitude of the lateral displacement of the sperm head about the axis of progression (ALH), a characteristic dependent upon the amplitude of the flagellar wave. Indeed, a small population of men exist whose motile spermatozoa are completely unable to penetrate into cervical mucus, or migrate through it, because of extremely small ALH values (for review see Mortimer, 1990).

In terms of fertility prediction, the pregnancy rate in couples with good Kremer-SMIT results was $> 10 \times$ higher than that for couples with poor Kremer-SMIT results (2.3% vs 29.0%: Eggert-Kruse *et al.*, 1989*b*). Furthermore, a study of Kremer-SMIT assessments on ejaculates provided for IVF, showed a close relationship between mucus penetrating ability and fertilizing ability (Barratt *et al.*, 1989).

There has also been considerable interest in using *in-vitro* tests of sperm migration in media other than cervical mucus to assess the quality of sperm motility and their ability to penetrate cervical mucus. Most recently, studies using migration media based upon sodium hyaluronate polymers have shown the greatest potential (for review see Mortimer, 1994). Such tests effectively assess the mucus penetrating potential of a semen sample without the need for large quantities of midcycle cervical mucus and can therefore augment (as an internal control), although not necessarily replace, the homologous Kremer-SMIT, thereby reducing the quantity of both patient and donor mucus needed for comprehensive crossed hostility format testing of sperm–mucus interaction. A standardized migration test can also be used as an independent *in vitro* test of sperm function.

Transport to the site of fertilization

A large study evaluating the value of LSR in infertility investigations in couples with idiopathic infertility showed that a positive LSR result had a good prognosis for a spontaneous pregnancy during a subsequent two-year, treatment-free, follow-up period (Templeton & Mortimer, 1982). At the same time, a negative LSR result had a poor prognosis for subsequent fertility. The overall rate of positive LSR findings was only of the order of 50% (with the admitted existence of some false negatives) which was considered to indicate that sperm transport failure may be a significant cause of human infertility. The concept that sperm dysfunction may be at least a partial explanation of this problem is supported by the association between sperm quality assessed by LSR and sperm fertilizing ability analysed using the zona-free hamster egg penetration test (Templeton *et al.*, 1982).

A recent study has reported that sperm recovery from the peritoneal cavity can be demonstrated in all patients, suggesting that sperm transport failure may not be an aetiological factor in infertility (Ramsewak *et al.*, 1990). However, this study used an endocrine synchronization of the women's cycles to facilitate scheduling LSR procedures which may well have impaired the test's independent diagnostic ability. None the less, this modified approach does retain its value for obtaining peritoneal spermatozoa for *in vitro* studies.

Conclusions

Although the transport of human spermatozoa through the female tract to the site of fertilization and the regulation of their fertilizing ability during this process remains poorly understood, critical reappraisal of data from our own species combined with extrapolation from reliable studies in other eutheria has allowed the formulation of a more integrated physiological hypothesis. This hypothesis must now be tested by appropriate *in vivo* observational studies and experimental studies to be carried out both *in vivo* and *in vitro*.

Further work on human sperm transport, although both clinically and ethically difficult, is crucial to developing a complete understanding of the human reproductive process. Knowledge of the mechanisms regulating sperm function *in vivo* will be vital for both the development of rational advanced diagnostic procedure and the improved application of assisted reproductive technology leading to the achievement of higher clinical success rates.

References

Ahlgren M, Boström K, Malmqvist R. Sperm transport and survival in women with special reference to the fallopian tube. In: Hafez ESE, Thibault CG, eds. *Sperm Transport, Survival and Fertilizing Ability in Vertebrates*. Paris: INSERM, 1974; Vol. 26: 183–200.

Barratt CLR, Bolton AE, Cooke ID. Functional significance of white blood cells in the male and female reproductive tract. *Human Reprod* 1990; **5**: 639–48.

Barratt CLR, Cooke ID. Sperm transport in the human female reproductive tract – a dynamic interaction. *Int J Androl* 1991; **14**: 394–411.

Barratt CLR, Osborn JC, Harrison PE, Monks N, Dunphy BC, Lenton EA, Cooke ID. The hypo-osmotic swelling test and the sperm mucus penetration test in determining fertilization of the human oocyte. *Human Reprod* 1989; **4**: 430–4.

Bedford JM. The significance of the need for sperm capacitation before fertilization in eutherian mammals. *Biol Reprod* 1983*a*; **28**: 108–20.

Bedford JM. Form and function of eutherian spermatozoa in relation to the nature of egg vestments. In: Beier HM, Lindner HR, eds. *Fertilization of the Human Egg* in vitro. *Biological Basis and Clinical Application*. Berlin: Springer-Verlag, 1983*b*: 133–46.

Burkman LJ. Hyperactivated motility of human spermatozoa during *in vitro* capacitation and implications for fertility. In: Gagon C, ed. *Controls of Sperm Motility: Biological and Clinical Aspects*. Boca Raton: CRC Press, 1990: 303–29.

Cohen-Dayag A, Ralt D, Tur-Kaspa I, Manor M, Makler A, Dor J, Mashiach S, Eisenberg M. Sequential acquisition of chemotactic responsiveness by human spermatozoa. *Biol Reprod* 1994; **50**: 786–90.

Cosson MP, Sperm chemotaxis. In: Gagnon C, ed. *Controls of Sperm Motility: Biological and Clincal Aspects*. Boca Raton: CRC Press, 1990: 103–35.

Croxatto HB, Faundes A, Medel M, Avendaño S, Croxatto HD, Vera C, Anselmo J, Pastene L. Studies on sperm migration in the human female genital tract. In: Hafez ESE, Thibault CG, eds. *Sperm Transport, Survival and Fertilizing Ability in Vertebrates*. Paris: INSERM, 1974; Vol 26: 165–82.

Drake TS, Tredway DR, Buchanan GC. A reassessment of the fractional postcoital test. *Am J Obstet Gynecol* 1979; **133**: 382–5.

Eggert-Kruse W, Gerhard I, Tilgen W, Runnebaum B. Clinical significance of crossed *in vitro* sperm–cervical mucus penetration test in infertility investigation. *Fertil Steril* 1988*b*; **52**: 1032–40.

Eggert-Kruse W, Leinhos G, Gerhard I, Tilgen W, Runnebaum, B. Prognostic value of in vitro sperm penetration into hormonally standardized human cervical mucus. *Fertil Steril* 1989*a*; **51**: 317–23.

Eliasson R, Lindholmer C. Effects of human seminal plasma on sperm survival and transport. In: Hafez ESE, Thibault CG, eds. *Sperm Transport, Survival and Fertilizing Ability in Vertebrates*. Paris: INSERM, 1974; Vol. 26: 219–30.

172   *D. Mortimer*

Griffith CS, Grimes DA. The validity of the postcoital test. *Amer J Obstet Gynecol* 1990;
    162: 615–20.

Hafez ESE. The cervix and sperm transport. In: Hafez ESE, ed. *Human Reproduction.*
    Conception and Contraception, 2nd edn. Hagerstown: Harper & Row, 1980: 221–52.

Horne HW, Thibault JP. Sperm migration through the human female reproductive tract.
    Fertil Steril 1962; **13**: 135–9.

Hunter RHF. Function and malfunction of the Fallopian tubes in relation to gametes,
    embryos and hormones. *Eur J Obstet Gynecol Reprod Biol* 1977; **7**: 267–83.

Hunter RHF. Human fertilization *in vivo*, with special reference to progression, storage and
    release of competent spermatozoa. *Human Reprod* 1987; **2**: 329–32.

Hunter RHF. Ovarian programming of gamete progression and maturation in the female
    genital tract. *Zool J Linn Soc* 1989; **95**: 117–24.

Hunter RHD, Cook B, Poyser NL. Regulation of oviduct function in pigs by local transfer
    of ovarian steroids and prostaglandins: a mechanism to influence sperm transport. *Eur
    J Obstet Gynecol Reprod Biol* 1983; **14**: 225–32.

Insler V, Glezerman M, Ziedel L, Bernstein D, Misgav N. Sperm storage in the human
    cervix: a quantative study. *Fertil Steril* 1980; **33**: 288–93.

Iwamoto T, de Lamirande E, Luterman M, Gagnon C. Influence of seminal plasma
    components on sperm motility. In: Gagnon C, ed. *Controls of Sperm Motility:*
    Biological and Clincal Aspects. Boca Raton: CRC Press, 1990: 331–9.

Jansen RPS. Cyclic changes in the human fallopian tube isthmus and their functional
    importance. *Amer J Obstet Gynecol* 1980; **136**: 292–308.

Katz DF, Drobnis EZ, Overstreet JW. Factors regulating mammalian sperm migration
    through the female reproductive tract and oocyte vestments. *Gamete Res* 1989; **22**: 443–69.

Katz DF, Morales P, Samuels SJ. Overstreet JW. Mechanisms of filtration of
    morphologically abnormal sperm by cervical mucus. *Fertil Steril* 1990; **54**: 513–16.

Kopf GS. The zona-pellucida-induced acrosome reaction: A model for sperm signal
    transduction. In: Bavister BD, Cummins J, Roldan ERS, eds. *Fertilization in Mammals.*
    Norwell: Serono Symposia, 1990: 253–66.

Kopf GS, Gerton GL. The mammalian sperm acrosome and the acrosome reaction. In:
    Wassarman P, ed. *Elements of Mammalian Fertilization. I. Basic Concepts.* Boca Raton,
    CRC Press, 1990: 153–203.

Kremer J. The *in vitro* spermatozoal penetration test in fertility investigations
    [Dissertation]. Groningen, The Netherlands: University of Groningen. 1968. 156 pp.

Mansour RT, Aboulghar MA, Serour GI, Abbas AM, Ramzy AM, Rizk B. *In vivo* survival
    of spermatozoa in the human Fallopian tube for 25 days: A case report. *J Assist
    Reprod Genet* 1993; **10**: 379–80.

Mattner P. The cervix and its secretions in relation to fertility in ruminants. In: Blandau RJ,
    Moghissi K, eds. *The Biology of the Cervix.* Chicago: The University of Chicago Press,
    1973: 339–50.

Mbizvo MT, Burkman LJ, Alexander NJ. Human follicular fluid stimulates hyperactivated
    motility in human sperm. *Fertil Steril* 1990; **54**: 708–12.

Meizel S, Pillai MC, Díaz-Pérex E, Thomas P. Initiation of the human sperm acrosome
    reaction by components of human follicular fluid and cumulus secretions including
    steroids. In: Bavister BD, Cummins J, Roldan ERS, eds. *Fertilization in Mammals.*
    Norwell: Serono Symposia, 1990: 197–222.

Morales P, Roco M, Vigil P. Human cervical mucus: Relationship between the biochemical
    characteristics and ability to allow migration of spermatozoa. *Hum Reprod* 1993; **8**: 78–83.

Mortimer D. Selectivity of sperm transport in the female genital tract. In: Cohen J, Hendry WF, eds, *Spermatozoa, Antibodies and Infertility*. Oxford & London: Blackwell Scientific Publications, 1978: 37–53.

Mortimer D. Sperm transport in the human female reproductive tract. In: Finn CA, ed, *Oxford Reviews of Reproductive Biology, Vol. 5*. Oxford: Oxford University Press, 1983: 30–61.

Mortimer D. Elaboration of a new culture medium for physiological studies on human sperm motility and capacitation. *Hum Reprod* 1986; **1**: 247–50.

Mortimer D. Objective analysis of sperm motility and kinematics. In: Keel BA, Webster BW, eds, *Handbook of the Laboratory Diagnosis and Treatment of Infertility*. Boca Raton: CRC Press, 1990: 97–133.

Mortimer D. *Practical Laboratory Andrology*. New York: Oxford University Press, 1994: 393 pp.

Mortimer D, Behaviour of spermatozoa in the human oviduct. *Arch Biol Med Exp* 1991; **24**: 339–48.

Mortimer ST, Mortimer D. Kinematics of human spermatozoa incubated under capacitating conditions. *J Androl* 1990; **11**: 195–203.

Overstreet JW, Katz DF. Interaction between the female reproductive tract and spermatozoa. In: Gagnon C, ed. *Controls of Sperm Motility: Biological and Clinical Aspects*. Boca Raton: CRC Press, 1990: 63–75.

Pandya IJ, Cohen J. The leukocytic reaction of the human cervix to spermatozoa. *Fertil Steril* 1985; **43**: 417–21.

Ralt D, Goldenberg M, Fetterolf P, Thompson D, Dor J, Mashiach S, Garbers DL, Eisenbach M. Sperm attraction to a follicular factor(s) correlates with human egg fertilizability. *Proc Natl Acad Sci USA* 1991; **88**: 2840–4.

Ralt D, Manor M, Cohen-Dayag A, Tur-Kaspa I, Ben-Shlomo I, Makler A, Yuli I, Dor J. Blumberg S, Mashiach S, Eisenberg M. Chemotaxis and chemokinesis of human spermatozoa to follicular factors. *Biol Reprod* 1994; **50**: 774–85.

Ramsewak SS, Barratt CLR, Li T-C, Gooch H, Cooke ID. Peritoneal sperm recovery can be consistently demonstrated in women with unexplained infertility. *Fertil Steril* 1990; **53**: 1106–8.

Settlage DSF, Motoshima M, Tredway DR. Sperm transport from the external cervical os to the fallopian tubes in women: a time and quantitation study. In: Hafez ESE, Thibault CG, eds. *Sperm Transport, Survival and Fertilizing Ability in Vetebrates*. Paris: INSERM, 1974; Vol 26: 201–17.

Sobrero AJ, MacLeod J. The immediate postcoital test. *Fertil Steril* 1962; **13**: 184–9.

Suarez SS, Drost M, Redfern K, Gottleib W. Sperm motility in the oviduct. In: Bavister BD, Cummins J, Roldan ERS, eds. *Fertilization in Mammals*. Norwell: Serono Symposia, 1990: 111–24.

Tauber PF, Propping D, Schumacher GFB, Zaneveld LJD. Biochemical aspects of the coagulation and liquefaction of human semen. *J Androl* 1980; **1**: 281–8.

Templeton A, Aitken J, Mortimer D, Best F. Sperm function in patients with unexplained infertility. *Br J Obstet Gynaecol* 1982; **89**: 550–4.

Templeton AA, Mortimer D. The development of a clinical test of sperm migration to the site of fertilization. *Fertil Steril* 1982; **37**: 410–15.

Tredway DR, Buchanan GC, Drake TS. Comparison of the fractional postcoital test and semen analysis. *Am J Obstet Gynecol* 1978; **130**: 647–52.

Tredway DR, Settlage DS, Nakamura RM, Motoshima M, Umezaki CU, Mishell DR.

Significance of timing for the postcoital evaluation of cervical mucus. *Am J Obstet Gynecol* 1975; **121**: 387–93.

Wallace-Haagens MJ, Duffy BJ, Holtrop HR. Recovery of spermatozoa from human vaginal washings. *Fertil Steril* 1975; **26**: 175–9.

Wehner AP, Hall AS, Weller RE, Lepel EA, Schrimer RE. Do particles translocate from the vagina to the oviducts and beyond? *Food Chem Toxicol* 1985: **23**: 367–72.

Williams M, Barratt CLR, Hill CJ, Warren MA, Dunphy B, Cooke ID. Recovery of artificially inseminated spermatozoa from the Fallopian tubes of a women undergoing total abdominal hysterectomy. *Hum Reprod* 1992; **7**: 506–9.

Williams M, Hill CJ, Scudamore I, Dunphy B, Cooke ID, Barratt CLR. Sperm numbers and distribution within the human Fallopian tube around ovulation. *Hum Reprod* 1993*a*; **8**: 2019–26.

Williams M, Thompson LA, Li TC, Mackenna A, Barratt CLR, Cooke ID. Uterine flushing: A method to recover spermatozoa and leucocytes. *Hum Reprod* 1993*b*; **8**: 925–8.

Yanagimachi R. Mammalian fertilization. In: Knobil E, Neill JD, Ewing LL, Markert CL, Greenwald GS, Pfaff DW, eds, *The Physiology of Reproduction, Volume 1.* New York: Raven Press, 1988: 135–85.

Zinaman M, Drobnis EZ, Morales P, Brazil C, Kiel M, Cross NL, Hanson FW, Overstreet JW. The physiology of sperm recovered from the cervix: acrosomal status and response to inducers of the acrosome reaction. *Biol Reprod* 1989; **41**: 790–7.

9

Clinical disorders affecting semen quality

A. M. JEQUIER

Introduction

There are many causes of infertility in the male which will be associated with abnormalities in the seminal fluid and indeed it is often these abnormalities, rather than any coital difficulty, that are frequently the direct cause of a couple's inability to conceive. However, it must be remembered that the changes that may occur in seminal fluid arise as a consequence of the disorder causing the infertility and these changes in the semen are not always diagnostic of any one condition; semen abnormalities usually only give a measure of the severity of infertility rather than any indication of its cause. Thus in many male patients with infertility, no diagnosis can be made simply from the examination of a sample of semen. As in the female patient, a history and examination are required to make a diagnosis of the cause of the infertility.

It must also never be assumed that abnormalities in semen if present are the sole cause of a couple's infertility. Such abnormalities may form only a part of an amalgam of both male and female disorders that will result in childlessness for a couple. Certainly, the more severe the abnormality present in the semen, the more likely it will be that this abnormality is the major and even the only cause of infertility. Nevertheless, even when a condition such as obstructive azoospermia, which will cause total sterility is present, female factors that are severe enough in themselves to cause infertility, may be found in 20% of their female partners (Jequier, 1986). Investigation of the female partner is always essential to provide a full understanding of the reasons for the childlessness. Infertility must be seen as a disorder of a couple even when an abnormality of the male is clinically obvious.

Examination of the semen, however, does not simply consist of counting the number of sperm, of examining the quantity and the quality of sperm movement and of evaluating the morphological abnormalities that may be seen among the sperm present in an ejaculate. There are many other methods of examining semen and these include the assessment of the physical features of seminal fluid, the estimation of the biochemical constituents of semen and also the microbiological examination of the ejaculate.

The determination of the presence of anti-sperm antibodies both in the blood and the semen is also of great diagnostic importance in the management of male infertility (see Chapter 12).

The application of the electron microscope to the ultrastructure of the sperm is also of value diagnostically in some patients where abnormalities particularly of the axoneme and disorders of the fibrous sheaths in the mid piece may give a clear indication of the cause of the sperm immobility.

Disorders of the functional capacity of sperm are also a feature of male infertility and tests of sperm function thus form an important part of the analysis of semen among men with infertility (Chapter 4). There is a wide variety of different sperm function tests that can be used in the clinical evaluation of the infertile male, and some of the more useful tests will be discussed in relation to the many disorders that can cause abnormalities in the seminal fluid. Sperm function tests include the standard post-coital test, the hypo-osmotic swelling test (Rogers & Parker, 1991), the hamster egg penetration test (Rogers, 1985) and the recently developed acrosome reaction ionophore challenge test (Cummins et al., 1991) (Chapter 4).

It may also be necessary diagnostically for the patient to produce the semen sample in a special way. The production of a split ejaculate (Eliasson & Lindholmer, 1976) can be very useful diagnostically as it allows the microbiological and the biochemical analysis of a part of the ejaculate that is predominantly derived from one source, and for this reason can be of great value in pin-pointing the source of a micro-organism within the ejaculate or for the demonstration of the defective function of one of the accessory glands.

Sperm from sources other than that of a simple sample of semen may need to be examined. In men with retrograde ejaculation, emission results in the ejaculate entering the bladder and for this reason examination of a post-micturition sample of semen will be required.

The human ejaculate

The human ejaculate varies considerably in volume between individuals but is usually between 2 and 6 millilitres in volume. The pH of fresh semen lies between 7.9 and 8.1. Unlike some other mammals such as the bull and the ram, human semen coagulates on ejaculation but liquefaction of the gel-like clot should normally have occurred within 20 minutes.

In order to be able to understand the changes that occur in seminal fluid in

Table 1. *The secretions that make up the ejaculate*

Source of secretion	% of ejaculate
Testes	5
Seminal vesicles	46–80
Prostate	13–33
Bulbo-urethral and urethral glands	2–5

From Lundquist, 1949.

the different lesions that cause infertility, it is important to understand the different sites from which the ejaculate is formed and their proportionate contribution to the ejaculate (Lundquist, 1949).

The testicular component of the ejaculate is made up of the spermatozoa themselves, the rete testis fluid and the very small volumetric contribution from the epididymis. Together, these contributions form some 5% of the total ejaculate. Thus exclusion of the testicular component of the ejaculate, as will occur in intra-testicular, epididymal or vasal obstruction, will make no obvious difference to the ejaculatory volume (Table 1).

The seminal vesicles, however, make up around 40–80% of the total ejaculatory volume and the exclusion of this component, as will occur in ejaculatory duct obstruction, will produce a very great reduction in the volume of a semen sample.

The prostatic contribution to semen makes up around 10–30% of the total ejaculatory volume. Total exclusion of the prostatic contribution almost never occurs as prostatic fluid is secreted through a number of ducts that open into a relatively large area of the prostatic urethra.

Lastly, the bulbo-urethral and urethral glands also secrete a small amount of mucus that forms around 2–5% of the total ejaculate.

Each of these components has biochemical markers that allows them to be distinguished individually and which provide a measure of their abnormality or their absence within an ejaculate.

The most obvious marker of the testicular component is the presence of spermatozoa but, in the absence of spermatogenesis, substances that are produced by the Sertoli cells such as androgen binding protein (Hansson *et al.*, 1974), inhibin (Burger, 1991) and transferrin (Holmes, Lipschultz & Smith, 1982) have been used to identify rete testis fluid and epididymal secretions within an ejaculate. Epididymal markers that have been used diagnostically in this way include carnitine, inositol and a variety of proteins (Table 2).

The major marker of the seminal vesicular secretions is fructose (Mann &

Table 2. *The important biochemical markers from which one can identify the presence of the different components of the ejaculate within a sample of semen*

Source	Biochemical markers
Testes	Androgen binding protein
	Transferrin
	Inhibin
	Testosterone
Epididymal ducts	Carnitine
	Inositol
	Glycerophosphorylcholine
Seminal vesicles	Fructose
	Prostaglandins
Prostate	Acid phosphatase
	Citrate
	Calcium, zinc
	Spermine
	Vesiculase
Bulbo-urethral and urethral glands	Mucoproteins
	IgA

Rottenberg, 1966) and the seminal vesicles are also the major source of prostaglandin synthesis (Eliasson, 1959). The seminal vesicles also produce an enzyme that induces clotting. The pH of seminal vesicular fluid is alkaline and so, if the seminal vesicular secretions are excluded from an ejaculate, the pH of semen falls.

The prostate produces a number of substances that can be used diagnostically and these include the enzyme acid phosphatase, citric acid, zinc, vesiculase and spermine. The pH of prostatic fluid is acid and thus exclusion of the seminal vesicular component will reduce the pH of the ejaculate as a whole.

The secretions of the bulbo-urethral and urethral glands consist entirely of muco proteins but some IgA is also present.

Against this background one can discuss the different causes of infertility in the male and examine the changes that may occur in the semen in men with these disorders.

Obstruction of the ductal system of the male genital tract

Obstructive lesions may occur at any point along the ductal system of the male genital tract. These lesions can be bilateral, or unilateral and can be either complete

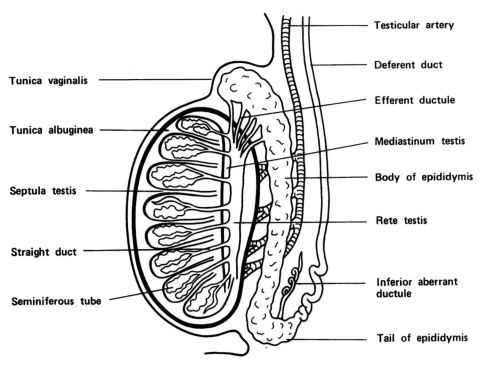

Fig. 1. Diagrammatic representation of the excurrent ducts of the testis in the human.

or incomplete. They may involve the proximal duct system of the male genital tract, or also can be seen much more distally where they can cause blockage of the distal vasa deferentia as well as the ejaculatory ducts. Thus obstruction in the male genital tract can now be divided into proximal and distal obstruction. This division is useful clinically owing to the differing presentations of the two lesions and also because the changes in the seminal fluid induced by the two types of lesions are very different.

Ductal obstruction can occur within the testis and thus be intra-testicular and may involve the seminiferous tubules or the rete testis. However, these obstructive lesions are also seen in the immediate excurrent ducts of the testes and may also involve the efferent ductules as well as the epididymal ducts or the vasa deferentia (Fig. 1).

Obstruction of the distal vasa and the ejaculatory ducts is much less common than epididymal obstruction but is certainly a well-known cause of obstructive azoospermia (Fig. 2).

If the post-vasectomy patients are excluded, the most common site for obstruction in the male genital tract is the epididymis in which more than two

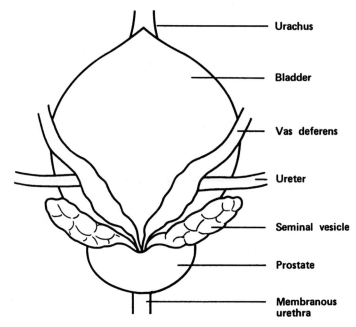

Fig. 2. Drawing showing the relationship of the distal vasa deferentia, the ejaculatory ducts and the accessory glands of the male genital tract.

thirds of all obstructive lesions are found. However, as the requests for vasectomy reversal approach 10% of all the vasectomies that are carried out (Baker, 1991), in practice, vasectomy is now rapidly becoming the most common cause of obstructive azoospermia presenting in an infertility clinic.

Proximal lesions

The hypercurvature syndrome

This condition was first described over 15 years ago (Averback & Wight, 1979) and there is still considerable controversy over whether it is a true clinical entity. It is said to be due to excessive coiling of the seminiferous tubules and can be diagnosed by finding increased numbers of tangentially cut tubules on testicular biopsy. The obstruction that it causes is never complete, and thus this condition will present with semen samples that show reduced numbers of sperm of reduced motility.

Rete testis obstruction

This lesion was first demonstrated histologically by Guerin and colleagues (1981) who reported a total obliteration of the rete by fibrous tissue. This lesion is

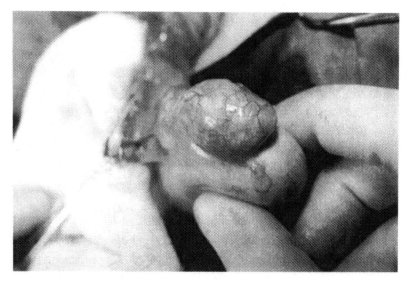

Fig. 3. Upper epididymal obstruction. The distended caput epididymis proximal
to the obstruction is clearly seen.

therefore complete but can be either unilateral or bilateral and may present with
either azoospermia or oligozoospermia. A feature of this condition is the high
titres of antisperm antibodies that may be present in both the blood and the
semen of patients (Hendry *et al.*, 1982) and these antibodies may, in themselves,
cause infertility even in men with a unilateral lesion and a good sperm count.
As these lesions are inoperable, unilateral orchidectomy has even been carried
out as a means of lowering the titre of the anti-sperm antibodies and achieving
fertility (Hendry *et al.*, 1982).

Non-junction of the efferent ductules and the epididymal duct

This is an uncommon but nevertheless well-recognized cause of obstruction
(Hodges & Hawley, 1966). It is always complete and bilateral and presents with
azoospermia. It is commonly associated with testicular maldescent (Heath, 1984)
and so patients with these lesions will often have an associated reduction in
spermatogenesis.

Epididymal obstruction

This is now the most common site of spontaneously occurring obstructive lesions
and these obstructions most commonly affect the region of the upper and the
middle thirds of the epididymis (Fig. 3). The distended upper epididymal caput

that is seen in these epididymal obstructive lesions can often be palpated on clinical examination, a finding known as Bayle's sign. Epididymal obstructive lesions may be the result of trauma both accidental and surgical or of epididymitis. However, in a number of these patients, no specific cause can be determined.

In around 25% of all men with upper epididymal obstruction, there is an associated problem of bronchiectasis and sinusitis to form the condition known as Young's Syndrome (Young, 1970). As these obstructive lesions are usually bilateral, the semen will be azoospermic.

Vasal obstruction

Due to the frequency of requests for vasectomy reversal, vasal obstruction is a common reason for attendance at an infertility clinic. Unintended vasal occlusion is otherwise most commonly due to infection or to inadvertent past surgical damage which is frequently related to the operation of herniotomy in childhood.

Semen abnormalities in men with proximal ductal obstruction

In the few patients who are deemed to have infertility due to the Hypercurvature Syndrome where the obstruction is incomplete, the semen will contain reduced numbers of sperm. The volume and the pH of the semen will be normal in these patients.

The seminal fluid in all the cases of complete obstruction of the proximal duct system will also be of normal volume and of normal pH. The only abnormality seen in the ejaculate in these cases will be the absence of sperm. In patients with rete testis or epididymal obstruction, the markers that are associated with the rete testis fluid will be absent. The biochemical markers from the epididymis are largely secreted into the distal end of the epididymal duct and thus these will only be reduced or absent in men with distal epididymal obstruction or proximal vasal obstruction (Amelar & Hotchkiss, 1963).

Congenital absence of the vasa deferentia

This is a surprisingly common cause of obstruction in which there is aplasia of all or of part of the vasa deferentia. This lesion may be present either unilaterally or bilaterally but it is usually only the bilateral lesions that present at the infertility clinic. Frequently associated with the absence of the vasa deferentia, is an aplasia of part of the epididymis (Fig. 4). The presence of the cystic fibrosis gene is evident in some men with this condition. In up to two-thirds of the patients with this anomaly, the seminal vesicles are also either aplastic or hypoplastic. On clinical

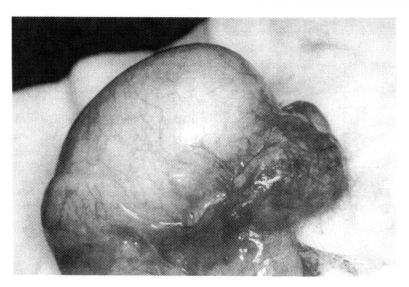

Fig. 4. Photograph of the testis in a man with congenital absence of the vasa deferentia in whom the lower half of the epididymis is also aplastic.

examination, the vasa cannot be palpated and a variable length of the epididymis will be distended.

Semen abnormalities in men with congenital absence of the vasa deferentia

In the case of bilateral congenital absence of the vas, the semen will be azoospermic. As the seminal vesicles are so often either absent or hypoplastic, the seminal volume in these men is frequently reduced and the seminal fructose also either absent or reduced (Amelar & Hotchkiss, 1963). In the total absence of seminal vesicular secretion, the pH may also be lowered. As the seminal vesicular component is not present as a diluent, the concentration of acid phosphatase and, indeed, of all the biochemical markers in prostatic fluid will be raised.

If there has been no surgical intervention on this lesion, anti-sperm antibodies are frequently absent both from the blood and in the semen.

The distal lesions

Distal obstructive lesions involving the ejaculatory ducts are a less common cause of obstruction than are the lesions that occur in the epididymis and the vasa deferentia. Distal obstructive lesions make up only some 2% of all obstructive lesions in the male genital tract (Jequier, 1986).

Table 3. *The biochemical abnormalities that may be seen in the semen in the three major types of ductal obstruction*

Abnormality	Volume	pH	Sperm	Fructose	Citrate
Complete proximal obstruction	Normal	Normal	Absent	Normal	Normal
Congenital absence of the vas	Usually reduced	Usually reduced	Absent	Usually reduced or absent	Raised
Ejaculatory duct obstruction	Reduced	Reduced	Absent	Absent	Raised

Ejaculatory duct obstruction may be the result of a congenital stricture or an aplasia of the duct system. It can also be the result of trans-urethral surgery, of urethral trauma, or of infection. Ejaculatory duct obstruction will thus exclude the testicular, epididymal and seminal vesicular components from the ejaculate and profound changes to the ejaculate will result from these lesions.

Semen abnormalities in men with ejaculatory duct obstruction

As the seminal vesicular fluid is absent, the ejaculate will be of low volume and have a somewhat acid pH. Fructose will be unmeasurable and the ejaculate will be azoospermic. Due to the absence of the dilutional effect of the seminal vesicular secretions, the concentrations of acid phosphatase and of citrate will be raised.

The changes that may be seen in the semen in patients with obstructive lesions are summarized in Table 3.

Partial or incomplete obstruction   A situation may occur in which the obstruction is incomplete, and semen samples from such patients will show a reduced sperm count rather than the total absence of sperm that will result from a bilateral complete obstruction. In such patients, oligozoospermia and a marked reduction of sperm motility will be seen (Jequier, Crich & Holmes, 1983).

Unilateral obstruction   The condition in which ductal obstruction may be unilateral rather than bilateral was first described by Hendry and colleagues (Hendry *et al.*, 1982). This problem is characterized by the presence of oligozoospermia and by the presence of high titres of anti-sperm antibodies which are most frequently directed against the head and the tail regions of the spermatozoa. In such situations, the site of the obstruction must be identified and the obstruction overcome by remedial surgery. If the obstruction cannot be by-passed or overcome and the antibody titre is very high, it has even been suggested that the drastic operation of orchidectomy may be the only way in which the infertility can be remedied (Hendry *et al.*, 1982).

Post-vasectomy reversal Vasectomy reversal is now a common operation and is frequently carried out in patients entering a second marriage or relationship. The prognosis for vasectomy reversal, especially in the long term, is not nearly as satisfactory as the operation of female sterilization reversal that is carried out on women who have been sterilized using the modern tubal clips. The prognosis for a normal semen analysis post-vasectomy reversal decreases significantly if the period of vasectomy exceeds 5 years. The prognosis for fertility is also related to the age of the patient. As daily sperm production and sperm quality deteriorates with age (Neaves *et al.*, 1984), vasectomy reversal in a man of 50 years or more carries a reduced prognosis for fertility.

Following vasectomy reversal, a variety of different problems can be seen in the semen. First, the vasectomy reversal operation can fail and this can be due to either a stenosis at the site of the vaso-vasostomy or it can also be due to the failure to diagnose a concomitant epididymal obstruction recognized by an epididymal 'blowout' that is so commonly associated with long-term vasectomy (Silber, 1984).

The second common problem is the presence of a low sperm count, and this can be the result of either a unilateral stenosis or of an incomplete stricture at the site of the reversal. Another problem is the presence of poor sperm motility and this may well be the result of epididymal distension and functional damage resulting from long-term vasectomy.

A low sperm count may also be due to the presence of additional pathology resulting in a low sperm count even in the absence of the previous vasectomy. Some argue that a testicular biopsy may be valuable at the time of vasectomy reversal. Vasectomy reversal carries a reasonable prognosis provided that the period of vasectomy has not exceeded five years and that the patient is under the age of 50 years.

Primary testicular disease (spermatogenic failure)

A primary disorder of the testis resulting in a disturbance in spermatogenesis is a very common cause of infertility in the male (Hargreave & Jequier, 1978) and is often known as spermatogenic or seminiferous tubular failure. Although in the majority, a cause for spermatogenic failure is not identified, endocrine hypogonadism may be seen in up to 10% and congenital or chromosomal problems in an equivalent number (Nieschlag & Behre, 1992). Other known aetiologies include testicular maldescent, trauma, cancer chemotherapy and X irradiation and viral infections such as mumps orchitis. The histological changes that are seen on testicular biopsy that may be performed on patients with this condition are very variable. Even within one testis the histological picture can vary at different sites indicating that these pathological changes can be focal within each testis and thus may not represent the overall pattern of sperm production within both testes.

There are three major types of change that can be seen histologically in patients. The most common of these is an arrest of spermatogenesis which frequently but not always is seen at the secondary spermatocyte stage and which is commonly described simply as a 'maturational arrest'. The second common histological change that may be seen is a change known as germinal aplasia where there is a total loss of all the gametogenic elements in the spermatogenic epithelium. Thirdly, a total obliteration of the tubules may also be seen in situations where the damage to the testes has been severe. Interestingly, the Leydig cells are much more resistant to damage than is the spermatogenic epithelium but, in the more severe cases, there may also be endocrinological and even histological evidence of Leydig cell malfunction.

In many patients with primary testicular disease, some or all of these histological types may be identified within a testis. The semen analysis will thus reflect the overall sperm production capability of both testes rather than the sperm production associated with each individual histological type. For this reason the semen analysis often does not correlate well with the histological change seen on a small testicular biopsy as this biopsy may not reflect the other changes that may be seen in the spermatogenic epithelium in the remainder of the testis nor that in the ipsilateral testis.

If one examines the abnormalities in a group of oligozoospermic men all of whom are known to have some form of spermatogenic failure due to primary testicular disease, a variety of different abnormalities may be present in the semen none of which may be helpful diagnostically. The sperm numbers are usually reduced but the degree of oligozoospermia is dependent upon the percentage distribution of the various lesions that can be present in the testes of men with this condition. The most constant failure seen in these patients is both a quantitative and qualitative loss of sperm motility and in many patients there is an increase in the percentage of sperm showing abnormal morphology.

Varicocoele

The role of a varicocoele in the causation of infertility in the male is poorly understood and is the subject of considerable controversy (Baker *et al.*, 1985).

Not all investigators believe that a varicocele requires ligation. However, it is generally thought that large varicocoeles do indeed impair both sperm production and sperm function and may even reduce testosterone production by the Leydig cells. It is generally believed that, in men with either unilateral or bilateral varicocoeles, increased venous pressure, scrotal temperature and reduced removal of toxic substances cause a reduction in sperm numbers, a deterioration in sperm movement and an increase in the percentage of abnormal forms.

Seminal vesiculitis

Infections of the seminal vesicle are a well-known but uncommon cause of male infertility. Inflammatory change in the seminal vesicles can result in a reduced semen volume and a reduction in the production of the biochemical compounds that are produced by the seminal vesicular epithelium. As a consequence, there may be a marked reduction in fructose concentration in the ejaculate and this will result in a serious loss of motility by the sperm. Clotting of the seminal fluid may also be inhibited. The identification of the organism causing the infection and its eradication with the appropriate antibiotic will resolve this problem and restore the semen biochemistry to normal.

The presence of white blood cells in the semen

A small number of white blood cells may be seen in normal semen. However, when their concentration exceeds 5 million per ml or when they are seen to be in numbers greater than 5 per high power field, an abnormality, in particular an infection, may be present. The presence of an infecting organism in semen may damage fertility in several different ways. First, the organism may cause structural damage to the sperm surface, and *E. coli* has been shown to act in this way. If the infection damages the function of the accessory glands, then the biochemical secretions of these glands may be impaired. This will give rise to abnormalities in the semen biochemistry and, as a consequence, an impairment in sperm function may occur. The presence of white cells is also likely to increase the concentration, in semen, of reactive oxygen species which are produced in large amounts by all white and red blood cells. Reactive oxygen species are known to be highly toxic to sperm (Aitken, 1989) (Chapter 11). The presence of both these types of cells in semen, and especially when infection may also result in active bleeding within the male genital tract, is very likely to cause a severe deterioration in sperm function. Treatment of the infection and the disappearance of the white blood cells will improve sperm function.

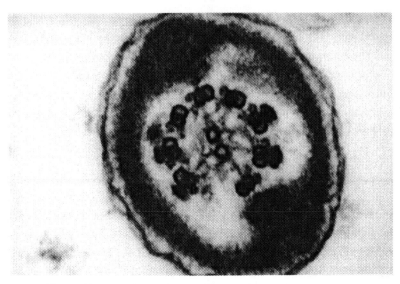

Fig. 5. Electron photomicrograph showing an absent doublet.

Polyzoospermia

Polyzoospermia, or the presence of a high concentration of sperm in the semen, is a rare but nevertheless well-recognized cause of infertility in the male (Amelar *et al.*, 1979). Polyzoospermia may be defined as semen containing a concentration of more then 350 million sperm per millilitre. The cause of this condition is unknown. The sperm show a progressive reduction of sperm movement following ejaculation owing to the rapid utilization of the fructose in the semen by the large numbers of sperm in the semen sample. In patients with this condition, the seminal fructose concentrations will therefore be very low. Treatment of the semen with glucose will restore sperm movement very promptly.

Ultrastructural abnormalities of the sperm

There are a large number of ultrastructural abnormalities that may be seen on the electron microscroscopy of infertile sperm. These abnormalities include the absence of the acrosomal cap (Holstein *et al.*, 1973), abnormalities of the fibrous sheaths of the mid piece or most commonly may involve the complex structure that makes up the axoneme. The axonemal abnormalities may involve a partial or a total loss of the doublets (Fig. 5) or, as occurs in the immotile cilia syndrome (Eliasson *et al.*, 1977), there may be an absence of the dynein arms that are normally seen between each of the nine peripheral doublets in the axoneme. Sperm with these abnormalities frequently show reduced movement on a semen

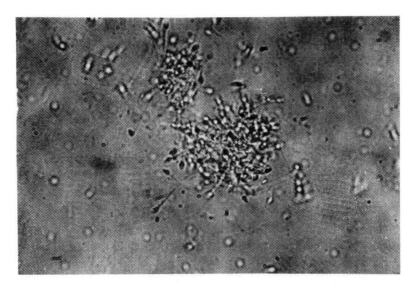

Fig. 6. Agglutinated sperm in the ejaculate of a man with a high titre of anti-sperm antibodies in his seminal fluid.

analysis. If there is no other explanation for poorly moving sperm in an infertile man, an electron microscopic examination of the sperm can be diagnostically helpful.

Sperm auto-immunity

The presence of anti-sperm antibodies in semen can only be detected with any certainty by specific tests (Chapter 12). In some patients with anti-sperm antibodies in their semen, an agglutination of large numbers of sperm occurs and can be seen soon after ejaculation (Fig. 6). However, it must be remembered that, in the semen of the majority of the patients with high titres of anti-sperm antibodies in the seminal fluid, no sperm agglutination will be seen. In many of the patients in whom the sperm autoimmunity is not associated with obstruction, no other abnormality may be detected in sperm numbers, sperm motility or sperm morphology. Thus the presence of sperm autoimmunity cannot be excluded simply by an absence of spontaneous sperm agglutination.

Abnormalities of ejaculation

Abnormalities of ejaculation can often result in infertility. The two main disorders of ejaculation that are seen in an infertility are discussed below.

Retrograde ejaculation is a condition where the semen is not expelled down the urethra but passes backwards into the bladder. Such a functional abnormality can have no known cause but is often to be seen in men with many different types of neurological disturbance including spinal injury. Retrograde ejaculation may also occur following bladder neck or urethral surgery and is a common complication of transurethral resection of the prostate. This abnormality is also very common among diabetics. The ejaculate is virtually absent and consists only of the mucus that is normally secreted into the ejaculate by the bulbo-urethral and urethral glands.

Retrograde ejaculation is diagnosed by finding large numbers of spermatozoa in a specimen of urine taken post-coitally. Urine rapidly ablates sperm movement and thus renders the ejaculate infertile (Crich & Jequier, 1978).

Ejaculatory failure is a much more serious disorder of ejaculation and is often associated with a severe neurological disorder such as spinal injury or the demyelinating diseases as exemplified by disorders such as multiple sclerosis. In this condition, no ejaculate is produced and there is thus no semen to examine.

Conclusions

Semen analysis is an important investigation in the evaluation of the infertile male but alone it is often of little value diagnostically; the diagnosis usually has to be made from the clinical history and the examination of the patient. The application of physical, biochemical microbiological and immunological methods of semen analysis aids diagnosis very greatly as does the use of the electron microscope enhance one's ability to examine the morphology of the spermatozoa. Most important of all is the use of semen analysis in conjunction with sperm function tests, as these can provide a much more accurate assessment of fertility and can thus provide the patient with a prognosis.

Treatment, however, must depend upon an accurate diagnosis, and this can only be obtained from the clinical assessment of the patients and by the judicious use of the many ways now available to us for the investigation of these patients and of their semen.

References

Aitken RJ. The role of free oxygen radicals and sperm function. *Int J Androl* 1989; **12**: 95–7.

Amelar RD, Dubin L, Quigley MM, Schonfield C. Successful management of infertility due to polyzoospermia. *Fertil Steril* 1979; **31**: 521–4.

Amelar RD, Hotchkiss RS. Congenital aplasia of the epididymes and vasa deferentia: effects on semen. *Fertil Steril* 1963; **14**: 44–8.

Averback P, Wight DG. Seminiferous tubule hypercurvature: a newly recognised common syndrome of human male infertility. *Lancet* 1979; **i**: 181–3.

Baker HWG. Failed vasectomy reversal: an epidemic of preventable infertility. In: *Fertility Society of Australia*. Lorne, Victoria, Australia: 1991: 18.

Baker HWG, Burger HG, De Kretser DM, Hudson B, Rennie GC, Straffon WGE. Testicular vein ligation and fertility in men with varicoceles. *Br Med J* 1985; **291**: 1678–80.

Burger HG. Inhibin: clinical physiology and cancer diagnosis. *Reprod Fertil Dev* 1991; **3**: 227–31.

Crich JP, Jequier AM. Infertility in men with retrograde ejaculation: the action of urine on sperm motility and a simple method for achieving antegrade ejaculation. *Fertil Steril* 1978; **30**: 572–6.

Cummins JM, Pember SA, Jequier AM, Yovich JL, Hartmann PE. A test of the human sperm acrosome reaction following ionophore challenge (ARIC): relationship to fertility and other seminal parameters. *J Androl* 1991; **12**: 98–103.

Eliasson R. Studies on prostaglandin. Occurrence, formation and biological action. *Acta Physiol Scand* 1959; **46**: 1–73.

Eliasson R, Lindholmer C. Functions of the male accessory genital organs. In: Hafez ESE, eds. *Human Semen and Fertility Regulation in Men*. St Louis: Mosby, 1976: 44–50.

Eliasson R, Mossberg B, Camner P, Afzelius BA. The Immotile Cilia Syndrome. A congenital ciliary abnormality as an aetiologic factor in chronic airway disease and male infertility. *N Engl J Med* 1977; **297**: 1–6.

Guerin J-F, Czyba J-C, Perrin P, Rollet J. Les obstructions congenitales ou aquises de l'epididyme humain: étude de la mobilite des spermatoides en amont de l'obstruction. *Bull Ass Anat* 1981; **65**: 297–306.

Hansson V, Trygstad O, French FS *et al*. Androgen transport and receptor mechanisms in testis and epididymis. *Nature* 1974; **250**: 387–91.

Hargreave TB, Jequier AM. Can follicle stimulating hormone estimation replace testicular biopsy in the diagnosis of obstructive azoospermia? *Br J Urol* 1978; **50**: 415–18.

Heath AL. Epididymal abnormalities associated with maldescent of the testes. *J Ped Surg* 1984; **19**: 47–9.

Hendry WF, Parslow JM, Stedrowska J. Wallace DMA. Diagnosis of unilateral testicular obstruction in subfertile males. *Br J Urol* 1982; **54**: 774–9.

Hodges RD, Hawley HG. Epididymovasostomy: a microdissection of two cases. *Br J Urol* 1966; **38**: 534–41.

Holmes SD, Lipschyultz LI, Smith RG. Transferrin and gonadal dysfunction in man. *Fertil Steril* 1982; **38**: 600–4.

Holstein AF, Schirren C, Schirren CG. Human spermatids and spermatozoa lacking acrosomes. *J Reprod Fertil* 1973; **35**: 489–91.

Jequier AM. Obstructive azoospermia: a study of 102 patients. *Clin Reprod Fertil* 1986; **3**: 21–36.

Jequier AM, Crich JP, Holmes SC. Incomplete obstruction of the male genital tract: a cause of oligozoospermia. *Br J Urol* 1983; **55**: 545–6.

Lundquist F. Aspects of the biochemistry of human semen. *Acta Physiol Scand* 1949; **19**: 7–105.

Mann T, Rottenberg DA. The carbohydrate of semen. *J Endocr* 1966; **34**: 257–64.

Neaves WB, Johnson L, Porter JC, Parker CR, Pelly CS. Leydig cell numbers, daily sperm production and serum gonadotropin levels in aging men. *JCEM* 1984; **55**: 756–63.

Nieschlag E, Behre HM. Male infertility due to testicular dysfunction. In: Templeton AA, Drife JO, eds. Infertility, Springer-Verlag London 1992: 65–80.

Rogers BJ. The sperm penetration assay: its usefulness reevaluated. *Fertil Steril* 1985; **43**: 821–40.

Rogers BJ, Parker RA. Relationship between the human sperm hypo-osmotic swelling test and sperm penetration assay. *J Androl* 1991; **12**: 152–8.

Silber S. Microsurgery for vasectomy reversal in vasoepididymostomy. *Urology* 1984; **23**: 505–24.

Young D. Surgical treatment of male infertility. *J Reprod Fertil* 1970; **23**: 541–2.

10

Sperm storage

D. P. WOLF

Introduction

The storage of sperm for prolonged time periods with retention of function carries application in diverse areas, for instance, the propagation of domestic animals, the treatment of human infertility, and the preservation of endangered species. While it has been known for over 200 years that sperm from some mammalian species can survive transient exposure to temperature near freezing – first described by Spallanzani (1776) for human, stallion and frog sperm stored on snow for 30 minutes and rewarmed with motility recovery – the long term storage of sperm requires exposure to ultra-low temperatures and freezing. Typically, storage is accomplished at $-196\,^\circ\text{C}$ in liquid nitrogen; however, it is not the exposure to ultra-low temperatures *per se* that creates a survival problem but rather the events that occur while reaching the storage temperature or during rewarming, i.e. the temperature transitions required to get to and from $-196\,^\circ\text{C}$. At a very early stage in the development of the discipline of cryobiology, it was recognized that the ice crystal formation that occurs inside a cell during freezing or thawing results in cell death.

Following the early observations by Spallanzani, Mantegazza (1866) published some rather impressive insights concerning the benefits of sperm freezing in support of therapeutic insemination (TI) in domestic animals and in women. However, despite the awareness created by these observations, it has been only within the last 50 years or so that the importance of cryoprotectants was recognized. In fact, semen cryopresentation, high motility survival post-thaw, became a reality only after the serendipitous discovery of the cryoprotective properties of glycerol by Polge and coworkers in 1949. This discovery, made originally on fowl sperm, opened the floodgates and was followed by intensive activity in the cryopreservation of semen from domestic animal species and man.

The freezing protocols that have resulted and are currently available are often species specific based in large measure on experimental findings in the bull and to a lesser extent in man, undoubtedly reflecting the fact that sperm from these species are relatively resistant to the insults associated with cryopreservation.

Successful application of semen cryopreservation in the human was provided in 1953 when pregnancies were reported in patients, inseminated with sperm previously frozen and stored in dry ice ($-78\,^{\circ}C$) (Bunge & Sherman, 1953). A decade later, the liquid nitrogen vapour technique for the freezing of human semen with subsequent storage at $-196\,^{\circ}C$ was introduced and it is this technique with only minor variation that is in widespread use today (Sherman, 1963). The interested reader is referred to a number of recent review articles on the history and practice of human semen cryobanking (Sherman, 1986, 1990).

The recognized risk of infectious disease transmission associated with therapeutic insemination by donor has, over the last decade, led to the mandate that quarantined semen be employed for this purpose, i.e. that semen collected from a screened donor be stored for 6 months after which time the donor is rescreened before the sample is released for use. This approach is designed to prevent the use of samples from infected donors that tested seronegative initially but converted at a later time. Because of the need to quarantine and an increased incidence of infertility among American couples, there has been a dramatic increase in the cryopreservation of human semen with current estimates of children produced via TI by donor in the tens of thousands. In this review, I will focus on the application of cryopreservation in the human by providing an overview of the princlples of cryobiology, the protocols currently in use, prefreeze and post-thaw and semen/sperm assessments and clinical results following therapeutic insemination. Occasionally I will contrast the relatively high degree of success enjoyed in the human with the marked lack of success obtained to date in non-human primates.

Cryobiological principles

A cell's ability to survive freezing is related to its size and shape, hydration state and membrane permeability properties. Thus, a cell's response can often be predicted given information on its permeability coefficient, surface area, the osmotic gradient between outside and inside and the temperature (Mazur, 1984). Ongoing efforts to better understand membrane structural and functional relationships may ultimately provide additional insights into the events associated with cell freezing (Hammerstedt, Graham & Nolan, 1990). Additional factors as they relate specifically to sperm cryosurvival are considered below.

Temperature shock, seeding, cooling and warming rates

Temperature shock or damage induced in sperm during cooling to the freezing point, of minimal concern in man (Sherman, 1955), can be limiting in the low temperature storage of domestic animal sperm (Watson, 1990). Such damage may reflect transition changes in membrane lipids that are critical to cell survival.

Seeding or the induction of extracellular ice crystal formation in supercooled mixtures can be critical to the survival of large, hydrated cells such as eggs or embryos. The osmotic gradient created between the inside and outside of the cell allows the relatively slow cellular dehydration essential to freezing without significant intracellular ice crystal formation. Seeding is not commonly incorporated into sperm freezing protocols. In a recent report by Critser and coworkers (1987), seeding resulted in only modest enhancements in sperm cryosurvival.

The use of optimum cooling rates is also critical to cryosurvival for many cell types as it influences the extent and rate of dehydration; however, human sperm are tolerant of a wide range of cooling rates from 0.5 to 50 °C/minute. This tolerance means that relatively poorly controlled, fast cooling rates are effective as are the slower rates used with protocols designed for controlled rate freezing machines. The literature is indecisive on the best combinations of freezing and thawing rates for human semen (Taylor *et al.*, 1982). Normally samples are thawed at ambient temperature or in a 37 °C water bath.

Storage temperature

Semen storage at −80 to −85 °C, in a mechanical freezer, may be as efficacious as storage in liquid nitrogen at −196 °C based on motility recovery (Mahadevan & Trouson, 1984). Despite this finding, long-term semen storage usually is conducted at −196 °C in liquid nitrogen.

Duration of storage

Metabolic processes in cells stored in liquid nitrogen are slow to non-existent and the major risk of storage damage is restricted to the accumulated exposure to cosmic radiation. However, hundreds of years may be required before radiation damage becomes significant (Mazur, 1984). Nevertheless, the evidence and/or bias persists that a decline in sperm survival occurs over time of storage. If such a decline occurs, it may reflect improper storage, for instance, transient but repeated exposure to ambient temperature during sample accesssing. The judicious recommendation would, therefore, be that storage time is limited, perhaps to 10 years.

Semen collection, processing and quality

Semen collection is not a major variable in humans where masturbation following a timed interval of sexual abstinence is the normal routine. In non-human primates, semen collection is not a trivial issue. Rectal or penile probe electroejaculation is used in macaques and the inability to control abstinence time, the small semen volume, and the potential for nonsperm cell contamination markedly influences sample quality. On the other hand, one of the striking advantages seen in the macaque over the human is the highly uniform morphology and motility of seminal sperm (Lanzendorf *et al.*, 1990).

Human semen should be allowed to liquefy for 30–60 minutes prior to cryoprotectant addition. This approach contrasts with some domestic animals which benefit from a delay of several hours before cryoprotectant addition and freezing (Watson, 1990). The mechanism of action of cryoprotectants, which includes a lowering of the freezing point of the solution and cellular dehydration, is incompletely understood. Hammerstedt and coworkers (1990) discuss the concept that cryoprotectants also exert effects on membrane structure and function. Glycerol is more effective in buffering the effects of low temperature on human sperm than is dimethylsulfoxide or propanediol, yet the latter cryoprotectants also dehydrate and lower the solution freezing point. Parenthetically these latter two cryoprotectants are preferred in the cryopreservation of human one- to eight-cell stage embryos.

In general, seminal sperm are incapable of fertilization; these cells must first undergo a final maturation step called capacitation which occurs during sperm transit in the female reproductive tract or following sperm processing *in vitro*, i.e. after seminal plasma removal. Thus, the motile, seminal sperm population available for cryopreservation is in a noncapacitated state. Protocols for the cryopreservation of washed sperm are also available (Katz, 1980), although unproven in the context of a TI by donor programme.

With human sperm, initial semen quality is probably the most significant single factor in determining cryosurvival. There are two components to this issue, one is the motile sperm population *per se* and the other is the seminal plasma. The latter is recognized to be complex and variable between ejaculates and donors and is usually not well characterized prior to cryopreservation. After all, the parameters used by the World Health Organization to define human semen, apart from sperm motility, morphology and concentration, include only semen volume and viscosity. As an interesting example of how semen parameters can influence sperm quality, goat semen contains a phospholipase A activity which hydrolyses lecithin to produce fatty acids and lysolecithin, the latter of which is highly toxic to sperm. This means that the relative concentration of this enzyme may largely account for the differences seen in the fertility of cryopreserved goat semen (Watson, 1990).

In considering sperm cryosurvival, it seems obvious that highly viable cell populations are more capable of surviving the insults of cryopreservation than are their less viable counterparts. This is consistent with the generally accepted notion that the abnormal semen from infertility patients will cryopreserve poorly. It must be stressed, however, that cryosurvival varies even among pregnancy-proven donors and cannot be predicted solely on the basis of semen parameters (Beck & Silverstein, 1975). In our sperm bank at the Oregon Health Sciences University (OHSU), 10% of the potential sperm donors who present with acceptable semen quality fail our requirement of 50% post-thaw survival of the initial motile population. At present, relatively little is known about the molecular or cellular level events that dictate sperm cryosurvival.

Freezing primate sperm

Descriptions of human semen freezing protocols currently in use which involve exposure to liquid nitrogen vapours can be found in Sherman (1990) and for the protocol used at OHSU (Wolf, in press[*b*]). The steps in the protocol employed at OHSU are outlined in Fig. 1. While glycerol is the universal cryoprotectant for human sperm cryopreservation, glycerol toxicity at high concentrations can occur (Critser *et al.*, 1988). Such toxicity is of minimal concern when extenders are used, i.e. glycerol is first diluted in the extender, but special attention should be devoted to mixing with any direct glycerol addition approach. The final glycerol concentration may also contribute to cryosurvival although concentrations in the 5–10% range appear equivalent (Hammitt, Walker & Williamson, 1988). In addition to acting as dilutents, extenders, which are now conveniently available commercially, may contribute a minor cryoprotective effect. Semen is usually diluted with cryoprotectants while at room temperature and the mixture is transferred to storage containers, either straws or vials. Several different culture media have been used in human semen cryopreservation (Prins & Weidel, 1986) suggesting that medium requirements are probably of limited concern given adequate pH stability, ionic composition and energy sources. The protein additive used may be of comparable importance.

The low temperature storage of nonhuman primate semen has proven much more difficult than human semen storage even when comparable cryopreservation procedures are utilized. Live births have been reported following TI or intrauterine insemination (IUI) with cryopreserved semen in the gorilla, chimpanzee and cynomolgus macaque (for review, see Wolf *et al.*, 1990); however, the experience base in these cases is very limited. Success in semen cryopreservation is essential

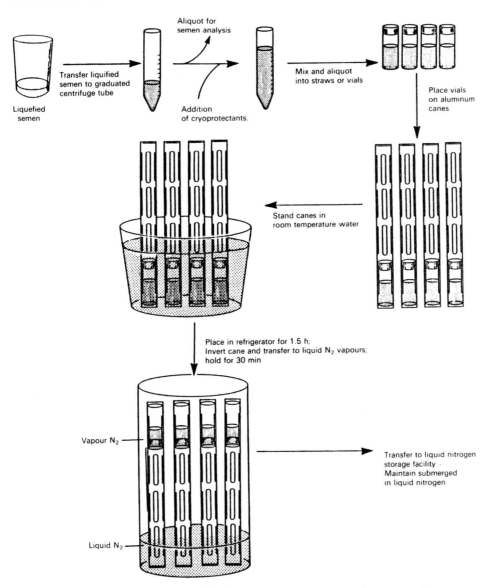

Fig. 1. Schematic outline of a human sperm cryopreservation protocol.

to the breeding management of primates and in strategies designed to preserve endangered species.

Post-thaw assessment and processing

While no entirely satisfactory laboratory method is available to measuring cryosurvival, the process is routinely assessed by post-thaw motility scores, determined in the presence of cryoprotectant. The premise, of course, is that the

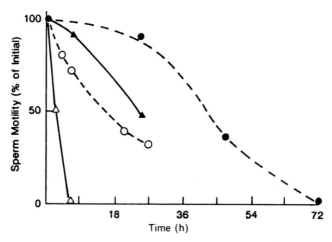

Fig. 2. Sperm survival in culture at 37 °C. Frozen (solid lines) and non-frozen (dashed lines) human (closed symbols) and rhesus monkey (open symbols) swim up sperm populations.

easily measured parameter of motility is reflective of fertility. A minimum standard of 50% survival of the initial motile sperm population is expected.

The kinetics of motility loss after thawing can also be used in cryosurvival evaluation. Such a stress test can be conducted directly on thawed semen or on sperm washed free of cryoprotectant and incubated in an appropriate medium at 37 °C for up to 24 hours. In contrast to simple exposure to cryoprotectant alone, freezing is usually associated with an immediate decline in the percentage of motile cells and time-dependent declines in curvilinear velocity and in the mean amplitude of lateral head displacement. Within 24 hours of thawing, the percentage of cryopreserved sperm that retain motility is low compared with survival in non-frozen controls (Fig. 2). These differences are even more dramatic if the quality of motility (progression) is also considered. For comparative purposes, the results of a stress test on frozen–thawed rhesus monkey sperm has also been included. The decline in motility is much more severe in monkey sperm, reflecting their inability to survive the rigours of cryopreservation. This increased lability of cryopreserved human sperm compared to their nonfrozen counterparts carries obvious implications to the timing of therapeutic insemination. Holt and coworkers (1989) used a 3.5-hour stress test on the post-thaw semen sample without sperm processing to compare two groups of TI donors, those that were pregnancy proven and those with low fecundities. The mean (SEM) velocities for the groups of 0 time were 65.9 (1.8) and 50.4 (3.2) and, after 2.5 hours, 42.1 (2.1) and 24.7 (5.7), respectively. The conclusion was reached that, despite the absence of significant differences in prefreeze semen parameters, washed sperm velocity differences post-thaw were diagnostically significant in fertility estimates.

With domestic animals, cryodamage is often monitored not only by motility measures but also by quantitative assessments of acrosomal status (Watson, 1990). Moreover, with non-human primate sperm, acrosomal damage is a major contributor to poor cryosurvival. Since acrosomal and plasma membrane damage also appears as a sequelae of human sperm cryopreservation (Mahadevan & Trounson, 1984; Cross & Hanks, 1991), this approach should be considered clinically. Indirect immunofluorescence assays for this purpose are readily available (Wolf, 1989).

The sperm penetration assay has been used by Critser and coworkers (1987) to evaluate cryosurvival; however, this assay is cumbersome and impractical as a routine test for large sample numbers.

Because of the increased lability of cryopreserved sperm, the method employed in sperm processing for TI may be critical. For an intracervical route of insemination, the sample can simply be thawed and used without processing. However, for an intrauterine insemination, the sample must first be processed to remove seminal plasma (reduce the antigenic load) and the cryoprotectant/extender and to concentrate the motile sperm population. Available techniques include centrifugation–resuspension with or without swim up, column separation and buoyant density centrifugation. The simple wash by repeated centrifugation– resuspension is employed in our protocol with the entire cellular fraction recovered in the final centrifugation used in the insemination. When a swim up procedure is imposed on this final cell pellet, the overall recovery of motile sperm is very low in the range of 5–7% (Graczkowski & Siegel, 1991), restricting this approach to samples with exceptionally high motile sperm poulations. It is, of course, recognized that improved methods to separate motile sperm from semen and cryoprotectant are needed. In an attempt to achieve this objective, a comparison of column, Percoll-separated and washed sperm has been made. Percoll-separated sperm showed decreased motility, viability and acrosomal integrity in comparison to sperm washed with or without Sephadex filtration (Drobnis, Zhong & Overstreet, 1991).

Another strategy to employ in the processing of cryopreserved sperm involves the *in vitro* stimulation of motility. Hammitt and coworkers (1989) tested caffeine, pentoxifylline, 2-deoxyadenosine, cyclic AMP, relaxin, adenosine, kallikrein and calcium and concluded that cryopreserved sperm were consistently stimulated (velocity and/or percentage motile) only by caffeine, pentoxifylline and 2-deoxyadenosine. When these chemical stimulants were examined in greater detail, pentoxifylline-treated sperm showed no reduction in fertilizing capacity in the sperm penetration assay and were concluded to be superior. It is important to note, however, that the efficacy of motility stimulants used either acutely or chronically in TI or the assisted reproductive technologies (ART) has yet to be established.

Clinical application of semen cryopreservation

Therapeutic insemination with either husband or donor sperm is a routine office procedure usually performed by an intracervical or an intrauterine route. In the former case, 1.5–2.5 ml of the thawed, semen–cryoprotectant mixture is used in our programme at OHSU (Patton *et al.*, in press). After placing a speculum into the vagina to expose the cervix, the exocervix is wiped with a cotton swab to remove vaingal secretions and excess cervical mucus. Semen is then delivered into the cervical canal with a syringe–cannula system, e.g. a 17 g Intracath-Deseret (Sandy, UT) and allowed to pool against the cervix for 20 minutes. IUI can be performed with the same syringe–cannula system also after vaginal–cervical preparation. In this case the flexible cannula is gently inserted through the internal cervical os into the upper fundal area of the uterine cavity before the suspension of washed sperm (0.25–0.4 ml) is slowly injected (30–60 seconds). The patient remains recumbent for 10–15 minutes before leaving the physician's office.

Homologous TI is of value when the principal indications are structural abnormalities of the vagina or cervix, abnormal postcoital testing and hence a suspected cervical factor, sexual dysfunction, immunologic infertility, abnormal semen parameters or idiopathic infertility. The TI in these cases would almost certainly involve non-frozen semen since infectious disease transmission is of minimal concern. Cryostorage in support of homologous TI is often considered before surgical, chemical or irradiation therapy which endangers the donor's reproductive potential, as a form of fertility insurance for the vasectomy candidate, as a back-up for couples participating in the ARTs and to support TI in the husband's absence. For heterologous TI with frozen, quarantined semen, indications would include a severe male factor or genetic problems, desired pregnancy by single women or, again, in support of the ARTs.

The monthly fecundity or probability of conception for therapeutic insemination is a function of a large number of parameters not the least of which is the quality and quantity of sperm delivered to the female reproductive tract. With low numbers, in the range of a few million motile cells, cycle fecundity will be near the spontaneous treatment-independent level. With increasing sperm numbers, cycle fecundity should increase until a plateau is attained at a threshold level of sperm. A similar argument can be made for sperm quality, although in TI by donor, quality should be relatively uniform since donors are highly selected on the basis of initial semen parameters and sperm cryosurvival results. The number of sperm required to achieve this hypothetical maximal or plateau level of fecundity is unknown for fresh, non-frozen as well as for cryopreserved specimens. Evidence is available, however, suggesting that a direct relationship exists between inseminating sperm numbers and cycle fecundity (Brown, Boone & Shapiro, 1988).

Parenthetically, in domestic species such as the bull, a threshold level of approximately 100 million progressively motile frozen–thawed sperm produced the highest nonreturn rates, i.e. fecundities (Watson, 1990).

In general, cycle fecundities in women, as established in the 1970s and 1980s with fresh (non-frozen) donor semen using an intracervical route of insemination, were in the range of 15–20%. Over and above sperm quantity and quality, factors that contribute to cycle fecundity determinations are multiple including, but not limited to, the ovulation detection method in use, whether single versus multiple inseminations are conducted, the type and severity of the infertility and the patient's age. With the transition to the exclusive use of quarantined, cryopreserved semen, cycle fecunidty levels, in general, have declined although several reports are available citing results within the fresh semen range quoted above when multiple intracervical inseminations are performed (Holt *et al.*, 1989; Centola, Mattox & Raubertas, 1990). In the limited number of studies which have compared intracervical insemination with IUI, the latter is clearly superior in a single timed insemination with donor semen or the washed sperm from semen (Byrd *et al.*, 1990; Patton *et al.*, in press). Of note also is the increasing use of controlled ovarian hyperstimulation in conjunction with TI.

Guidelines for the use of semen in TI by donor have been established by the Center for Disease Control, the American Fertility Society and the American Association of Tissue Banks. A detailed description of the management of a donor insemination programme can be found in Hummel & Talbert (1989) with specific reference to the programme at OHSU (Wolf, in press[*a*]). Of course, the major impetus behind the relatively recent but widespread cryopreservation of human semen is the risk of infectious disease transmission. The human immunodeficiency (HIV) and hepatitis C viruses can, along with a number of other infectious agents, be transmitted heterosexually. In 1988, and again in 1990, the American Fertility Society published revised guidelines which mandated the exclusive use of frozen semen that had been quarantined for 180 days. Thus, semen collected from a donor who was seronegative initially could not be released for TI until the sample had been held for at least 180 days and the donor had been retested and found to be seronegative for HIV. This recommendation revolutionized the TI process and, in the time frame of 1988–1990, many TI programmes could not be sustained for lack of quarantined sperm. A careful history of other sexually transmitted diseases must also be obtained; in fact, current testing should be considered minimal with the caveat that additional screens for infectious diseases will be added as they become available and/or necessary. Hummel & Talbert (1989) provide additional details to consider in the microbiological, medical and genetic screening of prospective sperm donors.

Quarantined donor semen is available from a number of sperm banks, a listing of which is maintained by the Americal Fertility Society in Birmingham, Alabama. The American Association of Tissue Banks also maintains a list of member banks. Sperm from donors representing widely diverse backgrounds or characteristics can be accessed through the collective sperm banking activity in the United States. Samples may be shipped in liquid nitrogen transport tanks by overnight or two-day delivery using one of several available express carriers. Dry ice transport is not considered as reliable and, therefore, is not recommended. Advance notice to sperm banks is judicious when timed inseminations are conducted and local liquid nitrogen storage is unavailable.

Quality control/assurance

Quality control and quality assurance programmes are essential to the delivery of high quality medical care and general laboratory guidelines or standards are available that apply to the andrology/sperm banking laboratory, e.g. Joint Commission on Accreditation of Hospitals or the College of American Pathologists in USA and Human Fertilisation and Embryology Authority in UK. A joint committee from the American Fertility Society and the College of American Pathologists has been formed to prepare for the accreditation of both human embryology and andrology laboratories including sperm storage facilities. This committee will address the unique activities of these speciality laboratories. Most notable of the quality assurance features in human sperm storage is the need to quarantine semen and to conduct trial thaws on banked specimens for use in a TI by donor program. In the latter case, an aliquot from each semen sample (ejaculate) stored in the sperm bank must be set aside, subjected to the same cryopreservation protocol as the banked specimen, and, prior to release of any sample for insemination, thawed for a quality check. Only samples with trial thaws meeting acceptable, pre-established post-thaw thresholds can be released for use. Both prefreeze and post-thaw semen parameters should be included along with identifying information for all specimens leaving the laboratory for therapeutic use.

Troubleshooting semen cryopreservation

Sperm storage by freezing requires a high degree of precision and problems capable of influencing outcome can arise during any phase of the procedure. The importance of storage containers, cryoprotectants, freezing machines, if used, cooling or warming rates and cryoprotectant removal has been discussed adequately by Kuzan & Quinn (1988) as they relate to embryo freezing. Moreover, some of the controversies in human sperm storage have been described recently by Sherman (1990). Other potential problems that may arise in sperm cryopreservation include low post-thaw motilities or fecundities in TI secondary to microbial contamination of the initial sample, transient but repeated sample exposure to room temperature during storage, or improper sample handling after thawing and processing before TI.

Acknowledgements

The author acknowledges the secretarial and editorial skills of Patsy Kimzey. This work was supported in part by National Institutes of Health grant RR00163. Publication No. 0000 of the Oregon Regional Primate Research Center.

References

American Fertility Society. Revised new guidelines for the use of semen–donor insemination. *Fertil Steril* 1988; **49**: 211.

American Fertility Society. New guidelines for the use of semen donor insemination: 1990. *Fertil Steril* 1990; **53** (suppl 1).

Beck WW Jr, Silverstein I. Variable motility recovery of spermatozoa following freeze preservation. *Fertil Steril* 1975; **26**: 863–7.

Brown CA, Boone WR, Shapiro SS. Improved cryopreserved semen fecundability in an alternating fresh–frozen artificial insemination program. *Fertil Steril* 1988; **50**: 825–7.

Bunge RG, Sherman JK. Fertilizing capacity of frozen human spermatozoa. *Nature* 1953; **172**: 767–8.

Byrd W, Braddhaw K, Carr B, Edman C, Odom J, Ackerman G. A prospective randomized study of pregnancy rates following intrauterine and intracervical insemination using frozen donor sperm. *Fertil Steril* 1990; **53**: 521–7.

Centola GM, Mattox JH, Raubertas RF. Pregnancy rates after double versus single insemination with frozen donor semen. *Fertil Steril* 1990; **54**: 1089–92.

Critser JK, Huse-Benda AR, Aaker DV, Arneson BW, Ball GD. Cryopreservation of human spermatozoa. I. Effects of holding procedure and seeding on motility, fertilizability, and acrosome reaction. *Fertil Steril* 1987; **47**: 656–63.

Critser JK, Huse-Benda AR, Aakar DV, Arneson BW, Ball GD. Cryopreservation of human spermatozoa. II. The effect of cryoprotectants on motility. *Fertil Steril* 1988; **50**: 314–20.

Cross NL, Hanks SE. Effects of cryopreservation on human sperm acrosomes. *Hum Reprod* 1991; **6**: 1279–83.

Drobnis EZ, Zhong CQ, Overstreet JW. Separation of cryopreserved human semen using Sephadex columns, washing, or Percoll gradients. *J Androl* 1991; **12**: 201–8.

Graczykowski JW, Siegel MS. Motile sperm recovery from fresh and frozen-thawed ejaculates using a swim-up procedure. *Fertil Steril* 1991; **55**: 841–3.

Hammerstedt RH, Graham JK, Nolan JP. Cryopreservation of mammalian sperm: what we ask them to survive. *J Androl* 1990; **11**: 73–88.

Hammitt DG, Walker DL, Williamson RA. Concentration of glycerol required for optimal survival and *in vitro* fertilizing capacity of frozen sperm is dependent on cryopreservation medium. *Fertil Steril* 1988; **49**: 680–7.

Hammitt DG, Bedia E, Rogers PR, Syrop CH, Donovan JF, Williamson RA. Comparison of motility stimulants for cryopreserved human semen. *Fertil Steril* 1989; **52**: 495–502.

Holt WV, Shenfield F, Leonard T, Hartman TD, North RD, Moore HDM. The value of sperm swimming speed measurements in assessing the fertility of human frozen semen. *Hum Reprod* 1989; **4**: 292–7.

Hummel WP, Talbert LM. Current management of a donor insemination program. *Fertil Steril* 1989; **51**: 919–30.

Katz DF. Freeze preservation of isolated populations of highly motile human spermatozoa. In: David G, ed. *Human Artificial Insemination and Semen Preservation*. New York: Plenum Press, 1980: 557–63.

Kuzan FB, Quinn P. Cryopreservation of mammalian embryos. In: Wolf DP, ed. *In vitro Fertilization and Embryo Transfer: A Manual of Basic Techniques*. New York: Plenum Press, 1988: 301–47.

Lanzendorf SE, Gliessman PM, Archibong AE, Alexander M, Wolf DP. Collection and quality of rhesus monkey semen. *Mol Reprod Dev* 1990; **25**: 61–6.

Mahadevan M, Trounson AO. Effect of cooling, freezing and thawing rates and storage conditions on preservation of human spermatozoa. *Andrologia* 1984; **16**: 52–60.

Mantegazza P. Sullo sperma umano. *Rendic reale Instit Lomb* 1866; **3**: 183.

Mazur P. Freezing of living cells: mechanisms and implications. *Am J Physiol* 1984; **247**: C125–42.

Patton PE, Burry KA, Thurmond A, Novy MJ, Wolf DP. Intrauterine insemination outperforms intracervical insemination in a randomized, controiled study with frozen, donor semen. *Fertil Steril* (in press).

Polge C, Smith AU, Parkes AS. Revival of spermatozoa after vitrification and dehydration at low temperatures. *Nature* 1949; **164**: 666.

Prins GS, Weidel L. A comparative study of buffer systems as cryoprotectants for human spermatozoa. *Fertil Steril* 1986; **46**: 147–9.

Sherman JK. Temperature shock in human spermatozoa. *Proc Soc Exp Biol Med* 1955; **88**: 6–7.

Sherman JK. Improved method of preservation of human spermatozoa by freezing and freeze-drying. *Fertil Steril* 1963; **14**: 49–64.

Sherman JK. Current status of clinical cryobanking of human semen. In: Paulson JD, Negro-Vilar A, Lucena E, Martini L, eds. *Andrology: Male Fertility and Sterility*. Orlando: Academic Press, 1986: 517–47.

Sherman JK. Cyropreservation of human semen. In: Keel BA, Webster BW, eds. *CRC Handbook of the Laboratory Diagnosis and Treatment of Infertility*. Boca Raton: CRC Press, 1990: 229–59.

Spallanzani L. Opuscoli di Fisica Animale, e Vegetabile, 2 vols, Opuscolo II: Osservazioni, e Sperienze intorno ai Vermicelli Spermatici dell' Uomo e degli Animali. Modena, 1776, Presso la Societa' Tipographica.

Taylor PJ, Wilson J, Laycock R, Weger J. A comparison of freezing and thawing methods for the cryopreservation of human semen. *Fertil Steril* 1982; **37**: 100–3.

Watson PF. Artificial insemination and the preservation of semen. In: Lamming GE, ed. *Marshall's Physiology of Reproduction; vol 2; Reproduction in the Male*. 4th edn. New York: Churchill Livingstone, 1990: 747–869.

Wolf DP. Acrosomal status quantitation in human sperm. *Am J Reprod Immunol* 1989; **20**: 106–13.

Wolf DP, Thomson JA, Zelinski-Wooten MB, Stouffer RL. *In vitro* fertilization-embryo transfer in nonhuman primates: the technique and its applications. *Mol Reprod Dev* 1990; **27**: 261–80.

Wolf DP. Cryopreservation of sperm. In: Wallach EE, Zacur HA, eds. *Reproductive Medicine and Surgery*. St. Louis: C.V. Mosby Company (in press[a]).

Wolf DP. Sperm cyropreservation. In: Keye WR, Chang RJ, Rebar RW, Soules MR, eds. *Infertility: Evaluation and Treatment*. Philadelphia: W.B. Saunders Company (in press[b]).

11

Cell biology of human spermatozoa

J. AITKEN

Introduction

The male factor is generally recognized as the single most significant cause of human infertility (Hull *et al.*, 1985), particularly amongst that cohort of patients for whom the current methods of infertility diagnosis and treatment are inadequate. Moreover, this high incidence of male infertility should be viewed in the context of a rising tide of male reproductive pathology which over the past four or five decades has seen progressive increases in the rates of testicular cancer and cryptorchidism in addition to the well-publicized decline in sperm counts (Østerlind, 1986; Carlsen *et al.*, 1992). In order to comprehend and address these changes in male reproductive function, there is a clear need to acquire a deeper understanding of the cellular mechanisms involved in the genesis, differentiation and function of human spermatozoa. This information will then provide a platform from which to develop an understanding of the mechanisms underlying specific pathologies of the male reproductive tract and thence engineer appropriate methods of treatment.

The responsibility for advancing our understanding of male reproductive physiology has fallen to the emerging clinical and scientific discipline of andrology, which has developed rapidly over the past 4–5 years. At a diagnostic level we have seen a change of emphasis from the descriptive criteria that underlies the traditional semen profile to the development of bioassays that ask questions about the functional competence of human spermatozoa rather than their appearance (Aitken, 1986, 1990; Aitken & Brindle, 1993; Aitken, Buckingham & Huang, 1993; Oehninger, 1992). With the aid of such bioassays we have begun to see the classification of male patients according to the functional defects in their spermatozoa and, from there, the first attempts to understand the loss of sperm function at the molecular level (Aitken & Clarkson, 1987; Alvarez *et al.*, 1987). In the light of such information, rational progress towards the treatment of the infertile male is becoming a feasible proposition. In the meantime, the major therapeutic thrust has been to make the optimal use of the spermatozoa that such patients produce, rather than try to improve the quality of spermatogenesis. This has largely been achieved through the refinement of *in vitro* fertilization (IVF) techniques to meet the special demands imposed by the spermatozoa of male factor patients, through the development of new range of micromanipulation techniques involving the sub-zonal insemination of the spermatozoa (Sakkas *et al.*, 1992) or the direct insertion of a single spermatozoon into the ooplasm (Palermo *et al.*, 1993) of the egg. The purpose of this review is to examine these developments and summarize the current state-of-the-art with respect to our knowledge of the cell biology of human spermatozoa, with emphasis on those aspects of this topic that might influence the diagnosis or treatment of the infertile male.

Sperm movement

An obvious and important feature of the human spermatozoon is the capacity of this cell for movement and, moreover, a capacity to exhibit specific patterns of movement that are exquisitely adapted to the particular needs of this cell at different stages of its life history. The advent of objective, computerized systems for monitoring the movement characteristics of human spermatozoa has greatly facilitated our capacity to analyse the complex relationships between the movement characteristics of human spermatozoa and their functional competence. For example, independent analyses of the ability of human spermatozoa to penetrate cervical mucus have repeatedly shown that the outcome of such tests is heavily dependent upon the concentration and morphology of the spermatozoa as well as their capacity for movement (Aitken *et al.*, 1985, 1992; Mortimer, Pandya & Sawers, 1986; Mortimer *et al.*, 1990). All of the various measures of sperm head velocity (curvilinear velocity, path velocity and progressive velocity) are positively correlated with cervical mucus penetration; however, it is the path velocity which is repeatedly selected as the most informative variable in stepwise multiple regression analyses (Fig. 1). A significant lateral displacement of the sperm head is also characteristic of spermatozoa with a capacity to penetrate cervical mucus. This is such a functionally important aspect of sperm movement that cases of infertility have been identified in which the only defect in the semen profile is a reduced amplitude of lateral sperm head displacement. In such patients, cervical mucus penetration cannot occur (Aitken *et al.*, 1985; Aitken, Warner & Reid, 1986; Feneux, Serres & Jouannet, 1985; Mortimer *et al.*, 1986) presumably because the insignificant amplitude of lateral sperm head displacement is reflective of a low amplitude flagellar wave (David, Serres & Jouannet, 1981) and it is the

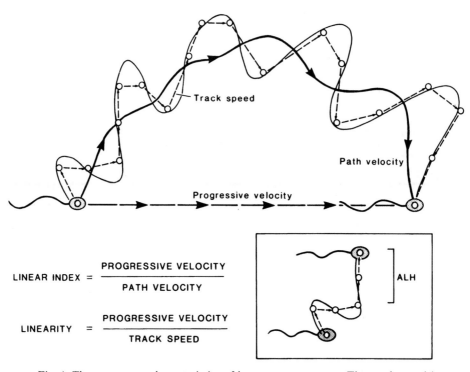

Fig. 1. The movement characteristics of human spermatozoa. The track speed is also known as the curvilinear velocity (VCL) and represents the total distance travelled by the sperm head in unit time; path velocity is also known as average path velocity (VAP) and represents the average path followed by the sperm head in unit time and is generally plotted as the 5 point running average; progressive velocity is also known as straight line velocity (VSL) and represents the straight line distance between the beginning and the end of the tract divided by the time elapsed; ALH represents the amplitude of lateral sperm head displacement and corresponds to the mean width of the lateral sperm head oscillation. Two measures of the linearity of sperm movement are: straightness (STR) calculated as STR = VSL/VAP and linearity (LIN) calculated as LIN = VSL/VCL.

latter that determines the propulsive force that can be generated by the spermatozoa at the cervical mucus interface.

The penetration of cervical mucus is not the only attribute of human sperm function dependent on movement. Another major physical barrier which spermatozoa must overcome in the process of fertilizing the egg is the zona pellucida, a translucent acellular structure that surrounds the oocyte. Zona penetration presents a different kind of physical challenge to the spermatozoa, necessitating the evolution of a second form of movement known as hyperactivation. As spermatozoa capacitate in the female reproductive tract, their changing physiological status results in a change in the flagellar beat characteristics such that the latter increases in amplitude and becomes progressively more asymmetrical.

The increase in beat amplitude seems to occur first, resulting in high amplitude sperm trajectories that are still progressive and characteristic of spermatozoa that have entered the transitional phase of hyperactivation (Burkman, 1990, 1991; Mortimer & Mortimer, 1990). Further capacitation of the cells results in an increasing asymmetry of the flagellar wave, so that the swimming trajectories become less progressive and may adopt a number of different configurations, variously described as helical, starspin or thrashing. Such highly motile non-progressive cells are fully hyperactivated and are generally regarded as having reached a terminal stage of capacitation (Fig. 2).

The high amplitude asymmetrical flagellar wave pattern that characterizes hyperactivated spermatozoa is thought to be a specific adaptation to penetration of the zona pellucida (Katz & Yanagimachi, 1980; Shalgi & Phillips, 1988) which is expressed by spermatozoa *in vivo* near the time of fertilization (Cooper, Overstreet & Katz, 1979; Cummins & Yanagimachi, 1982; Saurez, Katz & Overstreet, 1983; Suarez, 1987; Saurez & Osman, 1987). In contrast to laboratory species such as the hamster where the onset of hyperactivated motility is a synchronized activity expressed by 70% of the sperm population after 3 hours' culture *in vitro* (White & Aitken, 1989), this figure may range from 3 to 50% for suspensions of human spermatozoa (Burkman, 1990). In addition to the variable incidence of hyperactivation, recognition of this motility pattern in human spermatozoa is also hindered by two additional factors. First, within an individual sperm population there is considerable cell-to-cell variability in the kinetics of hyperactivation and secondly, human spermatozoa are capable of multiphasic behaviour and can spontaneously switch from one motility pattern to another (Fig. 3).

The analysis of hyperactivated motility and assessment of its functional significance has recently been facilitated by the development of computerized image analysis systems that may be programmed with threshold values for velocity, linearity and lateral sperm head displacement that are typical of hyperactivated cells. This facility therefore permits the automatic selection and quantification of hyperactivated cells within a given sperm population. However, it must be recognized that the threshold values for such automated sorting procedures are derived from the objective analysis of spermatozoa that have been subjectively classified as hyperactivated in the first instance. As a result there is considerable variation in the literature in terms of the threshold values that have been described for the classification of hyperactivated cells, because there is disagreement between individuals as to what constitutes a hyperactivated pattern of motility (Grunert, De Geyter & Nieschlag, 1990; Mortimer & Mortimer, 1990; Burkman, 1991). For some, only the completely non-progressive spermatozoon exhibiting a star-spin type motility is truly 'hyperactivated' whereas others

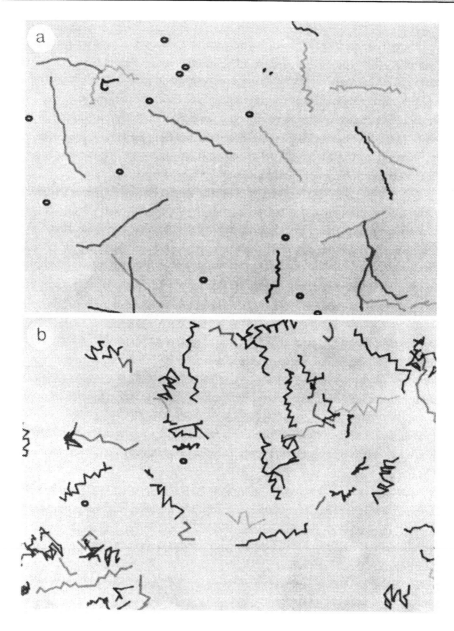

Fig. 2. Plots of sperm trajectories from spermatozoa in (a) an uncapacitated state in which the sperm tracks are linear, progressive and exhibit a moderate amplitude of lateral head displacement, and (b) a capacitated state in which the amplitude of lateral sperm head displacement has increased giving a transitional pattern of movement in cells that are still progressive and a hyperactivated pattern of movement in spermatozoa that have lost the capacity for forward movement due to the asymmetry of the flagellar beat pattern.

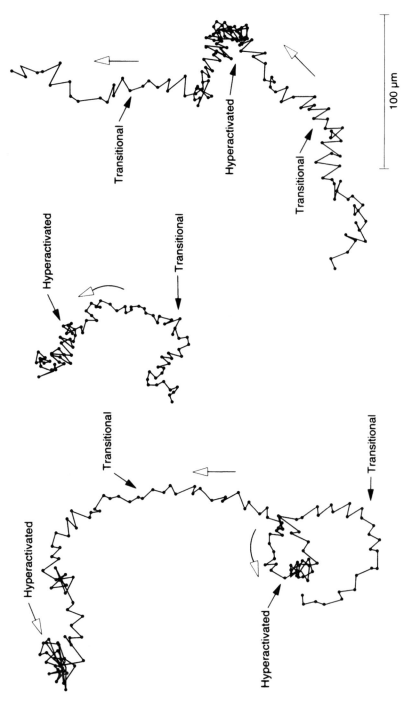

Fig. 3. Multiphasic activity by human spermatozoa during which these cells spontaneously switch from one form of movement (transitional) to another (hyperactivated).

Table 1. *Criteria for identifying hyperactivated and transitional spermatozoa in capacitating human sperm suspensions*

Classification	VCL (μm/s)	VSL (μm/s)	Straightness (%)	Linearity (%)	ALH (μm)
Hyperactivated	> 100	< 30	< 60	< 60	> 7.5
Transitional	> 100	> 30	> 60	> 60	< 7.5, > 5.0

Based on the work of Burkman (1991) and Mortimer & Mortimer (1990).

include transitional spermatozoa in this category. Clearly, the 'sort' criteria that are identified as a result of these various classification strategies will be quite different. A concensus is urgently needed in this field and it seems rational to this author to differentiate between these two types of movement, using criteria such as those indicated in Table 1.

The diagnostic value of estimating the hyperactivated status of human spermatozoa is based upon data suggesting that this pattern of motility reflects the capacitation status of the spermatozoa and thence their potential for fertilization. Thus, experiments have been conducted in which a combination of high osmolality, elevated pH and fetal cord serum was used to create conditions under which the level of sperm hyperactivation was elevated ($52.6 \pm 6.8\%$) relative to control cells maintained in medium BWW ($16.3 \pm 2.4\%$). This increase in hyperactivation rate was then found to be associated with a doubling in the rate of sperm–oocyte fusion from 28.9% to 69.4% (Burkman, 1990). Additional correlative evidence has also been obtained recently to suggest that hyperactivated movement is a prognostic indicator of IVF success, low levels of hyperactivation being associated with impaired fertility and poor zona binding (Mbizvo & Alexander, 1991).

Given the significance of sperm movement in defining the functional competence of these cells, it is clearly of interest to determine the biochemical basis of this activity. If we understood the molecular mechanisms responsible for controlling the flagellar wave form, then our understanding of sperm pathologies involving defects of sperm movement would be enhanced and the potential for designing rational therapeutic measures, facilitated. The beating of the sperm flagellum involves active sliding between the doublet microtubules within the axoneme, mediated by structures known as the dynein arms, which represent the sites of ATP hydrolysis (Warner, Satir & Gibbons, 1988). The congenital absence of dynein, observed in a condition known as Kartagener's syndrome, results in a triad of symptoms including chronic sinusitis, bronchiectasis, *situs inversus* and the complete absence of sperm motility. Despite this lack of sperm movement, spermatozoa from patients exhibiting Kartagener's syndrome are able to capacitate and acrosome react *in vitro* and will even fuse with the vitelline membrane of the oocyte, if micromanipulated into juxtaposition with this cell (Aitken, Ross & Lees, 1983).

The mechanisms by which the flagellar wave form is modified to generate the progressive motility associated with cervical mucus penetration or the hyper-activated movement associated with sperm capacitation has been the subject of considerable speculation. With regard to human spermatozoa, three regulatory factors have been identified to date including cAMP, calcium and intracellular pH. Support for the proposed importance of calcium has, for example, come from experiments in which progesterone-induced intracellular calcium transients have been shown to be associated with an increase in the incidence of hyperactivated motility (Mbizvo *et al.*, 1990; Mbizvo & Alexander, 1991). It has been proposed that the influx of calcium observed under such circumstances activates adenylate cyclase leading to an elevation in intracellular cAMP levels which, in turn, induces hyperactivation. Certainly, in animal models such as the mouse and hamster, there is good evidence to suggest that hyperactivation is calcium dependent (White & Aitken, 1989; Fraser & Monks, 1990) and data to indicate that calcium-regulated adenylate cyclase might be involved. Hence the capacitation of hamster spermatozoa is associated with clear temporal relationships between the progressive elevation of cytoplasmic calcium levels, the subsequent elevation of intracellular cAMP and the ultimate appearance of hyperactivated motility (White & Aitken, 1989). If calcium is omitted from the medium, the rise in intracellular calcium does not occur, cAMP levels do not become elevated and the spermatozoa fail to exhibit hyperactivated motility. Conversely, if the cAMP rise is promoted by the addition of phosphodiesterase inhibitors then the subsequent enhancement of cAMP levels is associated with an acceleration in the onset of hyperactivated motility (White & Aitken, 1989). The possibility that the hyperactivation of human spermatozoa is also associated with the elevation of cAMP levels is supported by the enhancing effect of phosphodiesterase inhibitors on the incidence of this motility pattern (Mbizvo, Johnston & Baker, 1993). However, the potential of such compounds to exert biological effects through their ability to increase intracellular pH, should cause us to exercise caution in interpreting such experiments.

In addition to calcium, intracellular pH and cAMP another potential regulator of hyperactivated motility has recently been discovered – the superoxide anion (De Lamirande & Gagnon, 1993). Using a free radical generating system comprising xanthine, xanthine oxidase and catalase, these authors have observed an enhancement of hyperactivated motility that could be reversed by the presence of superoxide dismutase. The mechanism by which the superoxide anion induces hyperactivated motility in populations of human spermatozoa is unknown. One possibility would be that superoxide, generated at intracellular sites or entering the cell through ion channels, would elevate intracellular pH as protons are consumed during the dismutation of this radical species to produce hydrogen peroxide.

Sperm–zona interaction

Hyperactivation is only one of a series of complex interactions between human spermatozoa and the zona pellucida during fertilization. Before spermatozoa can physically penetrate the zona pellucida, they must first recognize and bind to this structure. The act of sperm–zona recognition is an extremely important and specific event that initiates the cascade of intracellular changes that culminate in the fertilization of the oocyte. The specificity of this interaction is extremely important because a spermatozoon may make contact with thousands of different cells during its sojourn through the female reproductive tract, and yet must only recognize and respond to the presence of one specific cell – the egg. In order to accomplish this specificity, the spermatozoon has evolved surface receptors that will only bind to a unique protein on the surface of the zona pellucida, known as ZP3.

The nature of ZP3 receptors on the sperm surface is an extremely controversial area. Recent evidence involving the use of cross-linking agents in conjunction with mouse ZP3, have succeeded in identifying an $M_r = 56\,000$ sperm surface constituent with the properties of a primary zona-binding protein (Bleil & Wassarman, 1990; Wassarman, 1991). This protein (sp56) is located in the plasma membrane overlying the acrosomal region of acrosome-intact mouse spermatozoa but is lost following the acrosome reaction. The molecule binds tightly to ZP3 and, in keeping with data indicating that a terminal galactose residue is involved at the sperm binding site, sp56 has been found to bind to galactose affinity columns (Bleil & Wassarman, 1990).

An alternative model for sperm–zona interaction in the mouse, proposes the existence of a sperm surface β-1,4-galactosyl transferase enzyme that behaves like a lectin, binding to a specific glycoside substrate on ZP3 (Miller *et al.*, 1992). The specificity of this interaction is remarkable since the sperm galactosyl transferase binds to ZP3, but not to any of the other zona pellucida glycoproteins. The most significant difference between this protein and sp56 is that the latter is held to bind to galactose residues on ZP3 while the substrate for the galactosyl transferase is *N*-acetylglucosamine. According to a recent report (Miller *et al.*, 1992), if the Gal-transferase-binding sites on ZP3 are blocked by incubation with purified Gal-transferase and UDP-galactose, then ZP3 loses its biological activity.

Removal of the Gal-transferase binding sites with *N*-acetyl hexosaminidase also destroyed the ability of ZP3 to behave as a sperm receptor, while treatment with α-galactosidase had no effect, in contrast to the report of Bleil & Wassarman (1988). Following the acrosome reaction, spermatozoa lose their affinity for ZP3 and, in concert with this change, the Gal-transferase is thought to become relocated to a new membrane domain and lose its reactivity towards ZP3.

A third candidate for the sperm ZP3 receptor is the tyrosine kinase, p95, first identified on the surface of murine spermatozoa (Leyton & Saling, 1989*a*,*b*; Leyton *et al.*, 1992). Oligomerization of this receptor through the cross-linking activity of ZP3 leads to the phosphorylation of key tyrosine residues and initiation of a subsequent cascade of intracellular events leading to the activation of the spermatozoa and the induction of acrosomal exocytosis. Although a majority of these studies have used the mouse as an animal model, recent evidence has been obtained to suggest that human spermatozoa possess a homologous tyrosine kinase receptor, that might be involved in the mediation of sperm–zona interaction (Naz, Ahmad & Kimar, 1991).

The ZP3 molecule itself appears to be a ubiquitous constituent of the mammalian zona pellucida, with the primary amino acid sequence exhibiting around 60% homology in species as disparate as the mouse and the human (Kinloch *et al.*, 1988; Chamberlin & Dean, 1990; Wassarman, 1990). Human ZP3 comprises a 424 amino acid peptide including a 22 amino acid signal sequence which is proteolytically cleaved to yield a secreted protein of 402 amino acids, identical in length to marmoset and mouse ZP3 (Kinloch *et al.*, 1988; Ringuette *et al.*, 1988; Chamberlain & Dean, 1990; Thillai Koothan, van Duin & Aitken, 1993) and only two amino acids longer than the 400 amino acid ZP3 protein of the hamster zona pellucida. (Kinloch, Ruiz-Seiler & Wassarman, 1990; Moller *et al.* 1990). The characteristic features of the secreted protein include an abnormally high number of serine/threonine and proline residues and a highly conserved group of cysteine residues. In the human there is also good evidence to suggest that a second polymorphic locus for ZP3 exists, which has the potential to produce a truncated protein of 372 amino acids as the result of a single base insertion and a frame shift leading to the generation of a premature stop codon (van Duin *et al.*, 1992). The expression of this mutant form of ZP3 may have implications for the aetiology of human infertility involving a failure of sperm–egg interaction.

There is good evidence to suggest that such failures of sperm–zona interaction are commonplace in the population of patients whose infertility involves an inability to conceive. This evidence has come about as a result of the development of bioassays designed to measure the effectiveness of sperm binding to the zona pellucida. The development of such bioassays has been facilitated by the discovery that the ability of the human zona pellucida to bind homologous spermatozoa can be preserved indefinitely, if the ova are stored in high salt solutions containing 1.5 M magnesium chloride and 0.1% dextran (Yanagimachi *et al.*, 1979). As a consequence, unfertilized ova rejected from IVF programmes can be preserved and reused to test the functional competence of patients' spermatozoa. One of the major problems with this approach is that the sperm binding capacity of the zona pellucida shows variation from patient to patient and even between ova from the same patient. At least part of the reason for this variation in the biological properties of the zona pellucida derives from the fact that the sperm binding capacity of this structure varies with the state of oocyte maturation. Hence, significantly higher binding is observed to the zonae pellucidae surrounding metaphase II oocytes, compared with prophase I ova still containing a germinal vesicle (Oehninger *et al.*, 1991). Such data suggest that, as the human ovum approaches maturity, the zona pellucida undergoes subtle changes in its biochemical composition leading to increases in its capacity to bind, and be penetrated by, spermatozoa (Tesarik, Pilka & Traunik, 1988*a,b*; Oehninger, 1992).

In order to overcome this problem of inter-zona variability, two alternative strategies have been developed for diagnostic purposes. One employs two different fluorescent probes, rhodamine and fluorescein, to label spermatozoa from fertile donors and patients, respectively. These sperm populations are then mixed in equal proportions and used to inseminate human zonae pellucidae. By using the appropriate fluorescence filters, the ratio of donor to patient spermatozoa on the zonae pellucidae can be determined and thereby give an indication of the relative binding capacity of the patient's gametes (Liu *et al.*, 1988*a,b*). An alternative solution to this problem of inter-zona variability has been to use each zona as its own control, as in the 'hemi-zona' assay (Burkman 1990; Franken *et al.*, 1991; Coddington *et al.*, 1991; Oehninger, 1992). In this procedure each zona pellucida is cut into two equal halves using a micromanipulator; one half is then incubated with control spermatozoa from a donor of proven fertility, while the remaining half is placed with a sperm sample from a patient of unknown fertility status. The spermatozoa are prepared at a fixed concentration of 500 000/ml and incubated with the hemi-zonae for 4 hours at 37 °C. Thereafter each hemi-zona is pipetted five times in fresh medium to remove loosely adherent spermatozoa and then the number of spermatozoa tightly bound to each hemi-zona is calculated. The ratio of the number of spermatozoa bound to each hemi-zona then gives an indication of the functional competence of the patients' spermatozoa.

The kinetics of sperm binding in the hemi-zona assay have been monitored in small cohorts ($n = 7$) of fertile donors and subfertile patients and shown to be similar, reaching a peak after 4–6 hours (Coddington *et al.*, 1991). However, the absolute numbers of spermatozoa bound were shown to be significantly different between these two groups of subjects, approximately six times more donor spermatozoa binding to the hemi-zonae compared with the patients. Moreover, the number of spermatozoa bound to the zonae appeared to reflect other aspects of sperm quality including their morphology and their capacity for hyperactivated movement (Menkveld *et al.*, 1991; Oeninger, 1992).

Sperm–zona interaction is, therefore, an extremely important aspect of sperm function that should be monitored when assessing the competence of patients' spermatozoa for fertilization. Now that the gene encoding human ZP3 has been cloned and sequenced (Chamberlin & Dean, 1990; van Duin *et al.*, 1992), it can only be a matter of time before biologically active recombinant human ZP3 is available, as has already been achieved for the mouse (Kinloch *et al.*, 1991; Beebe *et al.*, 1992). With the aid of this material it will be a relatively straightforward proposition to generate simple colorimetric assays to determine whether a given sperm preparation possesses the cell surface receptors for the zona pellucida. Thus, the advent of recombinant ZP3 material will obviate the need to obtain native human zonae pellucidae for diagnostic purposes and also open up the way for a new generation of functional tests to monitor the fertilizing capacity of human spermatozoa. The emphasis on recombinant ZP3 in the future development of sperm function tests stems from the fact that the zona pellucida is not just the site at which sperm–zona recognition occurs. It is also the site at which the spermatozoa become activated and induced to undergo an important secretory event known as the acrosome reaction.

The acrosome reaction

The acrosome reaction is an exocytotic secretory event involving the fusion of the plasma and outer acrosomal membranes and the release of the acrosomal contents. This event may occur spontaneously, when spermatozoa are incubated for prolonged periods of time *in vitro*, or may be induced by reagents such as progesterone or A23187, that elevate the levels of intracellular calcium (Aitken *et al.*, 1984; Osman *et al.*, 1989; Blackmore *et al.*, 1990; Morales *et al.*, 1992). Stimulation of a calcium influx certainly apears to be the key to a wide variety of different treatments that stimulate the acrosome reaction. Low intracellular calcium levels are normally maintained in mammalian spermatozoa by virtue of a plasma membrane calcium ATPase which constantly operates to remove excess calcium from the cell. Treatments that impede the activity of this ATPase result in an accumulation of intracellular calcium and, as a consequence, the acrosome reaction is induced. One of the simplest ways to achieve this end is to reduce the temperature of the incubation medium to a value to below the phase transition temperature (about 22 °C) for the sperm plasma membrane. As the temperature declines below this level, the ATPases are inhibited owing to the increase in membrane order, and the calcium content of the spermatozoa increases (Irvine & Aitken, 1986). When the spermatozoa are subsequently returned to 37 °C, they respond to the build-up of calcium by undergoing the acrosome reaction (Sanchez et al., 1991). In a similar vein, protocols have been described for the hamster oocyte fusion assay in which the preparation of the spermatozoa has included an overnight incubation at 4 °C, in order to stimulate the acrosome reaction, and hence high levels of sperm–oocyte fusion (Johnson et al., 1984). An alternative procedure for elevating intracellular calcium is to inhibit ATPase activity by depriving the cell of ATP. Using the guinea pig as an animal model and temporary glucose deprivation as a strategy for reducing intracellular ATP levels, acrosome reactions have been successfully induced using this approach (Santos-Sacchi & Gordon, 1982).

In a diagnostic context, the usual routes employed for assessing the capacity of a patient's spermatozoa to undergo the acrosome reaction, involve the stimulation of calcium influxes with reagents such as A23187 or follicular fluid. A23187, in particular, is a chemically defined reagent which is an extremely effective inducer of the acrosome reaction in populations of human spermatozoa (Russell, Peterson & Freund, 1979; Aitken et al., 1984; Byrd & Wolf, 1986; Byrd, Tsu & Wolf, 1989; De Jonge, Mack & Zaneveld, 1989; Mortimer et al., 1989; Ford et al., 1991). However, A23187 does not simply induce an influx of calcium, it is biologically active because it induces a second change in these cells that is crucial for the acrosome reaction to occur – alkalinzation of the cytoplasm.

The concept that changes in intracellular calcium and pH play a dual role in the induction of the acrosome reaction, is supported by experiments in which elevations of intracellular pH have been shown to accompany the induction of the acrosome reaction in bovine and murine spermatozoa following stimulation with solubilized zonae pellucidae (Florman et al., 1989; Lee & Storey, 1985). Moreover, alkalinization of human sperm cytoplasm by exposing these cells to media with an elevated pH (pH 8.0 or 8.6) induces a limited increase in acrosome reaction rates, without the need for a calcium signal (RJ Aitken, unpublished observations). While the regulation of cytoplasmic pH is important for the control of human sperm function, the mechanisms by which this is achieved are unknown. Evidence has been presented for an Na^+/H^+ exchange although, if such a mechanism exists, it is significantly different from the somatic counterpart since amiloride and related inhibitors have no effect on pH_i in these cells (Babcock & Pfeiffer, 1989). The bicarbonate anion is also known to be an important requirement for agonist-induced acrosome reactions in mouse and bull spermatozoa as well as the spontaneous acrosome reactions exhibited by guinea pig spermatozoa

(Lee & Storey, 1986; Florman & First, 1988; Bhattacharyya & Yanagimachi, 1989). Whether these observations relate to the apparent importance of bicarbonate ion in the stimulation of sperm adenlate cyclase (Okamura *et al.*, 1985) or to the involvement of a HCO_3^-/Cl^- exchanger in the regulation of intracellular pH, has yet to be determined (Florman & Babcock, 1991).

From a diagnostic viewpoint, a knowledge of the biochemical mechanisms involved in the induction of the acrosome reaction has been of value in shaping the protocols used to examine the ability of human spermatozoa to undergo this change. It is apparent that both the native agonist, ZP3, and the ionophore, A23187, use the same second messengers, calcium and pH, to induce acrosomal exocytosis. Thus, until such time as recombinant ZP3 becomes commercially available, A23187 constitutes a powerful, alternative stimulus for bioassays of the acrosome reaction that is biologically relevant and generates results that correlate with the fertilizing capacity of human spermatozoa *in vivo* and *in vitro* (Russell *et al.*, 1979; Aitken *et al.*, 1984; Byrd & Wolf, 1986; Irvine & Aitken, 1987; Byrd *et al.* 1989; Mortimer *et al.*, 1989; Aitken, Irvine & Wu, 1991; Cummins *et al.*, 1991). Although complex biological mixtures such as maternal cord serum or follicular fluid (Burkman, 1990) can also stimulate human spermatozoa to acrosome react, the impossibility of standardizing such reagents is a considerable impairment to their routine use.

The laboratory protocols that have been developed to monitor the acrosome reaction, have also been shaped by the fact that the acrosomal vesicle of the human spermatozoon is so small that it cannot be resolved at the light microscope level. As a consequence, it has become necessary to develop reagents, such as fluorescein conjugated lectins or monoclonal antibodies to probe this structure, so that its status can be easily monitored (Aitken & Brindle, 1993). However, identifying appropriate labels to determine the state of the acrosome is not the only problem to be addressed in developing a diagnostic test around this secretory event. A second issue concerns the viability of the spermatozoa, since the acrosome may not only be shed as a result of a biologically meaningful acrosome reaction but also as a consequence of cell senescence. It is therefore necessary to include some means of monitoring the viability of the spermatozoa in the diagnostic system so that pathological acrosome *loss* can be differentiated from a physiological acrosome *reaction*. Discrimination between the physiological and pathological event can, for example, be accomplished with DNA sensitive fluorochromes, such as H33258, which exhibit limited membrane permeability and only stain cells that have lost their membrane integrity and hence their viability (Cross *et al.*, 1986). Alternatively, the viability of the spermatozoa can be assessed using the hypo-osmotic swelling (HOS) test, which identifies living cells with an intact, fluid, plasma membrane by virtue of the coiled configuration adopted by the

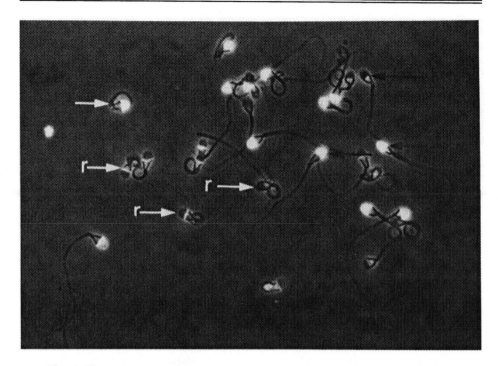

Fig. 4. Simultaneous use of the hypo-osmotic swelling test and a fluorescein conjugated lectin (*Arachis hypogaea*) to monitor the acrosome reaction in populations of human spermatozoa. Non-viable cells (black arrows) have straight tails and are excluded from the analysis. Viable cells have curled tails (white arrows) and may be classified as acrosome intact, if they possess a uniformly fluorescent acrosomal cap, or acrosome reacted, if the label has dissipated, usually being confined to the equatorial segment of the sperm head (r).

sperm tail when the spermatozoa are immersed in a hypo-osmotic medium (Jeyendran *et al.*, 1984). The simultaneous use of HOS medium and a fluorescent acrosomal probe, such as FITC-labelled peanut agglutinin, permits the simultaneous identification of acrosomal status and viability as indicated in Fig. 4.

In terms of the choice of probe to use for monitoring the acrosomal status of human spermatozoa, the monoclonal antibodies or lectins employed for this purpose may be directed against the acrosomal contents or the outer acrosomal membrane. With such reagents, the acrosome-intact cell exhibits a uniform bright fluorescence over the acrosomal region, but when the acrosome reaction occurs, the fluorescence gradually dissipates. Two of the most commonly used lectins are peanut agglutinin (*Arachis hypogaea*) which binds to carbohydrate residues on the outer acrosomal membrane (Mortimer, Curtis & Miller, 1988) and pea agglutinin (*Pisum sativum*) which binds to sites on the acrosomal matrix (Cross *et al.*, 1986). With both lectins, the acrosome reaction is associated with the appearance of a punctate pattern of labelling over the acrosome, followed by the restriction of the label to a band around the equatorial region of the sperm head. However, there is a considerable difference between these probes in the rates at which they are lost from the spermatozoa during the course of the acrosome reaction. Hence, using a dual labelling procedure during which the same spermatozoa are labelled with *Arachis hypogaea* and *Pisum sativum* lectins tagged with different fluorescent probes, the former can be shown to disperse from the spermatozoa at a much earlier stage of the acrosome reaction than the latter (Fig. 5). This must mean that, during the acrosome reaction, the outer acrosomal membrane is lost from the cells before those components of the acrosomal vesicle labelled with *Pisum sativum* lectin are dispersed. This observation has diagnostic implications since it clearly indicates that the *Arachis hyopogaea* lectin is a more sensitive probe for the acrosome reaction than that the equivalent reagent from *Pisum sativum* (Aitken & Brindle, 1993). In terms of fertilization biology, these results indicate that certain components of the acrosomal matrix must persist after the loss of the acrosomal cap in order to facilitate zona penetration. This 'secondary' phase of sperm–zona interaction is discussed below.

Secondary zona binding

Acrosomal exocytosis at the surface of the zona pellucida results in the release of the acrosomal contents and the initiation of a secondary phase of sperm–zona interaction. This event is associated with the tenacious binding of spermatozoa to the zona matrix and sperm penetration through to the perivitelline space. The mediators of this secondary phase of sperm–zona inrteraction are thought to be ZP2 on the part of the zona pellucida and an, as yet, uncharacterized component of acrosome-reacted spermatozoa. The most likely candidate for the ZP2 receptor at the present time is (pro) acrosin, an acrosomal constituent that expresses, in addition to its inherent proteolytic activity, a fucose binding domain that is capable of interaction with the zona pellucida (Töpfer-Petersen & Henschen, 1987). During the acrosome reaction, the alkalinization of the acrosomal contents leads to the autoactivation of proacrosin to generate acrosin through the modification of both the N-terminal and C-terminal ends of the protein (Fock-Nuzel *et al.*, 1984; Cechova, Töpfer-Petersen & Henschen, 1989; Baba *et al.*, 1989; Töpfer-Petersen *et al.*, 1990). The exposure of proacrosin/acrosin on the inner acrosomal membrane during the course of the acrosome reaction places this molecule in an ideal position to mediate the secondary phase of sperm–zona interaction (Töpfer-Petersen & Henshen, 1987). The nature of the binding site for proacrosin/acrosin on ZP2 is not known although the results of competition studies utilizing a variety of polysaccharides indicate that the presence of sulphate

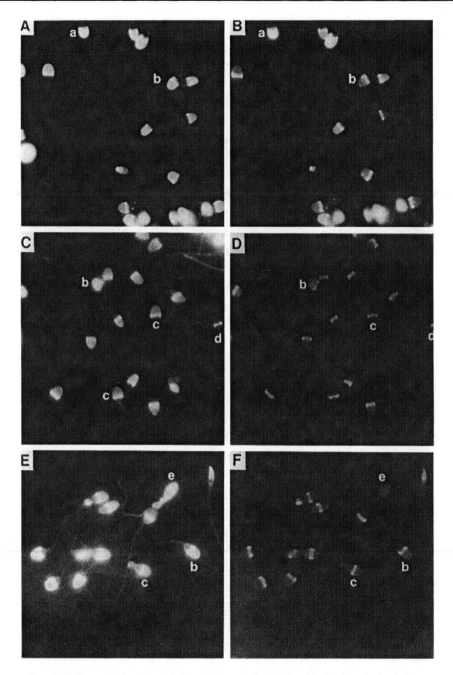

Fig. 5. Differences in the staining patterns observed with lectins derived from *Arachis hypogaea* and *Pisum sativum* using a double labelling technique. The panels designated A, C and E were stained with fluorescein-labelled *Pisum sativum* lectin while B, D and F were stained with rhodamine-labelled *Arachis hypogaea*. Within these panels it is possible to identify the following staining patterns: **a** acrosome intact spermatozoa that are uniformly labelled over the acrosomal region with

ester groups on the zona glycoproteins mediate interactions with basic residues on proacrosin/acrosin and that the density and location of sulphate groups along the polymer backbone are key determinants of biological activity (Jones, 1990). Thus, acrosin is an extremely important molecule in mediating the secondary phase of sperm–zona interaction, achieving both the binding of spermatozoa to the zona pellucida and the proteolytic cleavage of the zona matrix during sperm penetration. These processes are accomplished using a bind-and-cut mechanism that utilizes the diverse biochemical properties expressed by different regions of the same, exquisite molecule. The importance of acrosin in sperm–zona interaction has been further emphasized by the suggestion that acrosin activity is expressed on the surface of the plasma membrane during an early stage of the acrosome reaction and thereby mediates the primary, as well as the subsequent secondary, binding of spermatozoa to the zona pellucida (Tesarik, Drahorad & Peknicova, 1988*a*).

Sperm–oocyte fusion

Once the acrosome reacted human spermatozoon has penetrated through the zona matrix into the perivitelline space, it is in a position to initiate fusion with the occyte. This fusion event is possible because, concomitant with the acrosome reaction, the spermatozoon suddenly acquires a capacity to recognize and fuse with the vitelline membrane. This change is localized to a narrow band of plasma membrane around the equatorial segment of the sperm head, which initiates the fusion process. Recent studies employing the guinea pig as an animal model have shed some light on the molecular basis of this event. Employing a monoclonal antibody that blocks sperm–oocyte fusion, Blobel *et al.* (1992) have succeeded in cloning and sequencing a sperm surface component, PH-30, that appears to mediate both the recognition and fusion components of sperm–oocyte interaction.

Caption for fig. 5 (*cont.*)

> both lectins; **b** spermatozoa that still appear to be acrosome intact when stained with *Pisum sativum* lectin and yet display dissipation of the *Arachis hypogaea* labelling, indicating the initiation of the acrosome reaction; **c** spermatozoa in which the acrosomal contents appear to be dispersing, as indicated by a the reduction in *Pisum sativum* staining, while the labelling pattern observed with *Arachis hypogaea* is confined to the equatorial segment. In such cells the acrosomal membranes have been lost although elements from the acrosomal contents are still present. **d** Spermatozoa in which the labelling of the spermatozoa is confined to the equatorial segment with both lectins and in which both the acrosomal contents and membranes have dispersed and **e** morphologically abnormal spermatozoa characterized by an intense staining with *Pisum sativum* but lacking the target sites for *Arachis hypogaea* (× 400).

The molecule consists of a heterodimeric complex, comprising α- and β-subunits, both of which are type-1 integral membrane glycoproteins. The α-subunit comprises an open reading frame of 289 amino acids, with a single transmembrane domain and a relative molecular mass of 60 000 on reducing SDS gels. A putative viral fusion peptide has been identified in this subunit, which appears to exhibit some similarities to the viral fusion peptide on the rubella virus. An important feature of the α-subunit is its hydrophobicity which, in conjunction with the transmembrane anchoring segment on the same subunit, permits this molecule to act as a bridge between the sperm and oocyte plasma membranes. The α-subunit viral fusion motif is also characterized by the presence of a 'sided' α-helical structure in which most of the hydrophobic residues are to be found on one surface. It is easy to visualize how such a hydrophobic structure could readily assimilate into the oolemma and promote membrane fusion.

The β-subunit of the PH-30 complex is charged with the responsibility for recognizing the surface of the oolemma and thereby bringing the plasma membranes of the spermatozoon and oocyte into close apposition. The β-subunit contains a 353-amino acid peptide core, a single membrane spanning domain and an integrin-binding 'disintegrin' domain. The latter is thought to bind to integrin-like receptors on the surface of the oocyte and thereby effect sperm–oocyte recognition and adhesion (Bronson & Fusi, 1990*a,b*). An important feature of the PH-30 complex is that it is generated as a large precursor protein that becomes modified by proteolytic cleavage during the testicular differentiation and epididymal maturation of the spermatozoa (Blobel *et al.*, 1992). Since these cells only gain the capacity to recognize and fuse with the vitelline membrane of the oocyte following the acrosome reaction, it is tempting to speculate that the final processing of PH-30 is achieved through the action of proteases that are released from the acrosomal vesicle during the acrosome reaction.

Evaluation of the capacity of human spermatozoa to acrosome react and fuse with the vitelline membrane of the oocyte is achieved using the zona-free hamster oocyte penetration assay. In 1976, Yanagimachi, Yanagimachi & Rogers (1976) discovered that the oocyte of the golden hamster, once stripped of its zona pellucida, can fuse with spermatozoa from a wide variety of different mammalian species, providing they have previously undergone the acrosome reaction. The condition that fusion depends upon the previous occurrence of the acrosome reaction, suggests that the process of sperm–oocyte fusion in this heterologous model is physiologically meaningful. Moreover, the ultrastructural details of membrane fusion in this system appear to reflect the biological situation in that this process is initiated by the plasma membrane overlying the equatorial segment of the sperm head (Koehler *et al.*, 1982).

Since the original description of this interspecies *in vitro* fertilization assay as a means of monitoring human sperm function, the technique has been modified in a number of minor ways by independent research groups, in order to optimize penetration rates. In order to bring an element of standardization to this assay, the World Health Organization convened a consultation to establish a consensus protocol for this procedure (Aitken, 1986). The methodology established as a result of this consultation involves the overnight incubation of human spermatozoa in a simple defined salt solution, supplemented with energy substrates and a protein source such as bovine serum albumin (World Health Organization, 1987). Although this protocol has the dual advantages of being simple and readily standardized, it suffers from a major drawback in that it is entirely dependent upon the occurrence of spontaneous acrosome reactions within the sperm suspension being tested. Unfortunately the incidence of spontaneous acrosome reactions observed with human spermatozoa *in vitro* is generally less than 10% (Stock & Fraser, 1987) and, as a consequence, the rates of sperm–oocyte fusion recorded in this assay are poor even with the normal fertile samples (Aitken *et al.*, 1982). As we have already discussed in the context of the acrosome reaction, the ultimate solution to this problem will be to simulate human spermatozoa with recombinant human ZP3. In the meantime, the divalent cation ionophore A23187, represents a rational and effective stimulus for sperm–oocyte fusion (Aitken *et al.*, 1984, 1993*b*) which utilizes the same second messenger systems (pH and calcium) as ZP3 itself. In the presence of this reagent, high rates of sperm–oocyte fusion are observed with spermatozoa from the normal fertile population, giving penetration rates of 70–100%. In contrast, spermatozoa from subfertile males, such as the oligozoospermic population, exhibit penetration values of less than 10% after stimulation with A23187, with about half of such patients failing to fuse with any oocytes whatsoever (Aitken *et al.*, 1984). Most importantly, the A23187-stimulated version of this assay has been shown to be of significant prognostic value for predicting the fertilizing potential of human spermatozoa *in vitro* and *in vivo* (Aitken *et al.*, 1987, 1991) in situations where the conventional criteria of semen quality (sperm count, motility and morphology) were of little, or no, diagnostic significance.

Despite its apparent diagnostic value, an inherent problem with this bioassay is its complexity, as a consequence of which it must be carefully quality controlled if the results are to prove meaningful (see Aitken, 1986). In the long run, the real value of this bioassay may be as a research tool in studies designed to understand the reasons for impaired sperm–oocyte fusion at the molecular level. Once this level of understanding has been achieved, it should prove possible to use biochemical criteria to monitor the functional competence of human spermatozoa without the need to perform labour intensive, complex bioassays such as the zona-free hamster oocyte penetration test.

Biochemical criteria of sperm quality

The intrinsic advantages of biochemical techniques for assessing the functional competence of human spermatozoa is that such methods should be readily standardized and automated for routine use. The major problem with this approach is that our knowledge of the biochemical mechanisms that control human sperm function are still rudimentary and, as a consequence, only a limited number of biochemical markers of human sperm function have been identified. However, the cell biology of human of spermatozoa is a very rapidly developing field and a number of recent studies have succeeded in identifying biochemical markers of human sperm function such as creatine phosphokinase (Huszar, Corrales & Vigue, 1988*a*, Huszar, Vigue & Corrales, 1988*b*, 1990), acrosin (Goodpasture *et al.*, 1982; Francavilla *et al.*, 1993), lactic acid dehydrogenase (Casano *et al.*, 1991) or tysosine kinases (Naz *et al.*, 1991). Considerable interest has also been stimulated by an accumulation of evidence suggesting that oxidative stress plays a major role in the aetiology of defective sperm function (Jones, Mann & Sherins, 1979; Aitken & Clarkson, 1987; Alvarez *et al.*, 1987).

The fact that human spermatozoa can generate reactive oxygen species such as superoxide anion and hydrogen peroxide was published independently in 1987 by Aitken & Clarkson (1987) and Alvarez *et al.* (1987). The primary product of the spermatozoon's free radical generating system appears to be the superoxide anion, which dismutates to hydrogen peroxide under the influence of intracellular superoxide dismutase. The pathological significance of reactive oxygen species production by human spermatozoa was first indicated when chemiluminescent assays of this activity revealed an inverse relationship with functional competence, as measured by bioassays of sperm–oocyte fusion (Aitken & Clarkson, 1987; Aitken, Clarkson & Fishel, 1989; Aitken *et al.*, 1989, 1991). A specific example of this pathology is oligozoospermic patients, whose spermatozoa exhibit a median level of hydrogen peroxide generation which is about two log orders of magnitude greater than spermatozoa recovered from the normal fertile population (Aitken *et al.*, 1992*b*). In a separate study of oligozoospermic patients, approximately 50% of samples failing to exhibit sperm–oocyte fusion in response to A23187 were characterized by high levels of reactive oxygen species generation (Aitken *et al.*, 1989). Moreover, in a long-term prospective analysis, involving couples incorporating a normal female partner, a significant inverse relationship was observed between the level of reactive oxygen species generated by the washed semen sample and the incidence of spontaneous pregnancy (Aitken *et al.*, 1991). Significantly, the conventional semen profile (sperm number, motility and morphology) was of no diagnostic significance whatsoever within the cohort of patients analysed in this prospective study.

The enhanced generation of reactive oxygen species by the spermatozoa leads to the functional demise of these cells as a consequence of an attack on the unsaturated fatty acids that abound in the sperm plasma membrane. Spermatozoa contain high concentrations of unsaturated fatty acids, particularly decohexanoic acid (Jones *et al.*, 1979), which renders the sperm plasma membrane particularly susceptible to oxidative attack. This vulnerability stems from the fact that the presence of one or more double bonds in the unsaturated fatty acids, weakens the CH bonds on the adjacent carbon atoms, rendering these molecules vulnerable to a peroxidative process that commences with the removal of a hydrogen atom and the creation of a lipid-free radical. The lipid radical will then react with molecular oxygen to generate lipid alkoxyl and peroxyl radicals which will, in turn, abstract hydrogen atoms from adjacent fatty acids in order to create the more stable, lipid hydroperoxides. As a result of this hydrogen abstraction process, yet more lipid radicals are formed and, in this way, a chain reaction is initiated that propagates the damage throughout the membrane, unless blocked by chain-breaking antioxidants such as vitamin E.

The lipid hydroperoxides generated by the peroxidation process persist within the spermatozoa for a relatively long period of time unless their breakdown is catalysed by the presence of transition metals such as iron or copper (Aitken, Harkiss & Buckingham, 1993*c*,*d*). This chemistry is exploited when measurements are made of the peroxidative status of human spermatozoa for diagnostic purposes. To this end, spermatozoa are incubated with a ferrous ion promoter (ferrous sulphate and ascorbic acid) which catalyses the breakdown of the lipid peroxides that have accumulated within these cells to yield small carbonyl compounds, such as malondialdehyde, that are easy to measure using spectro-fluorimetric or spectrophotometric techniques (Aitken *et al.*, 1993*c*,*d*). The use of ferrous ion promoters to induce the decomposition of accumulated lipid peroxides, gives an important insight into the amount of oxidative stress these cells have suffered during their life history. Using such assays, it has been possible to show an excellent relationship between the lipoperoxidative status of human spermatozoa and their functional competence, as indicated by their movement and their capacity for sperm–oocyte fusion (Aitken *et al.*, 1993*c*).

The mechanism by which lipid peroxidation impairs the functional competence of human spermatozoa probably involves a change in the physical properties of the plasma membrane, characterized by a loss of fluidity. Since membrane fluidity is essential for membrane fusion events such as the acrosome reaction or fusion with the oocyte, the loss of fluidity associated with lipid peroxidation results in a dramatic loss of fertilizing potential. It is because of this loss of membrane fluidity that the free radical-generating spermatozoa produced by oligozoospermic patients do not exhibit biological responses, even when the appropriate second messengers are induced with the divalent cation ionophore A23187 (Aitken *et al.*, 1984).

The susceptibility of human spermatozoa to oxidative stress is not only a consequence of their high content of unsaturated fatty acids but also their lack of a defence against this kind of attack. Although human spermatozoa do contain the usual cytoplasmic defensive enyzyme systems of catalase, glutathione peroxidase and superoxide dismutase (Alvarez *et al.*, 1987; Alvarez & Storey, 1989; Jeulin *et al.*, 1989), the lack of cytoplasm and the highly compartmentalized nature of these cells, imposes limits on the effectiveness of this defence. As a consequence, these cells are particularly susceptible to oxidative stress, with hydrogen peroxide being the major effector of such damage (Aitken, Buckingham & Harkiss, 1993*a*).

The oxidative stress that damages human spermatozoa may not only involve the excessive generation of reactive oxygen species by these cells. There are other cell types in the human ejaculate, particularly neutrophils, that may be an important source of reactive oxygen species. In a vast majority of cases the number of such cells is in the order of 20×10^4/ml (Aitken & West, 1990; Aitken *et al.*, 1992*b*) and only very rarely does the concentration exceed the 1×10^6/ml threshold established by the World Health Organization (1987) as the definition of leukocytospermia (Aitken & West, 1990). However, whether the presence of even high concentrations of neutrophils creates a state of oxidative stress is not certain. Within the ejaculate, the spermatozoa are protected by the powerful combination of antioxidants that are present in seminal plasma (Jones *et al.*, 1979) and although an association between leukocytospermia and impaired semen quality has been claimed (Wolff *et al.*, 1990), the possibility that such associations are an indirect consequence of the impact of infection on secondary sexual gland function cannot be ruled out (Gonzales *et al.*, 1992). Certainly, within our own data set we have not observed a negative impact of seminal leukocytes on semen quality, despite the presence of leukocytospermia in several cases.

In contrast, when the spermatozoa are washed out of the protective environment afforded by seminal plasma and are prepared as sperm suspensions in culture medium for the purpose of assisted conception, then the presence of leukocytes can have devastating effects on their functional competence. Whenever leukocytes are present in significant numbers ($>3 \times 10^4$ leukocytes per 10^7 spermatozoa) sperm–oocyte fusion is impaired (RJ Aitken, unpublished observations). Moreover, if unfractionated sperm suspensions are centrifuged in the absence of seminal plasma as part of a preparative technique, then any functionally competent cells present in the mixture may become damaged as a result of exposure to the reactive oxygen species generated by defective spermatozoa and leukocytes present in the same cell population. However, if the chain breaking antioxidant, vitamin E, is incorporated in to the culture medium, then the extent of such damage is significantly reduced (Aitken & Clarkson, 1988).

Conclusions

In conclusion, the clinical assessment of male fertility is entering a new and exciting phase of its development when improvements in our understanding of sperm cell biology are beginning to have an impact on the diagnosis and treatment of this condition. A knowledge of the second messenger systems (calcium, pH, cAMP, superoxide anion) involved in the regulation of sperm movement should, for example, provide us with a sound platform from which to investigate the causes of asthenozoospermia. Similarly, the realization that lipid peroxidation plays a key role in the mechanisms by which spermatozoa lose their capacity for sperm–oocyte fusion, should be of value in facilitating the design of simple biochemical assays which will be much easier to standardize and perform than any bioassay. Moreover, once the biochemical mechanisms underlying sperm dysfunction are understood, a rational approach to the design of appropriate therapies becomes possible. Thus, if lipid peroxidation is a major factor in the aetiology of failed fertilization in IVF programmes, then there may be significant benefits to be gained from incorporating antioxidants into the culture medium. Similarly, our awareness of the importance of cAMP in the control of sperm movement has stimulated a search for reagents to promote this activity which has resulted in the identification of compounds such as 2-deoxyadenosine and pentoxyfylline (Aitken, Mattei & Irvine, 1986; Yovich *et al.* 1994) which are already proving effective in the use of IVF therapy to treat male factor infertility. In the future, further therapeutic opportunities should present themselves if we can continue to develop our understanding of male reproductive physiology in general and the cell biology of spermatogenesis and fertilization, in particular.

References

Aitken RJ. The zona-free hamster oocyte penetration test and the diagnosis of male fertility. *Int J Androl* 1986; **6**: 1–199.

Aitken RJ. Evaluation of human sperm function. In: Edwards RD, ed. *Assisted Human Conception. Br Med Bull* 1990: 654–74. vol 46).

Aitken RJ, Best FSM, Richardson DW, Djahanbakhch O, Lees MM. The correlates of fertilizing capacity in normal fertile men. *Fertil Steril* 1982; **38**: 68–76.

Aitken RJ, Bowie H, Buckingham D, Harkiss, D, Richardson DW, West KM. Sperm penetration into a hyaluronic acid polymer as a means of monitoring functional competence. *J Androl* 1992a; **13**: 44–54.

Aitken RJ, Brindle JP. Comparison of probes targeting constituents of the outer acrosomal membrane and acrosomal vesicle for their ability to detect the acrosome reaction in human spermatozoa. *Hum Reprod* 1993; **8**: 1663–9.

Aitken RJ, Buckingham D, Harkiss D. Use of a xanthine oxidase oxidant generating system to investigate the cytotoxic effects of reactive oxygen species on human spermatozoa. *J Reprod Fertil* 1993*a*; **97**: 441–50.

Aitken RJ, Buckingham DW, Huang G-F. On the use of A23187 to stimulate human spermatozoa to undergo the acrosome reaction and exhibit sperm-oocyte fusion: protocols and interactions. *J Androl* 1993*b*; **14**: 132–41.

Aitken RJ, Buckingham D, West K, Wu FC, Zikopoulos K, Richardson DW. On the contribution of leucocytes and spermatozoa to the high levels of reactive oxygen species recorded in the ejaculates of oligozoospermic patients. *J Reprod Fertil* 1992*b*; **94**: 451–62.

Aitken RJ, Harkiss D, Buckingham D. Relationship between iron-catalysed lipid peroxidation potential and human sperm function. *J Reprod Fertil* 1993*c*; **31**: 531–7.

Aitken RJ, Harkiss D, Buckingham DW. Analysis of lipid peroxidation mechanisms in human spermatozoa. *Mol Reprod Dev* 1993*d*; **35**: 302–15.

Aitken RJ, Clarkson JS. Cellular basis of defective sperm function and its association with the genesis of reactive oxygen species by human spermatozoa. *J Reprod Fertil* 1987; **81**: 459–69.

Aitken RJ, Clarkson JS. Significance of reactive oxygen species and anti-oxidants in defining the efficacy of sperm preparation techniques. *J Androl* 1988; **9**: 367–76.

Aitken RJ, Clarkson JS, Fishel S. Generation of reactive oxygen species, lipid peroxidation and human sperm function. *Biol Reprod* 1989; **40**: 183–97.

Aitken RJ, Clarkson JS, Hargreave TB, Irvine DS, Wu FCW. Analysis of the relationship between defective sperm function and the generation of reactive oxygen species in cases of oligozoospermia. *J Androl* 1989; **10**: 214–20.

Aitken RJ, Irvine, DS, Wu FC. Prospective analysis of sperm-oocyte fusion and reactive oxygen species generation as criteria for the diagnosis of infertility. *Am J Obstet Gynecol* 1991; **164**: 542–51.

Aitken RJ, Mattei A, Irvine S. Paradoxical stimulation of human sperm-motility by 2-deoxyadenosine. *J Reprod Fertil* 1986; **78**: 515–27.

Aitken RJ, Ross A, Lees MM. Analysis of sperm function in Kartagener's syndrome. *Fertil Steril* 1983; **40**: 696.

Aitken RJ, Sutton M, Warner P, Richardson DW. Relationship between the movement characteristics of human spermatozoa and their ability to penetrate cervical mucus and zona-free hamster oocytes. *J Reprod Fertil* 1985; **73**: 441–9.

Aitken RJ, Ross A, Hargreave T, Richardson D, Best F. Analysis of human sperm function following exposure to the ionophore A23187. Comparison of normospermic and oligozoospermic men. *J Androl* 1984; **5**: 321–9.

Aitken RJ, Thatcher S, Glasier AF, Clarkson JS, Wu FCW, Baird DT. Relative ability of modified versions of the hamster oocyte penetration test, incorporating hyperosmotic medium or the ionophore A23187, to predict IVF outcome. *Hum Reprod* 1987; **2**: 227–31.

Aitken RJ, Warner P, Reid C. Factors influencing the success of sperm-cervical mucus interaction in patients exhibiting unexplained infertility. *J Androl* 1986; **7**: 3–10.

Aitken RJ, West KM. Analysis of the relationship between reactive oxygen species production and leucocyte infiltration in fractions of human semen separated on Percoll gradients. *Int J Androl* 1990; **13**: 433–51.

Alvarez JG, Storey BT. Role of glutathione peroxidase in protecting mammalian spermatozoa from loss of motility caused by spontaneous lipid peroxidation. *Gamete Res* 1989; **23**: 77–90.

Alvarez JG, Touchstone JC, Blasco L, Storey BT. Spontaneous lipid peroxidation and production of hydrogen peroxide and superoxide in human spermatozoa. *J Androl* 1987; **8**: 338–48.

Baba T, Kashiwabara, S. Watanabe K, *et al.* Activation and maturation mechanisms of boar acrosin zymogen based on deduced primary structure. *J Biol Chem* 1989; **264**: 11920–7.

Babcock DF, Pfeiffer DR. Independent elevation of cytosolic [Ca^{2+}] and pH of mammalian sperm by voltage-dependent and pH sensitive mechanisms. *J Biol Chem* 1989; **262**: 15041–50.

Beebe SJ, Leyton L, Burks ED, *et al.* Recombinant mouse ZP3 inhibits sperm binding and induces the acrosome reaction. *Dev Biol* 1992; **151**: 48–54.

Bhattacharyya A, Yanagimachi R. Synthesis organic pH buffers can support fertilization of guinea pig eggs, but not as efficiently as bicarbonate buffers. *Gamete Res* 1989; **19**: 123–30.

Blackmore PF, Beebe SJ, Danforth SJ, Alexander N. Progesterone and 17α-hydroxy-progesterone. Novel stimulators of calcium influx in human spermatozoa. *J Biol Chem* 1990; **265**: 1376–80.

Bleil JD, Wassarman PM. Galactose at the nonreducing terminus of O-linked oligosaccharides of mouse egg zone pellucida glycoprotein ZP3 is essential for the glycoprotein's sperm receptor activity. *Proc Natl Acad Sci USA* 1988; **85**: 6778–82.

Bleil JD, Wassarman PM. Identification of a ZP3-binding protein on acrosome-intact mouse sperm by photoaffinity crosslinking. *Proc Natl Acad Sci USA* 1990; **85**: 6778–82.

Blobel CP, Wolfsberg TG, Turch CW, Myles DG, Primarkoff P, White JM. A potential fusion peptide and an integrin ligand domain in a protein active in sperm oocyte fusion. *Nature* 1992; **356**: 248–52.

Bronson RA, Fusi F. Sperm-oolemmal interaction: role of the Arg–Gly–Asp (RGD) adhesion peptide. *Fertil Steril* 1990a; **54**: 527–9.

Bronson RA, Fusi F. Evidence that an Arg-Gly-Asp adhesion sequence plays a role in mammalian fertilization. *Biol Reprod* 1990b; **43**: 1019–25.

Burkman LJ. Hyperactivated motility of human spermatozoa during *in vitro* capacitation and implications for fertility. In: Gagnon C, ed *Control of Sperm Motility: Biological and Clinical Aspects*. Boston: CRC Press, 1990: 303–31.

Burkman LJ. Discrimination between nonhyperactivated and classical hyperactivated motility patterns in human spermatozoa using computerized analysis. *Fertil Steril* 1991; **55**: 363–71.

Byrd W, Wolf DP. Acrosomal status in fresh and capacitated human ejaculated sperm. *Biol Reprod* 1986; **34**: 859–69.

Byrd W, Tsu J, Wolf DP. Kinetics of spontaneous and induced acrosomal loss in human sperm incubated under capacitating and noncapacitating conditions. *Gamete Res* 1989; **22**: 109–22.

Carlsen E, Giwercman A, Keiding N, Skakkebaek NE. Evidence for decreasing quality of semen during the past 50 years. *Br Med J* 1992; **205**: 609–13.

Casano R, Orlando C, Serio M, Forti G. LDH and LDH-X activity in sperm from normospermic and oligozoospermic men. *Int J Androl* 1991; **14**: 257–63.

Cechova D, Topfer-Petersen E, Henschen A. Boar proacrosin in a single chain molecule which has the N-terminus of the acrosin A-chain (light chain). *FEBS Lett* 1989; **241**: 136–40.

Chamberlin ME, Dean J. Human homolog of the mouse sperm receptor. *Proc Natl Acad Sci USA* 1990; **87**: 6014–18.

Coddington CC, Franken DR, Burkman LJ, Oosthuizen WT, Kruger T, Hodgen GD. Functional aspects of human sperm binding to the zona pellucida using the hemizona assay. *J Androl* 1991; **12**: 1–8.

Cooper GW, Overstreet JW, Katz DF. The motility of rabbit spermatozoa in the female reproductive tract. *Gamete Res* 1979; **2**: 35–42.

Cross NL, Morales P, Overstreet JW, Hanson FW. Two simple methods for detecting acrosome reacted human sperm. *Gamete Res* 1986; **15**: 213–26.

Cummins JM, Pember SM, Jequier AM, Yovich JL, Hartman PE. A test of the human sperm acrosome reaction following ionophore challenge (ARIC): relationship to fertility and other seminal parameters. *J Androl* 1991; **12**: 98–103.

Cummins JM, Yanagimachi R. Sperm-egg ratios and the site of the acrosome reaction during in vivo fertilization in the hamster. *Gamete Res* 1982; **5**: 239–56.

David G, Serres C, Jouannet P. Kinematics of human spermatozoa. *Gamete Res* 1981; **4**: 83–6.

De Jonge CJ, Mack SR, Zaneveld LJD. Synchronous assay for human sperm capacitation and the acrosome reaction. *J Androl* 1989; **10**: 232–9.

De Lamirande E, Gagnon G. Human sperm hyperactivation and capacitation as parts of an oxidative process. *Free Radicals Biol Med* 1993; **14**: 157–66.

Feneux D, Serres C, Jouannet P. Sliding spermatozoa: a dyskinesia responsible for human infertility? *Fertil Steril* 1985; **44**: 508–11.

Florman HM, Babcock DF. Progress toward understanding the molecular basis of capacitation. In: Wassarman PM, ed. *Elements of Mammalian Fertilization*. Boca Raton, Florida: CRC Press, 1991: 105–32.

Florman HM, First NL. The regulation of acrosomal exocytosis 1. Sperm capacitation is required for the induction of acrosome reactions by the bovine zona pellucida *in vitro*. *Dev Biol* 1988; **128**: 453–60.

Florman HM, Tombes RM, First NL, Babcock DF. An adhesion-associated agonist from the zona pellucida activities G protein promoted elevations of internal Ca^{2+} and pH that mediate mammalian sperm acrosomal exocytosis. *Dev Biol* 1989; **135**: 133–45.

Fock-Nuzal R, Lottspeich F, Henschen A, Muller-Esterl W. Boar acrosin is a two-chain molecule. Isolation and primary structure of the light chain; homology with the pro-part of other serine proteinases. *Eur J. Biochem* 1984; **141**: 441–6.

Ford WCL, Rees JM, McLaughlin EA, Goddard RJ, Hull MGR. The effect of A23187 concentration and exposure time on the outcome of the hamster egg penetration test. *Int J Androl* 1991; **14**: 127–39.

Franken DR, Windt ML, Kruger T, Oehninger S, Hodgen GD. Comparison of sperm binding potential of uninseminated, inseminated-unfertilized and fertilized, non-cleaved human oocytes under hemi-zona assay conditions. *Mol Reprod Dev* 1991; **30**: 56–61.

Francavilla S, Palermo G, Gabriele A, Cordeschi G, Poccia G. Sperm acrosin activity and fluorescence microscopic assessment of proacrosin/acrosin in ejaculates of infertile and fertile men. *Fertil Steril* 1993; **57**: 1311–16.

Fraser LR, Monks NJ. Cyclic nucleotides and mammalian sperm capacitation. *J Reprod Fertil* 1990; Suppl 42: 9–21.

Gonzales GF, Kortebani G, Mazzolli AB. Leukocytospermia and function of the seminal vesicles on semen quality. *Fertil Steril* 1992; **57**: 1058–65.

Goodpasture JC, Zavos PM, Cohen MR, Zaneveld LJD. Relationship of acrosin and proacrosin to semen parameters. 1. Comparisons between symptomatic men of infertile couples and asymptomatic men, and between split ejaculates. *J Androl* 1982; **3**: 151–6.

Grunert J-H, De Geyter C, Neischlag E. Objective identification of hyperactivated human spermatozoa by computerised sperm motion analysis with the Hamilton-Thorn sperm motility analyser. *Hum Reprod* 1990; **5**: 593–9.

Hull MGR, Glazener CMA, Kelly NJ. Population study of causes, treatment and outcome of infertility. *Br Med J* 1985; **291**: 1693–7.

Huszar G, Corrales M, Vugue L. Correlation between sperm creatine phosphokinase activity and sperm concentrations in normospermic and oligozoospermic men. *Gamete Res* 1988a; **19**: 67–75.

Huszar G, Vigue L, Corrales M. Sperm creatine phosphokinase quality in normospermic, variable spermic and oligospermic men. *Biol Reprod* 1988b; **38**: 1061–6.

Huszar G, Corrales M, Vigue L. Sperm creatine kinase activity in fertile and infertile oligospermic men. *J Androl* 1990; **11**: 40–6.

Irvine DS, Aitken RJ. Measurement of intracellular calcium in human spermatozoa. *Gamete Res* 1986; **15**: 57–72.

Irvine DS, Aitken RJ. Predictive value of *in vitro* sperm function tests in the context of an AID service. *Hum Reprod* 1987; **1**: 539–45.

Jeulin C, Soufir JC, Weber P, Laval-Martin D, Calvayrac R. Catalase activity in human spermatozoa and seminal plasma. *Gamete Res* 1989; **24**: 185–96.

Jeyendran RS, Van der Ven HH, Perez-Palaez M, Crabo BG, Zaneveld LJD. Development of an assay to assess the functional integrity of the human sperm membrane and its relationship to other semen characteristics. *J Reprod Fertil* 1984; **70**: 219–28.

Johnson AR, Syms AJ, Lipshultz LI, Smith RG. Conditions influencing human sperm capacitation and penetration of zone-free hamster ova. *Fertil Steril* 1984; **41**: 603–8.

Jones R. Identification and functions of mammalian sperm–egg recognition molecules during fertilization. *J Reprod Fertil* 1990; **42**: 89–105.

Jones R, Mann T, Sherins RJ. Peroxidative breakdown of phospholipids in human spermatozoa: spermicidal effects of fatty acid peroxides and protective action of seminal plasma. *Fertil Steril* 1979; **31**: 531–7.

Katz DF, Yanagimachi R. Movement characteristics of hamster spermatozoa within the oviduct. *Biol Reprod* 1980; **22**: 759–64.

Kinloch RA, Mortillo S, Stewart CL, Wassarman PM. Embryonal carcinoma cells transfected with ZP3 genes differentially glycosylate similar polypeptides and secrete active mouse sperm receptor. *J Cell Biol* 1991; **115**: 655–64.

Kinloch RA, Roller RJ, Fimiani CM, Wassarman DA, Wassarman PM. Primary structure of the mouse sperm receptor's polypeptide chain determined by genomic cloning. *Proc Natl Acad Sci USA* 1988; **85**: 6409–13.

Kinloch RA, Ruiz-Seiler B, Wassarman PM. Genomic organization and polypeptide primary structure of zone pellucida glycoprotein hZP3, the hamster sperm receptor. *Dev Biol* 1990; **142**: 414–21.

Koehler JK, Curtis I, Stenchever MA, Smith D. Interaction of human sperm with zona-free hamster eggs: a freeze fracture study. *Gamete Res* 1982; **6**: 371–8.

Lee MA, Storey B. Evidence for plasma membrane impermeability to small ions in acrosome-intact mouse spermatozoa bound to mouse zonae pellucidae, using an aminoacridine fluorescent probe: time course of the zona induced acrosome reaction monitored by both chlorotetracycline and pH probe fluorescence. *Biol Reprod* 1985; **33**: 235–46.

Lee MA, Storey BT. Bicarbonate is essential for fertilization of mouse eggs: mouse sperm require it to undergo the acrosome reaction. *Biol Reprod* 1986; **34**: 349–55.

Leyton L, Saling PM. Evidence that aggregation of mouse sperm receptors by ZP3 triggers the acrosome reaction. *J Cell Biol* 1989*a*; **108**: 2163–8.

Leyton L, Saling P. 95kd sperm proteins bind ZP3 and serve as tyrosine kinase substrates in response to zona binding. *Cell* 1989*b*; **58**: 1123–40.

Leyton L, LeGuen P, Bunch D, Saling PM. Regulation of mouse gamete interaction by a sperm tyrosine kinase. *Proc Natl Acad Sci USA* 1992; **89**: 11692–5.

Liu DY, Clarke GN, Lopata A, Johnston WIH, Baker GHW. A sperm–zona pellucida binding test and *in vitro* fertilization. *Fertil Steril* 1988*a*; **52**: 281–7.

Liu DY, Lopata A, Leung A, Johnston WIAH, Gordon Baker HW. A human sperm–zona pellucida binding test using oocytes that failed to fertilize *in vitro Fertil Steril* 1988*b*; **50**: 782–8.

Mbizvo MT, Alexander NJ. Functional changes during sperm transit; sites of acquisition and possible inhibition of fertilizing ability. In: Baccitti B, ed *Comparative Spermatology 20 Years After*. New York: Raven Press, 1991: 869–78.

Mbizvo MT, Johnston RC, Bader GHW. The effect of the motility stimulants caffeine, pentoxyfylline and 2-deoxyadenosine on hyperactivation of cryopreserved human sperm. *Fertil Steril* 1993; **59**: 1112–17.

Mbizvo MT, Thomas S, Fulgham DL, Alexander NJ. Serum hormone levels affect sperm function. *Fertil Steril* 1990; **54**: 113–20.

Menkveld R, Franken DR, Kruger TF, Oehinger S, Hodgen GD. Sperm selection capacity of the human zona pellucida. *Mol Reprod Dev* 1991; **30**: 357–62.

Miller DJ, Macek MB, Shur BD. Complimentarity between sperm surface β-1,4-galactosyltransferase and egg coat ZP3 mediates sperm–egg binding. *Nature* 1992; **357**: 598–602.

Moller CC, Bleil JD, Kinloch RA, Wassarman PM. Structural and functional relationship between mouse and hamster zona pellucida glycoproteins. *Dev Biol* 1990; **137**: 276–86.

Morales P, Llanos M, Gutierrez G, Kohen P, Vigil P, Vantman D. The acrosome reaction-inducing activity of individual human follicular fluid samples is highly variable and is related to the steroid content. *Hum Reprod* 1992; **7**: 646–51.

Mortimer D, Curtis EF, Camenzind AR, Tanaka S. The spontaneous acrosome reaction of human spermatozoa. *Hum Reprod* 1989; **4**- 57–62.

Mortimer D, Curtis EF, Miller RG. Specific labelling by sperm agglutinin of the outer acrosomal membrane of the human spermatozoon. *J Reprod Fertil* 1988; **81**: 127–35.

Mortimer ST, Mortimer D. Kinematics of human spermatozoa incubated under capacitating conditions. *J Androl* 1990; **11**: 195–203.

Mortimer D, Mortimer ST, Shu MA, Swart RA. A simplified approach to sperm-cervical mucus interaction testing using a hyaluronate migration test. *Hum Reprod* 1990; **5**: 835–41.

Mortimer D, Pandya IJ, Sawers RS. Relationship between human sperm motility characteristics and sperm penetration into human cervical mucus *in vitro*. *J Reprod Fertil* 1986; **78**: 93–102.

Naz RK, Ahmed K, Kimar R. Role of membrane phosphotyrosine proteins in human spermatozoal function. *J Cell Sci* 1991; **99**: 157–65.

Oehninger S. Diagnostic significance of sperm–zona pellucida interaction. *Reprod Med Rev* 1992; **1**: 57–81.

Oehninger S, Veeck LL, Franken D, Kruger TF, Acosta AA, Hodgen GD. Human preovulatory oocytes have a higher sperm-binding ability than immature oocytes under hemizona assay conditions: evidence supporting the concept of 'zona maturation'. *Fertil Steril* 1991; **55**: 1165–70.

Okamura N, Tajima Y, Soejima A, Masudo H, Sugita Y. Sodium bicarbonate stimulates the motility of mammalian spermatozoa through direct activation of adenylate cyclase. *J Biol Chem* 1985; **260**: 9699–707.

Olds-Clarke P. Motility characteristics of sperm from the uterus and oviducts of female mice after mating to congenic males differing in sperm transport and fertility. *Biol Reprod* 1986; **34**: 453–67.

Osman RA, Andria ML, Jones AD, Meizel M. Steroid induced exocytosis: the human sperm acrosome reaction. *Biochem Biophys Res Commun* 1989; **16**: 828–34.

Østerlind A. Diverging trends in incidence and mortality of testicular cancer in Denmark, 1943–1982. *Br J Cancer* 1986; **53**: 501–5.

Palermo G, Joris H, Derde M-P, Camus M, Devroey P, Van Steriteghem A. Sperm characteristics and outcome of human assisted fertilization by subzonal insemination and intracytoplasmic sperm injection. *Fertil Steril* 1993; **59**: 826–35.

Ringuette MJ, Chamberlin ME, Baur AW, Sobieski DA, Dean J. Molecular analysis of cDNA coding for ZP3, a sperm binding protein of the mouse zona pellucida. *Dev Biol* 1988; **127**: 287–95.

Russell L, Peterson RN, Freund M. Morphologic characteristics of the chemically induced acrosome reaction in human spermatozoa. *Fertil Steril* 1979; **32**: 87–92.

Sakkas D, Lacham O, Gianaroli L, Trounson A. Subzonal sperm microinjection in cases of severe male factor infertility and repeated *in vitro* fertilization therapy. *Fertil Steril* 1992; **57**: 1279–88.

Sanchez R, Toepfer-Petersen E, Aitken RJ, Schill W-B. A new method for evaluation of the acrosome reaction in viable human spermatozoa. *Andrologia* 1991; **23**: 197–203.

Santos-Sacchi J, Gordon M. The effect of ATP depletion upon the acrosome reaction in guinea pig spermatozoa. *J Androl* 1982; **3**: 108–12.

Shalgi R, Phillips DM. Motility of rat spermatozoa at the site of fertilization. *Biol Reprod* 1988; **39**: 1207–13.

Stock CE, Fraser LR. The acrosome reaction in human sperm from men of proven fertility. *Hum Reprod* 1987; **2**: 109–19.

Suarez SS. Sperm transport and motility in the mouse oviduct: observations *in situ*. *Biol Reprod* 1987; **36**: 203–10.

Suarez SS, Katz DF, Overstreet JW. Movement characteristics and acrosomal status of rabbit spermatozoa recovered at the site and time of fertilization. *Biol Reprod* 1983; **29**: 1277–87.

Saurez SS, Osman R. Initiation of hyperactivated flagellar bending in mouse sperm within the female reproductive tract. *Biol Reprod* 1987; **36**: 1191–8.

Tesarik J, Drahorad J, Peknicova J. Subcellular immunochemical localization of acrosin in human spermatozoa during the acrosome reaction and zone pellucida penetration. *Fertil Steril* 1988a; **50**: 133.

Tesarik J, Pilka L. Traunick P. Zona pellucida resistance to sperm penetration before the completion of human oocyte maturation. *J Reprod Fertil* 1988b; **83**: 487–95.

Thillai Koothan P, van Duin M, Aitken RJ. Cloning, sequencing and oocyte-specific expression of the marmoset sperm receptor protein, ZP3. *Zygote* 1993; **1**: 93–101.

Topfer-Petersen E, Henschen A. Acrosin shows zona and fucoze binding, novel properties for serine proteinase. *FEBS Lett* 1987; **226**: 38–42.

Topfer-Petersen E, Steinberger M, Ebner von Eschenbach C, Zucker A. Zona pellucida-binding of boar sperm acrosin is associated with the N-terminal peptide of the acrosin B-chain (heavy chain). *FEBS Lett* 1990; **265**: 51–4.

van Duin M, Polman JE, Verkoelen CC, *et al.* Cloning and characterization of the human sperm receptor ligand ZP3: evidence for a second polymorphic allele with a different frequency in the Caucasian and Japanese populations. *Genomics* 1992; **14**: 1064–70.

Warner FD, Satir P, Gibbons IR. Cell Movement. Volume 1. In: The Dynein ATPases. New York: Alan R Liss, 1988

Wassarman PM. Profile of a mammalian sperm receptor. *Development* 1990; **108**: 1–17.

Wassarman PM. Cellular and molecular elements of mammalian fertilization. In: Dale B, ed. *Mechanism of Fertilization*. Berlin: Springer-Verlag, 1991: 305–14.

White DR, Aitken RJ. Relationship between calcium, cyclic AMP, ATP and intracellular pH and the capacity of hamster spermatozoa to express hyperactivated motility. *Gamete Res* 1989; **22**: 163–77.

Wolff H, Politch JA, Martinez A, Haimovici F, Hill JA, Anderson DJ. Leucocytospermia is associated with poor semen quality. *Fertil Steril* 1990; **53**: 528–36.

World Health Organization. In: *WHO Laboratory Manual for the Examination of Human Semen and Semen–Cervical Mucus Interaction*. Cambridge: Cambridge University Press, 1987.

Yanagimachi R, Lopata A, Odom CB, Bronson RA, Mahi CA, Nicolson GL. Retention of biologic characteristics of zona pellucida in highly concentrated salt solution: the use of salt stored eggs for assessing the fertilizing capacity of spermatozoa. *Fertil Steril* 1979; **31**: 562–74.

Yanagimachi R, Yanagimachi H, Rogers BJ. The use of zona free animal ova as a test system for the assessment of the fertilizing capacity of human spermatozoa. *Biol Reprod* 1976; **15**: 471–6.

Yovich JM, Edirisinghe WR, Yovich JL. Use of the acrosome reaction to ionophore challenge test in managing patients in an assisted reproduction program: a prospective, double-blind, randomized controlled study. *Fertil Steril* 1994; **61**: 902–10.

12

Sperm antibodies: formation and significance

P. L. MATSON

Introduction

The presence of antibodies directed against sperm in either men, as an auto-immune phenomenon, or women can often be associated with a reduced fertility. This is of primary importance in the investigation and treatment of sub-fertile couples, as the identification of an immune disorder in these couples will have great bearing on the choice of an appropriate therapeutic option in their endeavours to achieve a pregnancy. However, the deliberate induction of antisperm antibodies can be used in the development of a contraceptive vaccine.

Before examining the production and clinical significance of these sperm antibodies, let us first consider some of the more fundamental aspects of the antibody–antigen interaction.

Antibodies

An immune response to an antigenic stimulus has two main components, namely a humoral and a cellular component. The former includes the production of antibodies and is the main topic of the present chapter, but the role of the lymphocytes in the cellular-mediated response should not be overlooked (Barratt, Bolton & Cooke, 1990).

The basic structural unit of an antibody molecule consists of four polypeptide chains, namely two identical light chains and two identical heavy chains, held together by a combination of non-covalent interactions and covalent bonds. Immunoglobulins have different regions which can be identified after the fragmentation of the molecule by the enzyme papain. The fragments or regions are known as the Fab (fragment antigen binding) fragments and the Fc fragment (so-called because of its ease of crystallization).

There are five different classes of antibodies, each with its own type of heavy chain, and these are IgA, IgD, IgE, IgG, IgM, although sperm antibodies are principally of the IgA, IgG and IgM classes. IgA is the major class of antibody in secretions, and is found either as a monomer or as a dimer. When found in secretions, it is usually as a dimer in which the two halves are joined by a J (joining) chain and a polypeptide known as the secretory component. The main class of antibody in the blood is that of IgG. It is often produced during a secondary immune response in which the Fc regions bind to specific binding sites on phagocytic cells, thereby increasing the efficiency of ingestion of antigenic cells which have antibody bound. IgM is the major class of antibody found in the early stages of a primary immune response. The antibody is secreted as a pentamer (i.e. five 4-chain units) and is a potent activator of the complement system.

Antigens

An antigen is any substance capable of eliciting an immune response. Spermatozoa are no exception in possessing a range of antigenic sites on their surface, being capable of stimulating antibody production in either the female partner of a couple or the man himself. There is an increased incidence of auto-antibodies in men with sperm antibodies which are specific to other tissues (Baker et al., 1985), and so a genetic predisposition to the development of sperm autoimmunity may exist.

To be clinically significant, antigens upon intact spermatozoa need to be on the surface of the cell for immunological recognition as opposed to being intracellular, so that any sperm antibodies in biological fluids may bind to the sperm and exert some effect. The method of preparation of sperm in any assay can markedly influence its antigenic appearance, with fixation of the sperm, in particular, causing dramatic changes. Therefore, when identifying the site of binding of antibodies upon prepared non-viable sperm, care should be taken in distinguishing between surface and intracellular antigens (Haas et al., 1988).

A number of antigens present upon spermatozoa have no significant role in regulating spermatozoal function, and so antibodies against these antigens have no effect upon fertility. Examples of such antigens include blood group antigens (Cooper & Bronson, 1990) and a number of antigens common to somatic cells (Naz & Menge, 1990). Nevertheless, antibodies against a number of important antigens have been identified in infertile couples and these are thought to reduce fertility. The antibodies are often directed against compounds involved in the fertilization process, such as acrosin (Howe et al., 1991), the fertilization antigen FA-1 (Bronson et al., 1989), galactosyltransferase (Humphreys-Beher, Garrison & Blackwell, 1990) and an antigen of approximately 80 kD (Haneji & Koide, 1990).

The antigenic appearance of spermatozoa is not always constant. Physiological changes occur in the antigenic appearance of sperm following capacitation and the acrosome reaction (Fusi & Bronson, 1990), prompting Monroe, Altenbaum & Mathur (1990) to suggest that biological fluids should be tested for the presence of antibodies using both fresh and capacitated sperm. Furthermore, they also found that antibodies from serum and seminal plasma did not bind in the same manner to husband's sperm compared to donor sperm. The possible limitation of assays using donor sperm in an uncapacitated state should therefore be remembered.

The detection of antispermatozoal antibodies

Choice of biological fluid

Sperm antibodies can be detected in blood of sub-fertile men and women (Clarke *et al.*, 1985*c*), but perhaps more relevantly in seminal plasma (Clarke, Elliott & Smaila, 1985*a*), cervical mucus (Clarke, 1984), follicular fluid (Kay *et al.*, 1985) and Fallopian tube fluid (Wong, 1979). The choice of fluid used when screening infertile couples is very important in avoiding erroneous results.

Blood has long been the fluid of choice for analysis because of its ease of collection from either partner of a couple in a clinic. Unfortunately, it is now realized that the most meaningful results are obtained in the secretions with which spermatozoa come into contact, since this is the only way the antibodies could exert some effect upon spermatozoal function. A good example of this is following vasectomy reversal where relatively high titres of antibody can be found in the blood of men after surgery, but the effects upon fertility only become apparent when the antibodies appear in the seminal plasma where the antibodies can bind to the sperm at ejaculation (Sutherland *et al.*, 1984).

Whilst the investigation of the male partner of an infertile couple is best done by examining the seminal plasma, the analysis of cervical mucus in the female is not so easy. Good mucus is only available at a limited time during the menstrual cycle, and the viscosity of the mucus means that it has to be digested enzymatically prior to analysis with possible changes in the antibody content (Ingerslev & Paulsen, 1980). Many clinics, therefore, still use blood as the medium for screening women, even though they are aware of the limitations. However, the antibody content of blood can now have direct relevance in certain situations, such as in an IVF programme where the serum is used as a supplement to the medium prepared for preparing and culturing the gametes.

Methods of detection

Although a wealth of information on sperm antibodies exists in the literature, the findings of different studies are often not comparable directly because of huge differences in methodology. Therefore, great care should be taken in reading the original articles and noting the method of detection used.

The three blood categories of tests used are those which either detect the agglutinating activity of the fluid, the complement-dependent immobilizing activity, or the specific class of immunoglobulin present.

Unfortunately, there is no reference method against which other methods can be compared. The fundamental principles of the three types of assay are very different, using different endpoints in the assay, and this makes the comparison of different studies very difficult. A good agreement is often seen when comparing the results obtained with the different methods (Linnett & Suonimen, 1987) although there are instances when the analysis of a single sample by any two methods will give different results. This may be due to the two methods detecting different things, or to the two methods having different sensitivities.

Detection of agglutinating activity

The original methods of detection were based upon the ability of samples to agglutinate donor spermatozoa, in a similar fashion to the agglutination of erythrocytes in the determination of blood groups. As such, the methods are always indirect since they cannot identify the presence of antibodies upon spermatozoa of the man under investigation, only agglutinating activity of donor sperm in his fluid. The tests can therefore be used in blood from both men and women, and seminal plasma. One limitation to these tests is their lack of specificity for immunoglobulins and so any substance causing the agglutination of sperm, whether immunological or not, will be detected (Boettcher *et al.*, 1971). The principal methods used are given below, although they have been summarized elsewhere (Adeghe, Barratt & Cohen, 1988):

Gelatin agglutination test (*Kibrick, Belding & Merriu, 1952*)   Also known as the Kibrick test. The method relies on the flocculation of donor sperm in a tube of gelatin, in the presence of serially diluted sample. The tubes of gelatin are held up to the light and inspected by eye. As such, no microscope is required but the type of agglutination cannot be identified and the test is insensitive to head–head agglutination. The result is then given as the highest dilution at which agglutination occurs. The test uses relatively large numbers of donor sperm per tube, and so the number of samples analysed at one time is relatively low.

Tray agglutination test (*Friberg, 1974*)   This is a micro-agglutination test using small volumes of serially diluted sample in tissue typing trays. Donor sperm are added to each droplet of diluted sample and the type of agglutination is observed directly using an inverted microscope. Again, the result is given as the largest titre causing agglutination, but the type of agglutination can also be given, e.g. head–head, tail–tail. Relatively large numbers of samples can be analysed on each occasion.

Complement-dependent immobilization

The main method is that of Isojima, Li & Ashtaki (1968) and determines the immobilizing activity of a sample in the presence of complement. It is generally thought that the test gives little diagnostic information over and above that of the agglutinating tests, although in theory it should be detecting different classes of antibody.

Detection of immunoglobulins

Specific immunoglobulins can be detected either directly upon a man's own spermatozoa, or indirectly in fluids following incubation with donor spermatozoa. The principal methods are:

MAR (mixed antiglobulin reaction) test It is based on the Coomb's reaction used in haematology, in which sensitized Group O Rh +ve erythrocytes are mixed with the test cells and a specific anti-human IgG antiserum. If the sperm cells carry IgG on their surface then mixed agglutination is observed. The method was first standardized by Jager *et al.* (1978) as a screening method for IgG antibodies bound to the sperm surface, but other workers have since adapted the method to detect IgA antibodies (Hendry *et al.*, 1982). The technique is best applied as a direct test on semen, but is limited by requiring the semen to have a good number of motile spermatozoa. Tests on samples with low spermatozoal concentrations or motility are not valid.

Immunobeads The immunobeads are produced commercially (Bio-Rad) for use in a range of immunological applications. However, they can be used to detect sperm antibodies (Bronson, Cooper & Rosenfeld, 1982). The beads can be used either directly or indirectly, and can detect IgA, IgG and IgM, as well as the site of binding upon the sperm. Again, motile spermatozoa are required in this test and so the direct method is not valid with oligozoospermic or asthenozoospermic samples. Whilst not perfect, this method is rapidly being accepted as the method of choice in characterizing samples.

Interpretation of results

For sperm antibodies to be regarded as clinically significant, an effect upon sperm function and fertility has to be demonstrated. However, before this can be done consideration should be given to the limits of sensitivity of the assay, i.e. the minimum level of antibody which can be detected. For tests detecting agglutinating activity of donor sperm, commonly used limits of detection are 1:4 in seminal plasma and 1:8 in serum although this will vary from laboratory to laboratory. Any agglutinating activity in sample diluted less than this is not reported as it may well be due to non-specific agglutination or other common substances (e.g. steroid hormones) which can cause sperm to agglutinate. Dilution of the sample eliminates this insignificant low-level activity. A second level of agglutinating activity then exists, at which the result is thought to be of clinical significance. Commonly used thresholds of clinical significance are $\geqslant 1:32$ in serum of either men or women, and $\geqslant 1:8$ in seminal fluid. Again these levels will vary, and so the level used by each laboratory should be checked.

Methods detecting specific immunoglobulins are subject to similar considerations, even though the methods may be more specific. This is clearly illustrated by those workers using immunobeads. An assay sensitivity at which either 10% (World Health Organization, 1987) or 20% (Clarke *et al.*, 1985*b*) of sperm are coated in beads is often used. However, levels of binding to be clinically significant varies enormously from 20% (Junk *et al.*, 1986) of sperm with beads attached to 50% (Barratt *et al.*, 1992) in blood, and even to 80% (Clarke *et al.*, 1985*b*) in semen.

Quality control

As with any assay, quality control is important in minimising inter-assay and intra-assay variation. A bank of sera is available from the World Health Organization, but most laboratories find the making of their own quality control samples much easier. Many commercial kits contain positive and negative sera. However, laboratories should collaborate and interchange samples wherever possible, particularly in the early stages of establishing a new test, to help maintain consistency of reporting between laboratories.

Clinical significance

The clinical significance of sperm antibodies is influenced by factors which affect their production, their prevalence in the sub-fertile population, and the way in which they affect spermatozoal function.

Antibody production

As with animal models, sperm antibodies can be induced by immunization with spermatozoa or testicular homogenates in either men (Mancini *et al.*, 1965) or women (Escuder, 1936). Differing effects can be seen, with the resulting antibodies causing aspermatogenic orchitis in the men whilst the female antibodies impair fertility, presumably by their action upon the partner's sperm. Such an approach was thought useful in the development of a contraceptive, given the anti-fertility effects of the antibodies produced, but it is now realized that the use of cellular preparations are insufficiently specific because of the several proteins on the sperm surface shared with other cells. The possible risk of side effects has therefore led to the search for specific antigens involved in fertilization (Naz & Menge, 1990).

Certain anatomical abnormalities of the genital tract in men can give rise to antibody production, and these are of particular significance in sub-fertile couples. Congenital absence of the vas (Girgis *et al.*, 1982) in the presence of normal spermatogenesis is often associated with antibody production because of the increased probability of spermatozoa entering the lymphatic system and triggering an immune response, although this is not always the case (Patrizio *et al.*, 1989). Antibody production can also be seen in men with unilateral testicular obstruction (Hendry *et al.*, 1982) for similar reasons. The presence of these antibodies, particularly in oligozoospermic men, can therefore be used as a diagnostic marker for unilateral obstruction. Antibodies may also be produced in cases with a varicocoele where there is injury to the seminal epithelium (Gilbert, Witkin & Goldstein, 1989).

In the infertile couple, sperm antibody production can be associated with infection by *Chlamydia* and mycoplasmas (Soffer *et al.*, 1990) and in cases of prostatitis (Fjallbrant and Obrant, 1968). The infection can therefore have a secondary effect upon fertility through the antibodies.

Antibody production which has subsequent inhibitory effects upon fertility may be induced iatrogenically. A good example is that of vasectomy reversal or vasovasostomy (Sutherland *et al.*, 1984) in which fertility is hopefully restored after reversal of the vasectomy. Many operations achieve patency of the vas and yet a pregnancy does not occur after unprotected intercourse. The irony is that the antibodies are often produced in the testis/epididymis (Linnet & Fogh-Andersen, 1979) and so that the more successful the operation in achieving patency of the vas, the higher the titre of the antibodies in the semen and the greater the inhibitory effect upon fertility (Sutherland *et al.*, 1984). Examples of antibody induction in the female partner during the course of infertility treatment include the placing of relatively large numbers of sperm high in the female reproductive tract by either intraperitoneal (Livi *et al.*, 1990) or intrauterine (Friedman,

Juneau-Norcross & Sedensky, 1991) insemination, although this is not always seen. Great care must therefore be taken to monitor those patients treated to ensure that the treatment does not actually compound their infertility, rather than help alleviate the problem.

Incidence

The true incidence of sperm antibodies in fertile and sub-fertile subjects is difficult to determine, as it depends on the source of the individuals screened. Very often, the fertile individuals studied are either sperm donors or female members of staff, and the sub-fertile individuals are seeking treatment at specialized centres selected during the referral process. Nevertheless, estimations in the general infertile population show an incidence of approximately 5–10% in women and the same in men (Ansbacher, Mararang-Panga, 1971; Ingerslev, Hjort & Linnet, 1979; Clarke *et al.*, 1985*a*; Junk *et al.*, 1986). Studies detecting the specific classes of antibody in the serum of men have found the main class to be IgG (Clarke *et al.*, 1985*c*; Junk *et al.*, 1986). However, there are conflicting results regarding the presence of IgM antibodies. For instance, Clarke *et al.* (1985*c*) and Junk *et al.* (1986) both saw an absence of IgM in the male serum, whereas Bronson *et al.* (1982) found antibodies of the IgM class in a high proportion of samples with immobilizing activity. The type of antibodies present in female serum gives a different profile, with all three main classes of antibody being found (Clarke *et al.*, 1985*c*; Junk *et al.*, 1986).

The incidence of sperm antibodies in various groups of individuals is very different, probably reflecting the different mechanisms of induction and susceptibilities of the individuals. For instance, sexually active homosexual men have a higher incidence of antispermatozoal antibodies, of around 25%, reflecting the immunological stimulus of spermatozoa presented during anal intercourse (Witkin *et al.*, 1983). Another group with a high incidence are men undergoing vasovasostomy, with the antibodies being produced in response to the surgery as described above. Estimates vary according to the methods used, but frequencies of between 30% and 60% of men have sperm antibodies in their semen after vasectomy reversal (Linnet, Hjort & Fogh-Andersen, 1981; Sutherland *et al.*, 1984; Matson *et al.*, 1989).

Effect upon sperm transport

Sperm antibodies may well exert part of their influence in reducing fertility by impeding the transport of sperm to the site of fertilization. The motility of sperm in semen may well be affected directly by antisperm antibodies (De Almeida *et al.*, 1991). However, the main way in which antibodies can affect sperm transport is by affecting sperm progression through cervical mucus. In this way, the transport of sperm within the female reproductive tract can be severely affected. Studies have shown impaired progression of sperm in mucus *in vivo* using the post-coital test (Bronson, Cooper & Rosenfeld, 1984; Eggert-Kruse *et al.*, 1991). In addition, other workers have systematically looked at the effects of the antibodies *in vitro*. Jager *et al.* (1981) showed that IgG could cause sperm to become bound within the mucus, resulting in a shaking motion or phenomenon. Furthermore, Clarke (1985) showed IgA capable of inducing the shaking phenomenon in mucus. More recently, Bronson *et al.* (1987) confirmed that both IgA and IgG could be involved in the impaired progression of sperm through mucus, and that the effects were mediated through the Fc region of the antibodies.

Effect upon fertilization

The effect of antibodies upon the fertilization process has been studied extensively using zona-free hamster ova. IgA antibodies seem to have the least effect, with the IgG and either IgG/IgA (Haas *et al.*, 1985) or IgG/IgM (Bronson, Cooper & Rosenfeld, 1983) antibodies significantly limiting the interaction of the sperm with the oocyte. Requeda *et al.* (1983) specifically looked at patients following vasovasostomy, and also showed a reduced fertilising ability in the presence of antibodies. However, whilst most antibodies have an adverse effect, Bronson *et al.* (1990) have identified some antibodies which actually promote the interaction of sperm and oocyte resulting in polyspermy.

In an attempt to study the sperm-oocyte interaction in a homologous system, Bronson *et al.* (1982) used oocytes taken from the ovaries of women undergoing surgery and, under experimental conditions, demonstrated that IgA or IgG antibodies directed against the head of sperm severely impair the binding of the sperm to the zona pellucida. Using aged oocytes from an IVF programme and a very elegant experimental design in which test and control sperm were labelled with different dyes in the same incubation droplet, Liu, Clarke & Baker (1991) have confirmed the reduced ability of sperm to bind to the zona pellucida, and also shown a reduced interaction with the vitelline membrane of zona-free human oocytes. Much information is now available from IVF laboratories, and the fertilization of oocytes is often reduced in couples in which the male partner has antibodies in his semen (Clarke *et al.*, 1985*b*; Matson *et al.*, 1988; De Almeida *et al.*, 1989).

Conclusions

Sperm antibodies can significantly reduce the fertility of couples by either affecting sperm transport to the site of fertilization, or by affecting the fertilization process itself. These antibodies occur in approximately 10% of infertile couples. However, great care must be taken in choosing the methodology for the detection of the sperm antibodies, and the body fluid chosen for analysis.

References

Adeghe JH, Barratt CLR, Cohen J. Principles and guidelines for antisperm antibody screening. In: Barratt CLR, Cooke ID, eds *Advances in Clinical Andrology*. 1988; pp 71–9. Lancaster: MTP Press.

Ansbacher R, Mararang-Panga S, Srivannaboon S. Sperm antibodies in infertile couples. *Fertil Steril* 1971; **22**: 298–302.

Baker HWG, Clarke GN, McGowen P, Hoon Koh S, Cauchi MN. Increased frequency of autoantibodies in men with sperm antibodies. *Fertil Steril* 1985; **43**: 438–41.

Barratt CLR, Bolton AE, Cooke ID. Functional significance of white blood cells in the male and female reproductive tract. *Hum Reprod* 1990; **5**: 639–48.

Barratt CLR, Dunphy BC, McLeod I, Cooke ID. The poor prognostic value of low to moderate levels of sperm surface-bound antibodies. *Hum Reprod* 1992; **7**: 95–8.

Boettcher B, Kay DJ, Rumke Ph, Wright LE. Human sera containing immunoglobulin and non-immunoglobulin spermagglutinins. *Biol Reprod* 1971; **5**: 236–45.

Bronson RA, Cooper GW, Margoliath EJ, Naz RK, Hamilton MS. The detection in human sera of antisperm antibodies reactive with FA-1, an evolutionary conserved antigen, and with murine spermatozoa. *Fertil Steril* 1989; **52**: 457–62.

Bronson RA, Cooper GW, Rosenfeld DL. Correlation between regional specificity of antisperm antibodies to the spermatozoa surface and complement-mediated sperm immobilization. *Am J Reprod Immunol* 1982; **2**: 222–4.

Bronson RA, Cooper GW, Rosenfeld DL. Sperm-specific isoantibodies and autoantibodies inhibit the binding of human sperm to the human zona pellucida. *Fertil Steril* 1982; **38**: 724–9.

Bronson RA, Cooper GW, Rosenfeld DL. Complement-mediated effects of sperm head-directed human antibodies on the ability of human spermatozoa to penetrate zona-free hamster eggs. *Fertil Steril* 1983; **40**: 91–5.

Bronson RA, Cooper GW, Rosenfeld DL. Sperm antibodies: role in infertility. *Fertil Steril* 1984; **42**: 171–83.

Bronson RA, Cooper GW, Rosenfeld DL, Gilbert JV, Plaut AG. The effect of an IgA_1 protease on immunoglobulins bound to the sperm surface and sperm cervical mucus penetrating ability. *Fertil Steril* 1987; **47**: 985–91.

Bronson RA, Fusi F, Cooper GW, Phillips DM. Antisperm antibodies induce polyspermy by promoting adherence of human sperm to zona-free hamster eggs. *Hum Reprod* 1990; **5**: 690–6.

Clarke GN. Detection of antispermatozoal antibodies of IgA, IgG and IgM immunoglobulin classes in cervical mucus. *Am J Reprod Immunol* 1984; **6**: 195–7.

Clarke GN. Induction of the shaking phenomenon by IgA class antispermatozoal antibodies from serum. *Am J Reprod Immunol Microbiol* 1985; **9**: 12–14.

Clarke GN, Elliott PJ, Smaila C. Detection of sperm antibodies in semen using the immunobead test: a survey of 813 consecutive patients. *Am J Reprod Immunol* 1985a; 7: 118–23.

Clarke GN, Lopata A, McBain JC, Baker HWG, Johnston WIH. Effect of sperm antibodies in males on human *in vitro* fertilization (IVF). *Am J Reprod Immunol Microbiol* 1985b; **8**: 62–6.

Clarke GN, Stojanoff A, Cauchi MN, Johnston WIH. The immunoglobulin class of antispermatozoal antibodies in serum. *Am J Reprod Immunol Microbiol* 1985c; 7: 143–7.

Cooper GW, Bronson RA. Characterization of humoral antibodies reactive with spermatozoa, N-acetyl galactosamine, and a putative blood group antigen in seminal plasma. *Fertil Steril* 1990; **53**: 888–91.

De Almeida M, Gazagne I, Jeulin C, Herry M, Belaisch-Allart J, Frydman R, Jouannet P. Testart J. *In vitro* processing of sperm with autoantibodies and *in vitro* fertilization results. *Hum Reprod* 1989; **4**: 49–53.

De Almeida M, Zouari R, Jouannet P, Feneux D. *In-vitro* effects of anti-sperm antibodies on human sperm movement. *Hum Reprod* 1991; **6**: 405–10.

Eggert-Kruse W, Hofsass A, Jaury E, Tilgen W, Gerhard I, Runnebaum B. Relationship between local anti-sperm antibodies and sperm–mucus interaction *in vitro* and *in vivo*. *Hum Reprod* 1991; **6**: 267–76.

Escuder CJ. Temporary biologic sterility of women produced by human sperm. *Am Fac Med Montevideo* 1936; **21**: 889–937.

Fjallbrant B, Obrant O. Clinical and survival findings in men with sperm antibodies. *Acta Obstet Gynaecol Scand* 1968; **47**: 451–68.

Friberg J. A simple and sensitive micro-method for demonstration of sperm agglutinating activity in serum from infertile men and women. *Acta Obstet Gynaecol Scand* 1974; suppl 36: 21–9.

Friedman AJ, Juneau-Norcross M, Sedensky B. Antisperm antibody production following intrauterine insemination. *Hum Reprod* 1991; **6**: 1125–8.

Fusi F, Bronson RA. Effects of incubation time in serum and capacitation on spermatozoal reactivity with antisperm antibodies. *Fertil Steril* 1990; **54**: 887–93.

Gilbert BR, Witkin SS, Goldstein M. Correlation of sperm-bound immunoglobulins with impaired semen analysis in infertile men with varicoceles. *Fertil Steril* 1989; **52**: 469–73.

Girgis SM, Ekladios EM, Iskander R, El-Dakhly R, Girgis FN. Sperm antibodies in serum and semen in men with bilateral congenital absence of the vas deferens. *Arch Ancrol* 1982; **8**: 301–5.

Haas GG, Ausmanus M, Culp L, Tureck RW, Blasco L. The effect of immunoglobulin occurring on human sperm in vivo on the human sperm/hamster ova penetration assay. *Am J Reprod Immunol Microbiol* 1985; 7: 109–12.

Haas GG, Debault LE, D'Cruz O, Shuey R. The effect of fixatives and/or air-drying on the plasma and acrosomal membranes of human sperm. *Fertil Steril* 1988; **50**: 487–92.

Haneji T, Koide SS. Identification of the sperm antigen interacting with antibodies in serum from an infertile woman. *Andrologia* 1990; **22**: 473–7.

Hendry WF, Parslow JM, Stedronska J, Wallace DMA. The diagnosis of unilateral testicular obstruction in subfertile males. *Br J Urol* 1982; **54**: 774–9.

Hendry WF, Stedronska J, Lake RA. Mixed erythrocyte-spermatozoa antiglobulin reaction (MAR Test) for IgA antisperm antibodies in subfertile males. *Fertil Steril* 1982; **37**: 108–12.

Howe SE, Grider SL, Lynch DM, Fink LM. Antisperm antibody binding to human acrosin: a study of patients with unexplained infertility. *Fertil Steril* 1991; **55**: 1176–82.

Humphreys-Beher MG, Garrison PW, Blackwell RE. Detection of antigalactosyltransferase antibodies in plasma from patients with antisperm antibodies. *Fertil Steril* 1990; **54**: 133–7.

Ingerslev HJ, Paulsen F. Bromelin for liquefaction of cervical mucus in sperm antibody testing: its effect on spermagglutinating immunoglobulin G. *Fertil Steril* 1980; **33**: 61–3.

Ingerslev HJ, Hjort T, Linnet L. Immunoglobulin classes of human sperm antibodies. *J Clin Lab Immunol* 1979; **2**: 239–43.

Isojima S, Li TS, Ashtaki Y. Immunologic analysis of sperm immobilizing factors found in sera of women with unexplained sterility. *Am J Obs Gynecol* 1968; **101**: 677–83.

Jager S, Kremer J, Kuiken J, van Slochteren-Draaisma T, Mulder I, de Wilde-Janssen IW. Induction of the shaking phenomenon by pretreatment of spermatozoa with sera containing antispermatozoal antibodies. *Fertil Steril* 1981; **36**: 784–91.

Jager S, Kremer J, van Slochteren-Draaisma T. A simple method of screening for antisperm antibodies in the human male. *Int J Fertil* 1978; **23**: 12–21.

Junk SM, Matson PL, O'Halloran F, Yovich JL. Use of immunobeads to detect human antispermatozoal antibodies. *Clin Reprod Fert* 1986; **4**: 199–206.

Kay DJ, Boettcher B, Yovich JL, Stanger JD. Antispermatozoal antibodies in human follicular fluid. *Am J Reprod Immunol Microbiol* 1985; **7**: 113–17.

Kibrick S, Belding DL, Merrill B. Methods for detection of antibodies against mammalian spermatozoa. II A gelatin agglutination test. *Fertil Steril* 1952; **3**: 430–8.

Koyama K, Kameda K, Nakamura N, Kubota K, Shigeta M, Isojima S. Recognition of carbohydrate antigen epitopes by sperm-immobilizing antibodies in sera of infertile women. *Fertil Steril* 1991; **56**: 954–9.

Linnet L, Fogh-Andersen P. Vasovasostomy: sperm agglutinins in operatively obtained epididymal fluid and in seminal plasma before and after operation. *J Clin Lab Immunol* 1979; **2**: 245–8.

Linnet L, Suonimen JJO. A comparison of eight techniques for the evaluation of the auto-immune response to spermatozoa after vasectomy. *J Reprod Immunol* 1987; **4**: 133–44.

Linnet L, Hjort T, Fogh-Andersen P. Association between failure to impregnate after vasovasostomy and sperm agglutinins in semen. *Lancet* 1981; **i**: 117–19.

Liu DY, Clarke GN, Baker HGW. Inhibition of human sperm–zona pellucida and sperm–oolemma binding by antisperm antibodies. *Fertil Steril* 1991; **55**: 440–2.

Livi C, Coccia E, Versari L, Pratesi S, Guzzoni P. Does intraperitoneal insemination in the absence of prior sensitization carry with it a risk of subsequent immunity to sperm? *Fertil Steril* 1990; **53**: 137–42.

Mancini RE, Andrada JA, Sarceni C, Bachmann AE, Lavieri JC, Nemirovsky M. Immunological and testicular response in men sensitised with human testicular homogenate. *J Clin Endocrinol Metab* 1965; **25**: 859–75.

Matson PL, Junk SM, Masters JRW, Pryor JP, Yovich JL. The incidence and influence upon fertility of antisperm antibodies in seminal fluid following vasectomy reversal. *Int J Androl* 1989; **12**: 98–103.

Matson PL, Junk SM, Spittle JW, Yovich JL. Effect of antispermatozoal antibodies in seminal plasma upon spermatozoal function. *Int J Androl* 1988; **11**: 101–6.

Meinertz H, Linnet L, Fogh-Andersen P, Hjort T. Antisperm antibodies and fertility after vasovasostomy: a follow-up study of 216 men. *Fertil Steril* 1990; **54**: 315–21.

Monroe JR, Altenbaum DC, Mathur S. Changes in sperm antibody test results when spermatozoa are subjected to capacitating conditions. *Fertil Steril* 1990; **54**: 1114–20.

Naz R, Menge A. Development of antisperm contraceptive vaccine from humans: why and how? *Hum Reprod* 1990; **5**: 511–18.

Patrizio P, Moretti-Rojas I, Ord T, Balmaceda J, Silber S, Asch RH. Low incidence of sperm antibodies in men with congenital absence of the vas deferens. *Fertil Steril* 1989; **52**: 1018–21.

Requeda E, Charron J, Roberts KD, Chapdelaine A, Bleau G. Fertilizing capacity and sperm antibodies in vasovasostomized men. *Fertil Steril* 1983; **39**: 197–203.

Soffer Y, Ron-El R, Golan A, Herman A, Caspi E, Samura Z. Male genital mycoplasmas and Chlamydia trachomatis culture: its relationship with accessory gland function, sperm quality and autoimmunity. *Fertil Steril* 1990; **53**: 331–6.

Sutherland PD, Matson PL, Masters JRW, Pryor JP. Association between infertility following reversal of vasectomy and the presence of sperm agglutinating activity in semen. *Int J Androl* 1984; **7**: 503–8.

Witkin SS, Bongiovanni AM, Yu IR, Goldstein M, Wallace J, Sonnabend J. Humoral immune responses in healthy heterosexual, homosexual and vasectomized men and in men with the acquired immune deficiency syndrome. *Aids Research* 1983; **1**: 31–44.

Wong WP. Sperm antibody activity in human fallopian tube fluid. *Fertil Steril* 1979; **32**: 681–4.

World Health Organization (1987). *Laboratory Manual for the Examination of Human Semen and Semen-Cervical Mucus Interactions*. Cambridge: Cambridge University Press.

13

Spermatogenesis

C. L. R. BARRATT

Background

Spermatogenesis is the process of cellular differentiation leading to the production of spermatozoa. This process, which is probably one of the most complicated mammalian cellular differentiation processes, occurs within the seminiferous tubules of the testis.

In mammals and birds there are two ovoid testes. Humans have quite small testes. Each testis is typically 15–20 ml in volume, 4 cm in length and weighs 10–15 g (less than 0.1% of the body weight). The size of the testis varies in part according to the race. The Chinese in particular are recognized as having smaller testes than Caucasians, although the relationship between testis size and body size is unclear (Glover *et al.*, 1990).

The testis is surrounded by a capsule which contains large arteries and veins (Fig. 1). Within the testis there are the seminiferous tubules in between which is the interstitial tissue. The seminiferous tubules are surrounded by myoid cells. The interstitial tissue contains blood vessels, nerves, Leydig cells, white blood cells and lymph vessels.

The ends of the seminiferous tubules open into the rete restis which is located near the epididymis in men and rodents. In bulls it is located in the centre of the testis. The ductuli efferenti lead from the rete testis into the epididymis where they form one single highly convoluted tubule that gives rise to the vas deferens (Fig. 1).

In man as well as many other mammals the testes descend into a scrotum during fetal or early post-natal life. This is particularly interesting as the majority of vertebrates have their testes normally situated in the abdomen (Glover *et al.*, 1990). In animals with a scrotum, the temperature of the testis and the epididymis is slightly cooler than the body, usually between 6–8 °C in bulls and rams, although in man this temperature difference is not so great (2 °C). It is therefore apparent

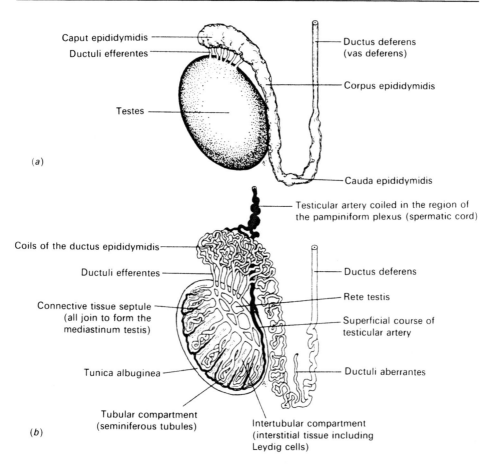

Fig. 1. The gross appearance of the testis and epididymis. (*a*) Outer appearance.
(*b*) inner appearance. (From Glover *et al.*, 1990.)

that the human testis is less sensitive to increased temperature than some
other animals. The reason why a lower temperature is required for efficient
spermatogenesis is not fully understood. It is known that body temperature can
be detrimental to sperm production, e.g. round spermatids are particularly
susceptible to body temperature. A lower temperature may be necessary for
sperm maturation in the epididymis, however, this hypothesis warrants further
investigation. Retention of one or more testes in the abdomen is termed
cryptorchidism. Bilaterally cryptorchid men are always infertile, but some men
with unilateral cryptorchidism can produce spermatozoa.

The spermatic cord contains the blood supply to and from the testis, as well
as the vas deferens, lymphatics and nerves. The pampiniform plexus is a complex
of veins which surround and intermingle with the testicular artery above the testis
and extends into the spermatic cord (see Fig. 1). In man and in many other

animals the pampiniform plexus consists of a complex vascular system involved in thermoregulation. This is an efficient countercurrent exchange system to cool the blood before it enters the testis and warm the blood before it returns to the body. This system also acts to eliminate the pulse pressure from arterial blood going to the testis. The testicular veins have valves and frequently they become varicose (producing varicoceles). Varicoceles are often associated with the left testicle possible due to the acute angle that the left testicular vein enters into the left renal vein. Varicocele can often be associated with an increased intrascrotal temperature which, it is suggested, affects fertility. Until very recently, the relationship between varicocele and fertility remained highly controversial, however, the WHO recently published their data on over 9000 men clearly showing a significant association of varicocele with an abnormal semen profile. Varicocele was accompanied by a decrease in testicular volume and decline of Leydig cell secretion (see WHO, 1992).

Seminiferous tubules and spermatogenesis

Sertoli cells

These are diploid cells which extend from the periphery of the tubule to the lumen. They play a pivotal role in spermatogenesis. Their main function is to create a favourable environment for germ cell differentiation. They have contacts with all other cell types. Their basal portion rests on the boundary tissue which has direct access to substances from the general circulation. Spermatogonia lie in between the Sertoli cells and the boundary tissue, whereas other cells are sited in between other Sertoli cells or embedded in their cytoplasm (Fig. 2). This interaction can be likened to trees in an orchard (Sertoli cells) and corresponding fruit (germ cells) (see Setchell, 1982).

Sertoli cells have a complicated morphology. They have considerable amounts of smooth endoplasmic reticulum and have a distinct cytoskeleton in the form of a cluster of microfilaments. The most fascinating features of these cells are the specialized junctional complexes. They form many different types of junctional structures with the other cell types maintaining contact and cellular communication with the germ cells. The most important junction is probably that between each of the Sertoli cell which brings the cells very close to each other so that they block the penetration of substances such as horseradish peroxidase and lanthanum. There are therefore two compartments in the seminiferous tubules: a basal compartment between the boundary tissue and the junctions and an adluminal compartment above the junctions. This junction is called the blood–testis barrier (Fig. 2). Spermatogonia exist in the basal compartment and later spermatogenic cells in the adluminal compartment.

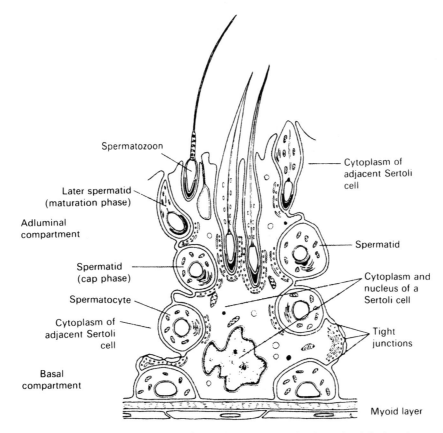

Fig. 2. Diagram of the seminiferous epithelium illustrating how the tight junctions between Sertoli cells divide the epithelium into basal and adluminal compartments. (From Glover *et al.*, 1990.)

Leydig cells

In man, these form into clusters especially around the blood vessels. They have an extensive smooth endoplasmic reticulum which is necessary for the production of steroids. In men, they have unique crystalline inclusions in their cytoplasm, which vary in size and shape (Reinke's crystals). Sometimes there are Leydig cells which lack these inclusions and they are usually considered as immature forms of the cell (Glover *et al.*, 1990). The Leydig cells are bound together by tight junctions.

Germ cells

Spermatogonia

The germ cells do not divide until after puberty. The spermatogonia, which are diploid, are situated close to the basement membrane and multiply mitotically either to produce other spermatocytes or enter differentiation to produce primary spermatocytes. The spermatogonia are divided into three types (A—A0 A1 A2 A3 A4, intermediate and B). Spermatogonial mitoses are either random (confined to A 0) or synchronized where the divisions are coordinated to the spermatogenic cycle. In these divisions, cytoplasmic links persist between daughter cells after each division. Type B spermatogonia are the ones which develop into spermatocytes. The mitotic kinetics of these divisions are complicated and still the subject of controversy (see DeRooij, Van Dissel-Emiliani & VanPelt, 1989 for further details).

Spermatocytes

Spermatocytes divide by meiosis to form four haploid spermatids. During these divisions, two important events occur which have major genetic consequences. First, there is the random separation of homologous chromosomes and secondly, there is the crossing over of genetic material. These two events product the genetic diversity required for survival of the species.

Prophase is very protracted and divides into stages: leptotene, zygotene, pachytene, diplotene and diakinesis. As the spermatocytes enter the leptotene stage of the first meiotic prophase they move away from the basement membrane towards the lumen. In the zygotene phase (where the homologous chromosomes, one from each parent, come together) they are separated from the basement membrane by the blood–testis barrier. Pachytene is the longest stage of meiosis and the stage where the spermatocytes are very susceptible to damage. It is during this stage that there is crossing over of genetic material (chiasma) (see Fig. 3). Each primary spermatocyte gives rise to two secondary spermatocytes. These secondary spermatocytes exist in a very short phase and each one divides to form two haploid spermatids. The behaviour of the sex chromosomes during meiosis is different from that of the other chromosomes in timing of DNA replication, condensation and transcription.

Spermatids

The development of spermatids from meiosis to detachment of the spermatozoa is known as spermiogenesis. This is a truly remarkable process during which the cell changes from a simple cell into a highly differentiated spermatozoon undergoing complex morphological, physiological and biochemical changes. This takes approximately 22 days in humans. The process by which this transformation occurs in poorly understood (Hamilton & Waites, 1990). One important feature is that of the many changes that take place during this time are unique events

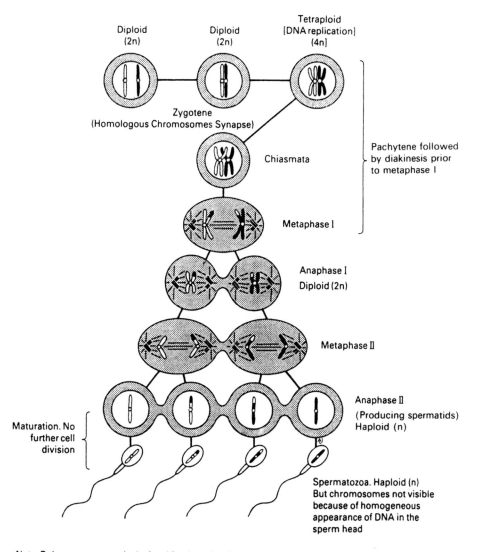

Note. Only one crossover is depicted for the sake of clarity and simplicity

Fig. 3. Chromosomal changes that occur in meiosis, e.g. during spermatogenesis.
(From Glover *et al.*, 1990.)

that do not occur in other cells. The process is tightly synchronized and integrated so that very small deviations are likely to lead to infertility, although the nature of these deviations are not yet certain.

In many animals, the young spermatids are associated with an older generation of spermatids formed one cycle earlier. At first the spermatid is a simple cell but many changes take place to form the basic cytoskeleton of the spermatozoon (see Fig. 4). The nuclear chromatin becomes more condensed. The cisternae of

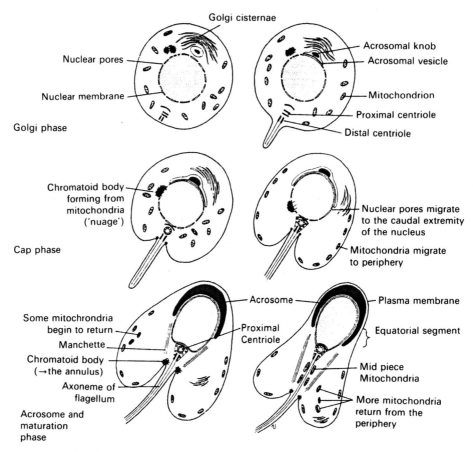

Fig. 4. Developmental changes in the spermatid that fashion the sperm head and
the beginnings of the tail. (From Glover *et al.*, 1990.)

the Golgi apparatus, which are more complex than in other cells, fuse to form
one acrosome which then migrates to the nucleus and spreads over the nuclear
surface developing into the acrosome system. The inner membrane of this is
closely associated with the nuclear envelope. This is one of the few secretory
structures which become so intimately associated with a nucleus. The two
centrioles migrate opposite to the developing acrosome, one assumes a radial
alignment and develops into the axoneme of the future tail, while the other, which
is located at right angles, forms the connecting piece which joins the tail to the
nucleus. The migration of the centrioles to the nucleus in spermatids is unique.
The axoneme of the tail elongates and at its base becomes attached to the annulus.
The mitochrondia divide, although the mechanism is unknown, and they
associate with the outer dense fibres to form a characteristic double helix. Several
structures appear and disappear during spermatogenesis including the manchette

and a chromatoid body. The latter may be associated with the storage of genetic material.

When spermatogenesis is complete, the cytoplasmic extensions with the Sertoli cells are broken and the spermatozoa are released. In some cases up to 70% of the cytoplasm of the mature spermatid is left behind and may be phagocytozed by the Sertoli cells.

Synthesis of nucleic acids, proteins and haploid gene expression

RNA and protein synthesis is maximal during meiosis and then decreases abruptly during early spermatogenesis to almost undetectable levels. During spermatogenesis the nucleus exchanges its somatic like nucleosome structure for the nucleoprotamine structure of the mammalian spermatozoon. The histones are replaced first with transition proteins which are in turn replaced by small basic proteins rich in arginine called protamines. The main role of these protamines appears to be to compact the nucleus to produce functional spermatozoa. Sperm DNA interacts with protamines to form linear side-by-side arrays of chromatin, whereas in somatic cells the DNA is coiled around the histones. Mammalian sperm DNA is the most tightly packed eukaryotic DNA, being at least six-fold more highly condensed than DNA in mitotic chromosomes, this allows the DNA to be compacted into a small volume (Ward & Coffey, 1991).

Haploid gene expression is where the unique genotype of a spermatozoon would be revealed in its structure or function. It is fair to say that the existence of haploid gene expression, despite the recent attention of several workers using sophisticated molecular biological techniques, is still controversial. Several putative haploid expressed gene products have been identified and are now under intensive investigation (Hecht, 1990; Johnson, 1991).

Probably the most widespread quoted example of haploid gene expression is thought to be the T locus mouse. The dominant T allele causes short tails in the homozygous, and it is lethal in the heterozygote. With several recessive T alleles it produces tail-less animals. When the heterozygous males for some T alleles are mated more than half of the offspring carry the T gene, i.e. transmission ratio distortion (TRD). The reason for this TRD is still uncertain, it has been suggested that the T spermatozoa have an advantage over other sperm (+) as very few + sperm can fertilize eggs *in vivo*. Interestingly, mice with both t/t spermatozoa are infertile, although they produce spermatozoa.

Despite considerable research, the mechanisms of this non Mendelian transmission and the relationship to expression of the haploid genome remain elusive. Interestingly, genetically distinct spermatids which develop in a syncytium have intercellular bridges (1 μm in diameter) which connect the cells ensuring synchronous development. It is now known that, in some cases, specific mRNA can move from spermatid to spermatid through these bridges; therefore products of all post meiotic genes may possibly be equally distributed amongst spermatids. This does not mean that all products are equally transported or shared but this interesting question warrants further investigation.

Diverse biochemical studies have identified and defined the time of expression of various testicular marker proteins. However, our understanding of the molecular biology of male germ cell maturation in mammals is limited and is continuously being refined (Johnson, 1991; Hecht, 1990; Ivel, 1992).

The spermatogenic cycle

In many animals, certain spermatogenic cells are only found in association with certain other cells. For example, in the mouse an A1 spermatogonium about to undergo its first synchronised division is always found in association with preleptotene and mature spermatids about to be released as spermatozoa. Each one develops in synchrony with the other so that, if one section of the seminiferous tubule could be watched over time, a series of different cell associations would be seen until the cycle was completed and the original cell association appeared again but with each cell one generation further advanced (Setchell, 1982). This association is termed the spermatogenic cycle. An analogy has been drawn between this and the recruitment and graduation of college students where once the process starts it continues at a defined rate such that cells (students) at a given developmental stage are almost always associated with other cells (students) at respective developmental stages, e.g. first-year, second-year and third-year college students (Johnson, 1990). There are differences, however, e.g. for each committed spermatogonium, a potential of 64 spermatozoa can be produced, whereas less than one student graduates per student entering college, the frequency of release is also greater in spermatogenesis where at least 20 committed spermatogonia are entering the process every second in humans such that there is a continual release of spermatozoa somewhere in the testis. The spermatogenic cycle must be repeated four to five times from the spermatogonium to the release of the spermatozoa derived from that particular cell. The length of each spermatogenic cycle is constant for any one species ranging between 8 and 16 days (8.9 days in mice to 16 days in humans).

Spermatogenic cycle in humans

In contrast to the regular pattern of seminiferous epithelium in many animals as described above, no such pattern is immediately obvious in the human. Many

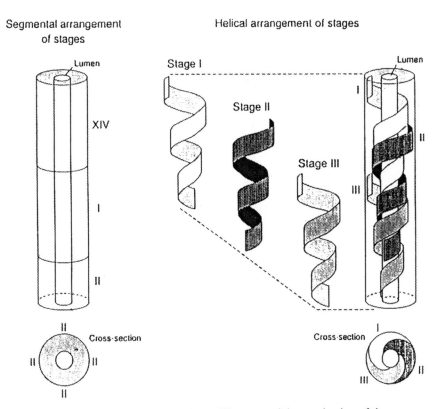

Segmental arrangement of stages

Helical arrangement of stages

Fig. 5. Diagrammatic illustration of the different spatial organization of the stages of the spermatogenic cycle along a short length of seminiferous tubule in the rat and human. The latter is based on the observations of Schulze and colleagues. (Taken from Sharpe 1994.)

irregularities occur such as the presence of more than one spermatogenic stage in tubular cross section and frequent inappropriate presence or absence of germ cells in typical cell associations. All this suggests that human spermatogenesis is irregular or at least subject to a lesser degree of coordination and synchronization. Recently, however, Schulze and colleagues provided strong evidence for the orderly sequencing of the seminiferous epithelium (Schulze & Rehder, 1984), suggesting that the stages of spermatogenesis are fitted helically into the longitudinal course of the seminiferous tubule. The seminiferous epithelium is therefore subject to a complex plan of organization based on the geometry of spirals which is a fundamental principle of growth and differentiation occurring ubiquitously in biology (Figs. 5 and 6). This work has mainly concentrated on the special arrangements of primary spermatocytes. The descriptions of the arrangements of cells are described in detail by Schulze & Rehder, 1984). Suffice to say that the spermatocyte populations of successive degrees of

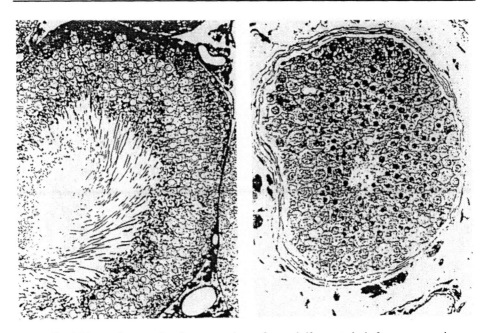

Fig. 6. Photomicrographs of cross-sections of a seminiferous tubule from a normal adult rat (left) and a normal adult man (right). Note that the epithelium of the rat tubule cross-section is homogenous (all at late stage VII/early stage VIII) whereas that for the human contains a mixture of stages. Refer also to Fig. 5. Photomicrographs were kindly supplied by Professor Jeffrey Kerr, Monash University. (Taken from Sharpe, 1994.)

development are arranged in helices that are contracted conically to the tubular lumen. This has been likened to the setting on of leaves (phyllotaxis) during plant growth. There is some evidence that type B and preleptotene spermatocytes are also arranged in this order. Thus the arrangement of the seminiferous epithelium in humans is not irregular or chaotic as once thought but shows a complex organisation. The mechanisms regulating this complex arrangement are largely unknown but paracrine and autocrine regulatory mechanisms are likely to be involved.

Interestingly, intermediate forms of organization between humans and rodents exists, e.g. in the crab-eating monkey where a helical arrangement and clear spermatogenic stages are seen. In these animals, there are tubular segments where stages occupy only small areas of spermatogenic tissue.

Efficiency of spermatogenesis

In all species studied to date, one common feature is that the majority of the germ cells *fail* to complete development. Degeneration of the majority of developing germ cells is thus a physiological phenomenon. There appear three critical phases of extensive cell loss: spermatogonial development, meiotic divisions and spermatogenesis. In rats, only 25% of the theoretically possible number of preleptotene spermatocytes are produced from the original population of A1 spermatogonia. Spermiogenic loss in meiotic divisions has been reported in mice, rats and bulls. In humans, using more sophisticated techniques, comparing the potential daily sperm production per gram of testis parenchyma with daily sperm production per gram testis parenchyma has shown that considerable degeneration occurs (Johnson, 1986). Johnson concluded that 50% of potential sperm production was lost during meiosis and that this loss was confined to the end of the second meiotic division (Johnson, 1986). Very little cell loss occurs during spermiogenesis in man, mice, rats or bulls. In seasonally breeding animals at sexual regression there is often a depletion of germ cells in the testis. Photoperiodicity and availability of food are important factors controlling this in seasonally breeding animals but the mechanisms of degeneration and wastage in the normal testis are still a matter of debate. Limiting factors such as the number of Sertoli cells are important.

Spermatogenesis is therefore not a very efficient process, humans having a low efficiency of spermatogenesis when compared to other species, being only 25% as efficient as that of rats and other primates (see Table 1).

In some T locus mice, which ejaculate low numbers of spermatozoa, there is an increase in germ cell loss in the testis at spermatogenesis. This greater than normal wastage of germ cells accounts for at least 20% of the reduction in numbers in the ejaculate, an increase in resorption in the epididymis accounting for the rest (80%) (Barratt & Cohen, 1986). This observation highlights an important question: can the low numbers of spermatozoa in the ejaculate of some men be accounted for by an increase in the wastage of germ cells at a particular stage of development? Oligozoospermia is present in up to 30% of the men attending our infertility clinic (Barratt, Bolton & Cooke, 1990) and accurate quantitative studies assessing germ cell wastage have not yet been performed. Such studies might help determine, at least in some of these men, if there is an increased wastage in the testis and at what stages this occurs. This interesting phenomenon requires further investigation because, if it proved possible to ascertain the mechanisms of this wastage, rational therapy might then be proposed. We may even be able to increase the sperm production in normal men!

There is an age-related reduction in daily sperm production in men which is associated with a loss of Sertoli cells. This usually results from an increase in germ cell degeneration during prophase of meiosis, i.e. loss of primary spermatocytes. There is also a reduction in the number of Leydig cells, non-Leydig interstitial cells, myoid cells and Sertoli cells.

Table 1. *Comparative efficiency of spermatogenesis in a number of mammals using either the elongate spermatid:Sertoli cell ratio (Mean ± SD) or the rate of daily sperm production (DSP) per gram of testis*

	Efficiency of spermatogenesis			
Species	Number of elongate spermatids per Sertoli cell	DSP per gram of testis (10^6/g)	Paired testis weight (g)	Total DSP (10^9/both testes)
Rabbit	12.2 ± 2.0	25	6.4	0.16
Hamster	10.8 ± 1.4	24	3	0.07
Rat	10.3 ± 1.6	24	3.7	0.09
Rhesus monkey	—	23	49	1.1
Boar	—	23	720	16.2
Ram	—	21	500	9.5
Bull (Charolais)	—	13	775	8.9
Cynomolgus monkey	8.2 ± 3.6	—	—	—
Orang-utang	5.7 ± 2.3	—	—	—
Human	3.9 ± 0.5	4.4	34	0.13[a]

[a]This is an average figure. It may range from 0.02×10^9–0.27×10^9/day.
Adapted from Sharpe (1994).

Endocrine and paracrine control of spermatogenesis

The secretion of the pituitary gonadotrophins, follicle stimulating hormone (FSH) and luteinising hormone (LH) are the main modulators of spermatogenesis. LH stimulates the Leydig cells in the interstitial tissue to increase androgen production, whose main site of action is the Sertoli cells. FSH acts on the germinal epithelium and Sertoli cells, and has only minor direct effects on androgen production. Complete qualitative spermatogenesis requires both FSH and LH.

The situation, however, is not as simple as this as a number of factors complicate the issue. First, there are clear species differences which make generalizations of this intricate control difficult. Secondly, much of the research has been done on animals, specifically the rat, thus limiting the value of extrapolation to the human. Thirdly, the testis cannot be regarded as homogenous in terms of its biochemical and physiological functions. Perhaps a more realistic way of understanding the endocrine/paracrine control of spermatogenesis is to view each segment of the tubule as a microcosm (De Kretser *et al.*, 1990).

The response of the seminiferous epithelium to exogenous stimuli (LH, FSH) is modulated by local testicular factors. The interaction between the endocrine and paracrine mechanisms determines the functions within the testis. However, the nature and mechanisms of these interactions are still a matter of controversy as, although a large number of potential paracrine factors have been identified, there is little direct evidence of their physiological role *in vivo* (Fritz, 1990; De Kretser *et al.*, 1990; Bellve & Zheng, 1989; Skinner, 1991).

The functions of all the different testicular cell types are interconnected, e.g. testosterone produced by Leydig cells acts on peritubular cells and Sertoli cells, and via this action maintains and drives germ cell development as well as exerting an effect on the vasculature (Sharpe, 1990). Testosterone thus primarily acts as a paracrine and not as an endocrine product in the testis (Sharpe, 1990).

The Sertoli cells can influence the Leydig cells and their precursors and this effect can be modulated by the germ cells. The mechanisms involved in germ cell–Sertoli cell interaction are incompletely understood but clear evidence exists that intact pachytene spermatocytes affect the Sertoli cells by stimulating the production of androgen binding protein and stimulating adenylate cyclase activity. These effects are cell specific as round spermatids have no stimulatory effect (Djakiew & Dym, 1988). Sertoli cells produce proteins including transferrin and insulin-like growth factor which also modulate intratesticular regulation. The production and effects of many of the paracrine regulators produced by the Sertoli cells are influenced by the stage of the cycle of the seminiferous epithelium, e.g. production by Sertoli cells of transferrin.

In conclusion, growth and differentiation of testicular germ cells involves a series of complex interactions between somatic and germinal elements (see reviews by Bellve & Zheng, 1989; Sharpe, 1990, 1992). These interactions are endocrine, paracrine and autocrine and may have several similarities to those which operate in the brain, pituitary and liver. These mechanisms obviously achieve a fine balance for the normal functions of the testis (see Sharpe, 1994).

Immune status of the testis: immunosurveillance

Spermatozoa, late pachytene spermatocytes and spermatids express unique antigens that have the potential to elicit an autoimmune response in the male. These antigens are not formed until puberty in man and therefore immune tolerance is not developed. Commensurate with the development of autoantigens is the development of the blood testis barrier (Fig. 2). Until recently it was thought that isolation of the autoantigens by the blood testis barrier prevented an immune response against these cells and that there was a paucity of immune competent cells in the testis to achieve an effective immune response. The testis is considered to be an immune privileged site, i.e. transplanted foreign tissue can survive for a period of time without immunological rejection. There are two other main areas of immune privilege in man, i.e. the anterior chamber of the eye and the brain. Although a deficient lymphatic drainage is one of the main features of this immune privilege in both the eye and brain this does not apply to the testis. Studies using monoclonal antibodies against the various white blood cells show clearly that there are numerous immunocompetent cells within the testis. It would appear that the blood–testis barrier is not an absolute barrier to the sequestration of antigens. The current consensus of opinion is that there is immune surveillance in the testis and the epididymis which shows an active immunoregulation to prevent autoimmune disease (Barratt et al., 1990, Mahi-Brown, Yule & Tung, 1988). These mechanisms are both systemic and local (Chapter 12).

Effects of vasectomy

The effects of vasectomy on spermatogenesis differ between species and individuals. Generally in mice there are some focal changes in tubules and a slight reduction in the number of spermatozoa produced (Barratt & Cohen, 1986, 1987, 1988). However, there is no effect on the cycle duration of spermatogenesis or on sperm transport to the caput epididymis (Barratt & Cohen, 1987, 1988). It is clear therefore, that spermatozoa are still produced; however, the testis of men and animals who have had a vasectomy do not expand or rupture. Thus the natural resorption mechanisms in the epididymis act to dispose of these extra spermatozoa (Barratt & Cooke, 1988; Barratt, Bolton & Cooke, 1990). There is a paucity of quantitative data available in men. Jarrow completed a semi-quantitative study on men after vasectomy and found that there was no correlation with amount of damage to the seminiferous epithelium and length of time since operation (Jarrow et al., 1985).

Testicular biopsy in men

Testicular biopsy was introduced as an additional investigative procedure for male infertility over 50 years ago. This investigation has been the subject of intense debate and, although popular and used indiscriminately in the past, it is now used only in certain circumstances. When performed with care it is associated with only a few complications. The needle biopsy can be used as an alternative and is performed as an office procedure under local anaesthesia. However, being a blind procedure, it can result in injury to the epididymis or the testicular artery and useful specimens are not always obtained. The main purpose of a testicular biopsy in infertility is to distinguish between obstructuve azoospermia and primary testicular failure. Biopsy is usually indicated when the FSH is normal, vas palpable, testis size normal and there is severe oligozoospermia or azoospermia (Magid, Cash & Goldtein, 1990). Flow cytometry can be used as an alternative method to routine histopathology to evaluate spermatogenesis. In flow cytometry, testicular cells are separated usually on their DNA content into (1) tetraploid representing primary spermatocytes (17%), (2) diploid composed of spermatogonia, secondary spermatocytes, Sertoli cells and Leydig cells (36%) and (3) haploid comprising spermatids and spermatozoa (45%) (Hellstrom *et al.*, 1989). Flow cytometry is a rapid, reproducible and objective method to determine the relative proportions of cells in the testis. Hellstrom and colleagues (1989) examined the use of this technique in men undergoing vasovasostomy and were able to identify 84% of men who would have sperm present in their semen post reversal. It may be possible to monitor spermatogenesis by examining marker substances in the blood which are a reliable indication of critical events in spermatogenesis, e.g. Sertoli cell proteins (Sharpe, 1994).

Effects of toxin, drugs and radiation

There are a wide range of known, and probably many unknown as yet, toxins which affect the testis. The most notable are cadmium salts, lead and drugs used for the treatment of cancer such as busulphan, methotrexate, vinblastine and vincristine.

The effects of these anti-cancer drugs are now well known and, prior to treatment, men can provide semen samples in a sperm bank (for cryopreservation in liquid nitrogen where the samples can be kept indefinitely) so that, if their fertility is not restored, they still have a chance of achieving pregnancy by using stored spermatozoa. Many testicular cancer patients have lower than average sperm counts prior to treatment. Testicular cancer itself may be deleterious to spermatogenesis. However, fertility trials are still in their infancy and more research needs to be performed. Although anti-cancer drugs are toxic to spermatogenesis fertility is often restored even after combinations of radiotherapy and chemotherapy. In fact, 40% of such patients father children after treatment (Berthelsen, 1987). Older treatment regimens were very toxic. However, modern treatment, e.g. radiotherapy, with low or therapeutic dosage regiments appear to do little permanent damage (Berthelsen, 1987; Fossa *et al.*, 1990).

Acknowledgements

The author wishes to acknowledge the financial support of the University of Sheffield and the Infertility Research Trust.

References

Barratt CLR, Cohen J. Fate of superfluous sperm products after vasectomy and in the normal male tract of the mouse. *J Reprod Fertil* 1986; **78**: 1–10.

Barratt CLR, Cohen J. Quantification of sperm disposal and phagocytic cells in the tract of short- and long-term vasectomised mice. *J Reprod Fertil* 1987; **81**: 277–84.

Barratt CLR, Cohen J. Quantitative effects of short and long-term vasectomy on mouse spermatogenesis and sperm transport. *Contraception* 1988; **37**: 415–25.

Barratt CLR, Cooke ID. *Advances in Clinical Andrology.* Lancaster: MTP Press, 120.

Barratt CLR, Bolton AE, Cooke ID. Functional significance of white blood cells in the male and female reproductive tract – a review. *Hum Reprod* 1990a; **5**: 639–48.

Barratt CLR, Cooke ID. Review: sperm transport in the human female reproductive tract – a dynamic interaction. *Int J Androl* 1991; **14**: 394–411.

Bellve AR, Zheng W. Growth factors as autocrine and paracrine modulators of male gonadal functions. *J Reprod Fertil* 1989; **85**: 771–93.

Berthelsen JG. Testicular cancer and fertility. *Int J Androl* suppl 1987; **10**: 371–80.

De Kretser DM, Sun YT, Drummond AE, Gonzales GF, Robertson DM, Riosberbriger GP. In: Asch RH, Balmaceda JP, Johnson I eds Serono Symposia USA, 1990: 19–30.

DeRooji DG, Van Dissel-Emiliani FMF, VanPelt AMM. Regulation of spermatogonial proliferation. In: Robaire B, Ewing LL, eds Regulation of testicular function signalling molecules and cell–cell communication. *Ann NY Acad Sci* 1989; **564**: 1140–53.

Djakiew D, Dym M. Pachytene spermatocyte proteins influence Sertoli cell function. *Biol Reprod* 1988; **39**: 1193–205.

Fossa SD, Theodorsen L, Norman N, Aabyholm T. Recovery of impaired pre-treatment spermatogenesis in testicular cancer. *Fertil Steril* 1990; **54**: 493–6.

Glover TD, Barratt CLR, Tyler JJP, Hennessey *Human Male Fertility and Semen Analysis.* London: Academic Press, 1990: 247.

Hamilton DW, Waites GMH. Cellular and Molecular events in spermiogenesis. *Scientific Basis of Fertility Regulation.* World Health Organization. Cambridge University Press 1990; 334.

Hecht NB. Regulation of 'haploid expressed genes' in male germ cells. *J Reprod Fertil* 1990; **88**: 679–93.

Hellstrom WJG, Deitch AD, DeVere White RW. Evaluation of vasovasostomy candidates by dexoribonucleic acid flow cytometry of testicular aspirates. *Fertil Steril* 1989; **51**: 546–8.

Ivel R. 'All that glistens is not gold' – common testis transcripts are not always what they seem. Editorial. *Int J Androl* 1992; **15**: 85–92.

Jarrow JP, Budin RE, Pym M *et al.* Quantitative pathologic changes in the human testis after vasectomy. A controlled study. *N Eng J Med* 1985; **313**: 1252–6.

Johnson L. Review article: Spermatogenesis and aging in the human. *J Androl* 1986; **7**: 331–54.

Johnson L. Spermatogenesis (animal species and humans). In: Ash RH, Balmaceda JP, Johnson I. eds *Gamete Physiology* Serono Symposia USA 1990: 3–18.

Johnson MD. Genes related to spermatogenesis: molecular and clinical aspects. *Seminars in Reproductive Endocrinology* 1991; **9**: 73–86.

Magid MS, Cash K, Goldtein M. The testicular biopsy in the evaluation of infertility. *Seminars in Urology* 1990; **8**: 51–64.

Mahi-Brown CA, Yule TD, Tung KSK. Evidence for active immunological regulation in prevention of testicular autoimmune disease independent of the blood testis barrier. *Am J Reprod Immunol Microbiol* 1988; **16**: 165–70.

Schulze W, Rehder U. Organisation and morphogenesis of the human seminiferous epithelium. *Cell and Tissue Research* 1984; **237**: 395–407.

Setchell BP. Spermatogenesis and spermatozoa. In: Austin CR, Short RV, ed. *Reproduction in Mammals: 1. Germ Cells and Fertilization.* Cambridge University Press 1982; 63–101.

Sharpe TM. Reivew: Intratesticular control of steroidogenesis. *Clinical Endocrinology* 1990; **33**: 787–807.

Sharpe RM. Editorial. Monitoring of spermatogenesis in man – measurement of Sertoli- or germ cell- secreted proteins in semen or blood. *Int J Androl* 1992; **15**: 201–10.

Sharpe RM. Regulation of spermatogenesis. In: Knobil E, Neill JD, eds. *Physiology of Reproduction.* 2nd edn. New York: Raven Press, 1994.

Skinner MK. Cell–cell interactions in the testis. *Endocrine Reviews* 1991; **12**: 45–77.

World Health Organization. The influence of varicocele on parameters of fertility in a large group of men presenting to infertility clinics. *Fertil Steril* 1992; **57**: 1279–93.

Ward WS, Coffey DS. DNA packaging and organisation in mammalian spermatozoa: comparison with somatic cells. *Biol Reprod* 1991; **44**: 569–74.

14

Sperm preparation for assisted conception

J. L. YOVICH

Human semen contains decapacitation factors from which the spermatozoa must be separated in order to proceed to the stages of capacitation followed by hyperactivation and the acrosome reaction which then enables zona binding and fertilization. Following coitus, these effects are achieved on spermatozoa which travel from the ejaculate into favourable fertile cervical mucus. In assisted reproduction, the various spermatozoal processes enabling fertilization must be achieved by *in vitro* techniques. Relatively simple successful methods have been developed for semen preparation from normospermic men with normal sperm function, but many cases of infertility are associated with abnormal semen parameters or abnormal sperm function. Such cases require rather specialized semen preparation techniques.

Not only must spermatozoa be separated from seminal plasma to achieve fertilizing capacity, but the process must be achieved rapidly, preferably within 30 min. It has been shown that longer exposures to seminal plasma *in vitro* can permanently diminish the fertilizing capacity of spermatozoa. For this reason as well as sperm sensitivity to temperature variations, seminal ejaculates should be collected in the immediate vicinity of the laboratory undertaking the preparation procedure for assisted reproduction effective sperm preparation procedures should also remove dead cells, debris, micro-organisms, non-spermatozoal cells (especially inflammatory cells), sperm precursors, immotile and most morphologically abnormal spermatozoa, as well as prostaglandins, other spasmogens and lytic enzymes carried within the plasma.

The range of clinical procedures requiring sperm preparation include intrauterine insemination (IUI), donor insemination, gamete intrafallopian transfer (GIFT) and *in vitro* fertilization (IVF) with uterine transfer of embryos (ET) or tubal transfer of either pronuclear stage oocytes (PROST) or cleaving embryo stages (TEST). The latter procedures are sometimes designated as zygote intrafallopian transfer (ZIFT). Other less well-established clinical procedures which require sperm preparations include direct intraperitoneal insemination (DIPI) and either peritoneal oocyte–sperm transfer (POST) or transcervical sperm–egg transfer (T-SET).

In clinical practice, sperm preparation techniques were originally developed for IVF where the underlying infertility problem was due to fallopian tube obstruction. The sperm preparation techniques of 'washing' with either over-layering of culture media or placement of the sperm pellet under culture medium (underlayering) followed by spermatozoal swim up and harvest, gave suitable 'sperm preps' for fertilization. However, as male factor infertility and other complex cases were included into the assisted reproduction programmes, these techniques were found to be inappropriate for many cases and often associated with failed fertilization in severe forms of oligo/asthenozoospermia. A variety of other sperm prep techniques have improved the prognosis for such cases and include the use of discontinuous Percoll gradients and sedimentation techniques, reducing or excluding centrifugation procedures when the spermatozoa are considered to be fragile.

Further specialized sperm preps have evolved to cope with specific conditions such as micromanipulation, microinsemination and spermatozoal microinjection; the presence of antispermatozoal antibodies; micro-epididymal sperm aspiration (MESA); and specific spermatozoal dysfunctions. Delicate preparation techniques are required along with substances designed to improve motility parameters, to induce the acrosome reaction or to suppress reactive oxygen species formation.

Swim-up procedures

An overlay technique which has proven suitable for normospermic cases with normal sperm function is schematically described in Fig. 1. It has also proved suitable for moderate oligozoospermic cases but only occasionally for severe cases, by adjustment of the final sperm concentration (Yovich & Stanger, 1984). The aim is to achieve between 50 000 to 100 000 motile spermatozoa as a 'clean' preparation, i.e. devoid of leukocytes, sperm precursors and immotile spermatozoa. Sometimes, larger numbers can be inseminated in IVF or GIFT to compensate for mild to moderate oligozoospermic cases with sperm dysfunction (Matson *et al.*, 1987). In IVF procedures, fertilization rates should exceed 70% of preovulatory oocytes inseminated. For IUI, at least 2 million spermatozoa, and usually 5–10 million where available, should be prepared in 100–200 μl for insemination.

Overlay techniques of sperm prep have been criticized because the centrifugation process may pack the useful spermatozoa into a tight pellet along with all the deleterious factors, including reactive oxygen species from immotile spermatozoa (Aitken & Clarkson, 1988), which are destined to be removed after the two-stage

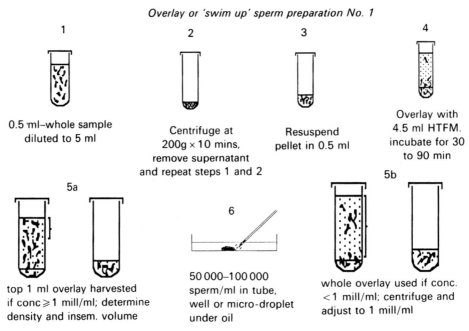

Fig. 1. Sperm preparation technique using washing process followed by centrifugation and overlayering of medium enabling 'sperm rise'. It is important not to exceed 200 g at centrifugation and to avoid tight sperm pellets. The loose pellets are fully resuspended in 0.5 ml medium before overlayering.

wash and centrifugation processes. However, this is not a problem in practice if centrifugation forces do not exceed 200 g; tight pellets are not created; and the loose pellets are fully resuspended in 0.5 ml of sperm prep medium. To avoid these potential problems, the most recent edition of the WHO laboratory manual (WHO, 1992) advises a preliminary swim up of overlayered semen to harvest a relatively clean motile fraction before the washing/centrifugation steps (Fig. 2).

A wide range of culture media appear to be suitable for sperm preps. In the author's experience HTFM (Table 1) or other modified Tyrode's solutions (Yovich & Grudzinskas, 1990) and supplemented Earle's medium (as described in Appendix XXIV of the third edition of the WHO manual (WHO, 1992)) have proved suitable. Culture media are usually supplemented with deactivated serum collected from the female partner after excluding the presence of antispermatozoal antibodies which may inhibit fertilization (Yovich *et al.*, 1984). Alternative protein sources include fetal cord serum, pooled human serum albumin and bovine serum albumin. The latter two are sometimes used in commercial media but serum-transmitted infections remain a serious potential consideration. One pooled human albumin source is Albuminar-20 which has been associated with satisfactory IVF results (Staessen *et al.*, 1990).

Table 1. *Human tubal fluid medium (HTFM)*

Component	Strength
NaCl	101.5 mM
KCl	4.69 mM
$MgSO_4 \cdot 7H_2O$	0.2 mM
KH_2PO_4	0.37 mM
Na lactate	21.4 mM
Glucose	2.78 mM
Penicillin	100 IU/ml
Streptomycin	50 g/ml
$NaHCO_3$	25 mM
Na pyruvate	0.33 mM
$CaCl_2 \cdot 2H_2O$	2.04 mM
Phenol red	0.001%

Osmolality is adjusted to 280 mOsmol and pH to 7.5 for sperm preps. See text reference for full preparation details.

Overlay or 'swim up' sperm preparation No. 2

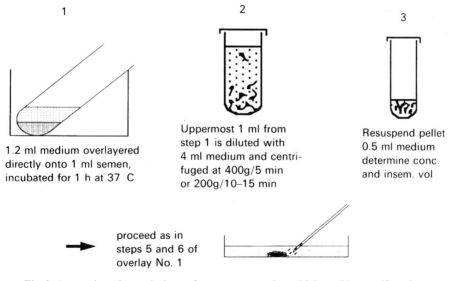

1   1.2 ml medium overlayered directly onto 1 ml semen, incubated for 1 h at 37 C

2   Uppermost 1 ml from step 1 is diluted with 4 ml medium and centrifuged at 400g/5 min or 200g/10–15 min

3   Resuspend pellet 0.5 ml medium determine conc. and insem. vol

proceed as in steps 5 and 6 of overlay No. 1

Fig. 2. An overlayering technique of sperm preparation which avoids centrifugation of diluted semen. The first step ensures that the majority of immotile sperm, other cells and debris are left behind when the sperm is subsequently washed, centrifuged and overlayered again. The method is intended to reduce reactive oxygen species from the sperm prep.

Individual sperm preparations

A number of variables within semen are known to correlate with poor fertilization rates and require individualized sperm preps.

Oligo/asthenozoospermia

This term describes semen with progressive motile numbers of spermatozoa < 10 million/ml. There is a steadily worsening state such that it is difficult to obtain fertilization with numbers < 1 million/ml. However, there is no absolute cut-off, and successful pregnancies have occasionally been generated from sedimentation techniques with motile numbers as low as 200 000/ml.

Teratospermia

Until recently the measurement of single sperm parameters has not shown high predictive values for fertilization *in vitro* although triple sperm defects (i.e. oligo/astheno/teratospermia) have tended to fare poorly. However, Kruger's strict morphology classification (Kruger *et al.*, 1986) does appear to be relevant, i.e. >86% abnormal forms including those with retained cytoplasmic remnants are associated with a poor fertilization rate. The revised WHO manual also embraces a more strict classification of spermatozoal abnormalities, particularly to include all neck and midpiece defects, and retained cytoplasmic droplets. This may provide a morphological correlation with two biochemical measures of sperm dysfunction within semen and which probably reflect the failure of sperm to shed cytoplasm completely, i.e:

(i) creatine phosphokinase (Huszar, Vigue & Morshedi, 1992)
(ii) reactive oxygen species (Aitken & West, 1990)

Leukocytospermia

Accurate assessment of the number of leukocytes in semen is very important, and detection methods have improved although the popular histological and biochemical methods detect fewer leukocytes than do techniques using monoclonal antibodies. A threshold normal level is difficult to define and appears to be up to 2 million/ml (WHO cut-off is 1 million per ml). Leukocytes will be most relevant if sperm have been exposed to them for a prolonged period and there are associated raised levels of reactive oxygen species (Aitken *et al.*, 1992).

Computer-defined motility dysfunction

After sperm preparation, fertilizing spermatozoa will exhibit more than 10% displaying hyperactivated motility patterns on computer assisted semen analysis (CASA). Hyperactivation is CASA-defined as spermatozoa with high curvilinear velocity, low linearity, and high amplitude of lateral head displacement (Burkman, 1990) along with high beat cross-frequency.

Acrosome reaction

After sperm preparation, at least 10% of sperm (for 85% specificity and 82% negative predictive value) should demonstrate a complete acrosome reaction following ionophore challenge (ARIC). The ARIC score is now used as the main guiding indicator for the use of enhancers of sperm motility such as pentoxifylline and 2-deoxyadenosine (Yovich, Edirisinghe & Yovich, 1994).

Antispermatozoal antibodies

Autoantibodies to spermatozoa will reduce the fertilization rate in direct proportion with the seminal or spermatozoal antibody titre. Special procedures are required to separate out free-swimming motile spermatozoa which may then lead to normal fertilization.

Reactive oxygen species

The superoxide anion, along with the hydroxyl radical and the dismutase-degenerated product hydrogen peroxide, constitute the reactive oxygen species. Their presence in semen may result from leukocytes secondary to genital tract infection, but may also be leukocyte independent. These reactive oxygen species probably cause peroxidation of unsaturated fatty acids in the acrosomal membranes. The ensuing damage may cause the plasma membrane to lose its responsiveness to the calcium influx signal which triggers the acrosome reaction. Sperm preps containing antioxidants such as pentoxifylline, may suppress the formation of reactive oxygen species (Gavella, Lipovac & Marotti, 1991; Yovich, 1993).

Unexplained sperm dysfunctions

Despite seemingly normal parameters, some sperm will persistently fail to fertilize eggs. This situation may be evaluated in a zona binding study, by hamster oocyte penetration (after induction of the acrosome reaction); or by electron microscopic study of the sperm. After exclusion of genetic disorders microinjection procedures will usually be required. Ethical considerations will also be required when undertaking fertilization with structurally abnormal spermatozoa such as that associated with Kartagener's syndrome (immotile cilia; absent dynein arms) and round-headed sperm disorders.

Specialized semen preparations

The principles of sperm preparation for specialized cases are to produce a seminal plasma-free suspension of highly motile sperm (ranging from progressive to hyperactivated motility) with mostly normal morphology, free from seminal debris and other cells. Depending upon the clinical circumstances and the fertilization culture system, the actual number of sperm required will range from as few as 250 up to as many as 150 000. The larger number is required for oocytes cultured in tubes containing 1 ml of medium; the smaller number for oocytes cultures in straws with as little as 5 μl medium. In each case the sperm concentration is similar. Most units dealing with large numbers of male-factor cases will prefer to culture in microdroplets of variable sizes under paraffin oil. Sperm microinjection procedures such as subzonal insemination and intracytoplasmic sperm injection entail the use of one to five sperm per oocyte, so that theoretically even fewer spermatozoa are required in the harvest for such cases. In normospermic cases good fertilization rates can be achieved with as few as 20 000 spermatozoa/ml in the insemination droplet. However in cases with dysfunctional sperm, particularly where the acrosome reaction rate is known to be very low, one may aim for higher insemination concentrations in order to compensate for the reduced proportion of fertilizing sperm present.

Viscous semen

Poorly liquefied and viscous semen may be an effect of infrequent ejaculation or a persisting unexplained feature in some men. Such samples can be difficult to handle and are best managed by adding culture medium to the semen and frequently pipetting the sample with an undrawn pipette. Severely viscous samples can be treated with enzymic digestion using α-amylase or chymotrypsin for 15–30 min. The common practice of drawing viscous semen through a fine-bore needle causes spermatozoal damage as well as a low yield of motile spermatozoa and should be discouraged. Centrifugation through discontinuous Percoll columns can be very effective (see below) but higher centrifugation forces may be required.

Two-layered Percoll preparation

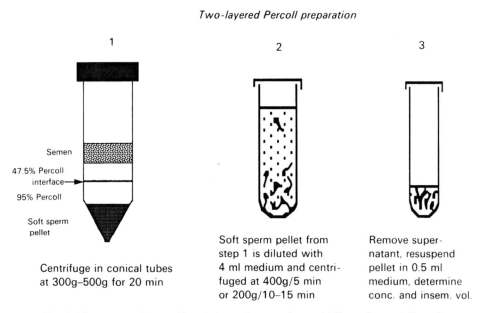

Fig. 3. Neat semen is centrifuged through a two-layered (discontinuous) Percoll column. The Percoll layers are prepared in culture medium and a soft sperm pellet containing mostly motile spermatozoa appears at the bottom of the conical tube, whence it is removed by pipette for subsequent washing, mainly to remove Percoll fragments. Most of the cellular debris and immotile sperm becomes trapped at the interface between the Percoll layers.

Discontinuous Percoll columns

Although many assisted reproduction units have now converted to two-layered Percoll for their routine preparations, the experience at PIVET has not been trouble-free, despite beginning to explore the use of Percoll from 1983. On several occasions fertilization problems have been traced back to Percoll, despite satisfactory results in the quality control system (sperm motility survival measured at 48 and 72 hours). Both IUI and IVF results have been more consistent since introducing routine filtration and re-sterilization of the Percoll in a dry heat oven (120 °C for 8 hours). Two-layered Percoll (e.g. 47.5%:95%) (Mortimer, 1990) or 40%:80% (WHO, 1992)) is used on moderate oligo/asthenospermic cases particularly where there is increased abnormal sperm (e.g. > 50%), high viscosity semen, raised leukocytes or high debris content (Fig. 3). Three-layered Percoll (mini-Percoll 50%:70%:95%) (Ord *et al.*, 1990) is used for MESA cases if the sperm is contaminated with blood cells and degenerate sperm (Fig. 4). Sometimes a single layer (70%) is used for preliminary cleanup of samples with a very high content of debris and degenerate sperm prior to sedimentation (see below).

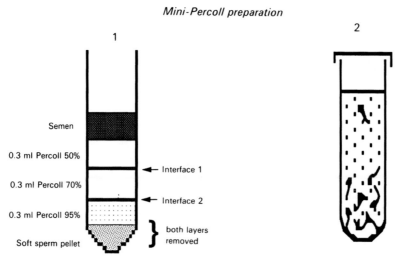

Fig. 4. The mini-Percoll technique involve a three-layered discontinuous column designed especially for small volume MESA aspirates. This entails small volumes in small tubes but the method can be adapted for other, larger volume situations where there is much cellular and particulate debris to be extracted. Such material will appear at the two interfaces and motile spermatozoa are removed from the bottom along with most of the 95% fraction where some motile spermatozoa will be suspended.

Sedimentation and migration techniques

Sedimentation methods (Cohen *et al.*, 1985) are applied for severely oligo/asthenozoospermic cases, i.e. < 5 million motile sperm/ml. Depending upon the severity, the following order may be applied:

(i) Single wash to remove most plasma (can be wash/spin or single layer Percoll 70%/spin), followed by sedimentation in Nunc four-well dish. Centrifugation forces should not exceed 200 g in poor quality sperm preps;

(ii) Overlayering of culture medium in tilted round-bottomed 15 ml Falcon tubes, frequent gentle agitation and allow to sediment, collecting small volumes of motile sperm occasionally over 2–2½ hours. Several tubes with a high medium/semen ratio are required (as in the first step of Fig. 2). However, no centrifugation is involved;

(iii) True sedimentation and migration techniques in Tea-Jondet glass tubes (Fig. 5) (Tea, Jondet & Scholler, 1983). This method is ideal for the worst semen samples. Again, no centrifugation is involved.

Sedimentation technique with Tea-Jondet tube

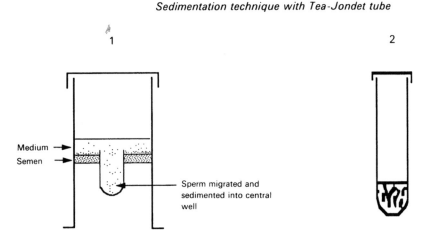

1

2

Medium →

Semen →

Sperm migrated and
sedimented into central
well

Tea-Jondet tube is incubated for 60 to
150 min at 37 °C. Sperm can be drawn
off intermittently from central well

Depending upon sperm
numbers, dilution, wash
or direct insemination
may be performed

Fig. 5. Tea–Jondet tubes comprise a small tube creating a well within a larger tube. Plastic models are commercially available or they can be hand made from borosilicate glass. They are particularly suited to high debris, oligo/asthenozoospermic cases and the central well can be aspirated intermittently over 2 to 3 hours if required until sufficient spermatozoa are recovered.

Antispermatozoal auto-antibodies

Useful samples can be achieved, even with high antibody levels. by receiving the semen sample immediately after it has been ejaculated directly into culture medium and submitting it to Immunobead separation (Grundy *et al.*, 1992). In this situation, it is imperative that the sperm collection facility is adjacent to the semenology laboratory, e.g. where semen samples can be received through a double door hatchway system with an alerting buzzer triggered by the patient.

Other sperm separation methods

A variety of other sperm separation methods have been reported but have not demonstrated any advantages over the aforementioned techniques and have not gained wide popularity. These include:

   (i) the Sperm Select System which has the benefit of simplicity and can generate a 'clean' sperm prep, but with a lower yield of motile spermatozoa;

  (ii) transmembrane migration where sperm travel into the culture medium across a nucleopore membrane filter. Again, yields are very low;

(iii) adherence techniques involving glass wool columns or glass beads which cause immotile spermatozoa to adhere to the glass surfaces whilst motile spermatozoa swim through the system; and

(iv) multilayered columns of albumin with varying densities have been applied for sex preselection with some reported success (Beernink, Dmowski & Ericsson, 1993).

Pentoxifylline

We have described the *in vitro* use of Pentoxifylline (PF: 1-9{5-oxohexyl}-3,7-dimethylxanthine), a phosphodiesterase inhibitor, to enhance spermatozoal motility and improve the fertilization rate of oocytes in male factor infertility treated by assisted reproduction. PF 1 mg/ml (3.6 mM) is incubated with the washed sperm preparation after sperm rise or sedimentation and subsequently eluted out prior to insemination of the partner's oocytes (Fig. 6) (Yovich *et al.*, 1988, 1990). The actions and applications of PF in assisted reproduction have recently been reviewed (Yovich, 1993) and can be summarized as follows:

(i) The acrosome reaction can be improved by PF in dysfunctional semen samples (Tesarik & Mendoza, 1993). The optimum indication is where the ARIC score is <10% but shows improvement with PF as this is usually the relevant end-point to be achieved (Yovich *et al.*, 1994). Low ARIC scores may be the consequence of high levels of reactive oxygen species and PF is known to suppress their formation.

(ii) Severe asthenozoospermia. PF has a variable effect on motility as measured by eye under light microscopy. However, CASA studies will often show PF to produce an improvement in the proportion of hyperactivated sperm (Tesarik, Thebault & Testart, 1992) and such cases will usually benefit by its addition in the sperm preparation.

(iii) Previous failed or poor fertilization. There are quite variable causes for this phenomenon and only some will be corrected by PF. It is wise to evaluate such cases carefully and be guided by PF enhancement of the ARIC score or hyperactivation. If one has the facility for measuring reactive oxygen species, this may be another group to benefit. Otherwise improvement should not be expected.

(iv) MESA. PF has proven invaluable in the preparation of epididymal sperm for fertilization (Ord *et al.*, 1992). It has sometimes stimulated motility in 'dormant' spermatozoa and has significantly enhanced the fertilization rate when added either before or after sperm cleanup with mini-Percoll or by

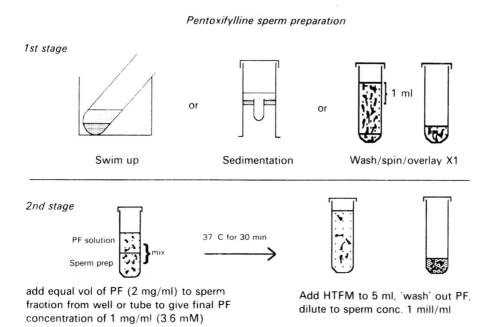

Fig. 6. Pentoxifylline is indicated on the basis of sperm function tests rather than semen analysis parameters. Therefore any appropriate sperm recovery technique is suitable for the first stage. Thereafter the sperm prep is incubated in 3.6 mM PF for just 30 mins prior to washout and immediate insemination. This provides better results than prolonged incubation; however MESA cases may require PF addition before the mini-Percoll stage to 'enliven' dormant sperm in some situations.

sedimentation. The addition of 2-deoxyadenosine often appears to be beneficial in MESA cases.

(v) Micromanipulation. Preparations for partial zona dissection, subzonal insemination and intracytoplasmic sperm injection have aimed to achieve small numbers of hyperactivated sperm in a very clean suspension on a cavity slide or in a culture well. PF, with or without added follicular fluid, can be beneficially used routinely to maximize the chance of inducing the acrosome reaction.

(vi) Caution is advised against the routine use of adding PF to all semen preparations. Normospermic cases will often show a reduced fertilization rate with PF, probably representing a burn-out phenomenon due to the raised intracellular cAMP levels adversely affecting processes which were already proceeding optimally. Some oligo/asthenozoospermics will also show an adverse response hence one should now be guided by the ARIC test and other preliminary studies.

Conclusions

The rationale behind the application of a range of sperm preparation techniques have been presented. These may all be part of daily routines in busy units which can apply flexible management protocols to achieve optimal results. However one must also caution against smaller units introducing this approach as the number of variables which may cause an adverse effect within the overall programme, increases markedly. Trouble-shooting with limited resources under these circumstances can be a tediously frustrating exercise. Many such units will therefore often settle for a standardised approach, e.g. two-layered Percoll sperm preps, aiming for consistent, albeit perhaps slightly suboptimal, results.

Acknowledgements

Over a 20-year period, numerous colleagues have, by direct personal association, suggested many useful ideas concerning sperm preparation techniques, and I am especially grateful to Ms Jeanne Yovich, BSc and Dr Rohini Edirisinghe, PhD who have undertaken numerous trials to develop the working protocols.

References

Aitken RJ, Buckingham D, West K, Wu FC, Zikopoulos K, Richardson DW. Differential contribution of leucocytes and spermatozoa to the generation of reactive oxygen species in the ejaculates of oligozoospermic patients and fertile donors. *J Reprod Fertil* 1992; **94**: 451–70.

Aitken RJ, Clarkson JS. Significance of reactive oxygen species and antioxidants in defining the efficiacy of sperm preparation techniques. *J Androl* 1988; **9**: 367–76.

Aitken RJ, West KM. Analysis of the relationship between reactive oxygen species production and leucocyte infiltration in fractions of human semen separated on Percoll gradients. *Int J Androl* 1990; **13**: 433–51.

Beernink FJ, Dmowski WP, Ericsson RJ. Sex preselection through albumin separation of sperm. *Fertil Steril* 1993; **59**: 382–6.

Burkman LJ. Hyperactivated motility of human spermatozoa during *in vitro* capacitation and implications for fertility. In: Gagnon C ed. *Controls of Sperm Motility: Biological and Clinical Aspects*. Boca Raton: CRC Press, 1990: 303–29.

Cohen J, Edwards R, Fehilly C, Fishel S, Hewitt J, Purdy J, Rowland G, Steptoe P, Webster J. *In vitro* fertilization: a treatment for male infertility. *Fertil Steril* 1985; **43**: 422–32.

Gavella M, Lipovac V, Marotti T. Effect of pentoxifylline on superoxide anion production by human sperm. *Int J Androl* 1991; **14**: 320–7.

Grundy CE, Robinson J, Guthrie KA, Gordon AG, Hay DM. Establishment of pregnancy after removal of sperm antibodies *in vitro*. *Br Med J* 1992; **304**: 292–3.

Huszar G, Vigue L, Morshedi M. Sperm creatine phosphokinase M-isoform ratios and fertilizing potential of men – a blinded study of 84 couples treated with *in vitro* fertilization. *Fertil Steril* 1992; **57**: 882–8.

Kruger TF, Menkveld R, Stander FSH, Lombard CJ, van der Merwe JP, Van Zyl JA, Smith K. Sperm morphological features as a prognostic favor in *in vitro* fertilization. *Fertil Steril* 1986; **46**: 1118–23.

Matson PL, Blackledge DG, Richardson PA, Turner SR, Yovich JM, Yovich JL. The role of gamete intrafallopian transfer (GIFT) in the treatment of oligospermic infertility. *Fertil Steril* 1987; **48**: 608–12.

Mortimer D. Semen analysis and sperm washing techniques. In: Gagnon C ed. *Controls of Sperm Motility: Biological and Clinical Aspects*. Boca Raton: CRC Press, 1990: 263–84.

Ord T, Marello E, Patrizio P. Balmaceda JP, Silber SJ, Asch RH. The role of the laboratory in the handling of epididymal sperm for assisted reproductive technologies. *Fertil Steril* 1992; **57**: 1103–6.

Ord T, Patrizio P, Marello E. Balmaceda JP, Asch RH. Minipercoll: a new method of sperm preparation for IVF in severe male factor infertility. *Hum Reprod* 1990; **5**: 987–9.

Staessen C, Van den Abbeel E, Carlé M, Khan I, Devroey P, Van Steirteghem AC. Comparison between human serum and Albuminar-20 (TM) supplement for *in-vitro* fertilization. *Human Reprod* 1990; **5**: 336–41.

Tea NT, Jondet M, Scholler R. A 'migration-gravity sedimentation' method for collecting motile spermatozoa from human semen. In: Harrison R, Bonnar J, Thompson W eds. In-vitro *Fertilization, Embryo Transfer and Early Pregnancy. Themes from the XIth World Congress on Fertility and Sterility*. Dublin: MTP Press Ltd, 1983: 117–20.

Tesarik J, Mendoza C. Sperm treatment with pentoxifylline improves the fertilizing ability in patients with acrosome reaction insufficiency. *Fertil Steril* 1993; **60**: 141–8.

Tesarik J, Thebault A, Testart J. Effect of pentoxifylline on sperm movement characteristics in normospermic and asthenospermic specimens. *Hum Reprod* 1992; **7**: 1257–63.

WHO. *WHO Laboratory Manual for the Examination of Human Semen and Sperm–Cervical Mucus Interaction*. 3rd edn. Cambridge: Cambridge University Press, 1992: 107.

Yovich JL. Pentoxifylline: actions and applications in assisted reproduction. *Hum Reprod* 1993; **8**: 1786–91.

Yovich JM, Edirisinghe WR, Cummins JM, Yovich JL. Preliminary results using pentoxifylline in a pronuclear stage tubal transfer (PROST) program for severe male factor infertility. *Fertil Steril* 1988; **50**: 179–81.

Yovich JM, Edirisinghe WR, Cummins JM, Yovich JL. Influence of pentoxifylline in severe male factor infertility. *Fertil Steril* 1990; **53**: 715–22.

Yovich JM, Edirisinghe WR, Yovich JL. Use of the acrosome reaction to ionophore challenge (ARIC) test in managing patients in an assisted reproduction program: a prospective, double blind, randomized controlled study. *Fertil Steril* 1993; 1994; **61**: 902–10.

Yovich JL, Grudzinskas JG. *The Management of Infertility: a Practical Guide to Gamete Handling Procedures*. London: Heinemann Medical Books, 1990: 276.

Yovich JL, Stanger JD. The limitations of *in vitro* fertilization from males with severe oligospermia and abnormal sperm morphology. *J In Vitro Fert Embryo Transf* 1984; **1**: 172–9.

Yovich JL, Stanger JD, Kay D, Boettcher B. *In vitro* fertilization of oocytes from women with serum antisperm antibodies. *Lancet* 1984; **ii**: 369–70.

15

Bioethics and the spermatozoon: reproductive destiny

R. P. S. JANSEN

Spermatozoa out: reproductive destiny

Most spermatozoa are made to be lost. From the time that spermatozoa are first released from a man's seminiferous tubules until disease or death puts an end to sperm production, a man with a typical sperm count will discharge more than a thousand thousand million sperm cells. Almost any of these cells, in the right place, can make him a father. Religious belief may or may not make it sinful to waste an ejaculation on purpose, but it is beyond argument that, with the thousands likely in a lifetime, not to waste all but a very few seminal emissions would cause a man to be sexually profligate, reproductively irresponsible, and genetically arrogant.

This chapter's purpose is to explore from biological and modern cultural perspectives the moral codes and ethical rules that society has developed and continues to develop to govern its exposure to human spermatozoa. My perspective is that the wisdom of ethical principles should be tested and that what is an ethical, moral or wise course of action or inaction should respond to evidence and, in principle, be alterable.

Sperm as reproductive property

Semen shares with blood the property of perpetual regeneration in the body. Semen, more so than blood, can be donated with inconsequential physical detriment to the donor (given that its emission is probably going to take place one way or another). The two tissues differ in other ways, because semen contains the male gametes – haploid packets of usable genetic information for sexual reproduction of the species. When semen, particularly its spermatozoa, is spilled in way that stops genetic information from finding expression, God may show displeasure (e.g. Genesis 38:9), but sperm soaked into the soil (or washed out of the linen, lost down the drain) troubles most people not one bit. No respondents in one recent survey, for example, expressed objections to artificial insemination simply because it involves masturbation (Rowland & Ruffin, 1983). The reason we do not care if semen is wasted (unless for some reason the sperm cannot be replaced) is that once lost in these ways the information the spermatozoa contain is not usable (Jansen, 1985): it will not find genetic expression: it will not mix with an oocyte's chromosomes to produce a new individual: we can forget about it.

Some contentious matters among the new reproductive technologies may be clarified if we accept that, whether from intuition or thoughtfulness, men have a legitimate and persisting concern for their genetic expression among offspring, whatever the social or medical circumstances are that govern the impregnation. Agencies engaged in these technologies should recognize this lasting dominion or provenance that sperm providers have over their gametes, otherwise these special ethical tensions will be added to the moral milieu that already confuses application of the technologies. (The concerns of men over their genetic destiny may mirror similar concerns among women: a female perspective is discussed in a companion chapter on the oocyte in Volume 2 of this series; in many respects the differentiation of these two chapters is artificial and I encourage readers both to make their own philosophical integrations and to excuse inadvertent nonbiological distinctions of gender.)

Can there be biological or cultural doubt about the importance men feel towards genetic expression among offspring?

Paternity

Paternity is biologically uncertain compared with maternity. There are three levels of insecurity. Firstly, there may be doubt about paternity itself: in monogamous species there is physical competition between males for female attention and choice. Secondly, there is the need to ensure that the female is brought securely to the end of gestation. Thirdly, the family must be brought safely to the point where the offspring are independent and are themselves sexually competent. Throughout the animal kingdom, therefore, males exhibit social behaviour that monopolises female attentions and rewards female fidelity. In contrast, when males are driven from their mates by invaders, the new males displace not just their immediate rivals, but their offspring too, with actions directed at abortion and infanticide.

Among a range of species, evidence shows that the less certainty there is between impregnation and the reaching of reproductive age among the offspring the more male care of progeny predominates over female care. Among lower animals, exclusive male care tends to happen when there is external fertilisation (Clutton-Brock, 1991), with male stickleback fish, for example, accepting responsibility for guarding spawned eggs till they hatch. Popular theories propose that among prehistoric evolving hominids, as the vulnerable time spent in preadolescence and childhood lengthened, it was the evolution of mutually pleasurable sexuality that kept male–female relationships monogamous, division of labour efficient, and paternity certain (Lovejoy, 1981; Morris, 1986; Foley & Lee, 1989).

How natural is male or female fidelity among men and women? Behaviour among non-human primates is so varied that more recent information than that provided by comparative primatology is needed from which to draw a moral hypothesis. None the less a study of the semen of great apes provides an interesting starting point.

Gorillas are four times the size of chimpanzees, but their testes weigh just one-fourth that of their fellow apes (Short, 1979; Harvey & May, 1989). Whereas gorillas are mostly monogamous, female chimpanzees will accept several males during one ovulation, producing intense competition among sperm from different males for genetic expression through fertilization of the oocyte. Because the production of sperm per unit volume of testicular tissue is essentially constant, testicular weight is proportional to sperm production over time. In nature those primates that have evolved high sperm production rates also have high sperm concentrations and high sperm motility in the ejaculate (Moller, 1988). Primate sperm counts thus may owe much to genetic, evolutionary influences. As it turns out, the environmental pressure that governs this evolution is the pattern of female mating behaviour (Harvey & May, 1989). Table 1 compares observed 'fidelity' and average sperm counts among the males of different primates. The data support the idea that humans have evolved away from profligacy and towards faithfulness (Foley & Lee, 1989), albeit incompletely (Morris, 1986; Parker, 1989).

Lineage

Matrifocal groups predominate among the non-human primates (Fleagle, 1988). Prehistorically, human societies may have been matrilineal in inheritance more often than in modern times, at least in Europe and India (Darlington, 1969). Patrilineal descent then became virtually exclusive, perhaps as the experience of animal husbandry taught that sexual intercourse causes pregnancy and that male as well as female traits are able to be inherited. For example, in leviate marriage among the ancient Hebrews, expression of male lineage was important enough to compel the surviving brother of a deceased husband to impregnate the dead brother's wife (Deuteronomy 25: 5-10). This is what made Onan uncomfortable (though worse was to come). It was such a forced set of

Table 1. *Comparison of mating system, relative testicular weight and total motile sperm number in representative monkeys, apes and man*

Species	Mating system	Testes wt.	Body wt.	Ratio (/1306)	Motile sperm (/ejaculate)
Rhesus monkey (*Macaca mulatta*)	polygamous	46 g	9.2 kg	5	472×10^6
Baboon (*Papio cynophalus*)	polygamous	52 g	24.3 kg	2.1	232×10^6
Gibbon (*Hylobates lar*)	monogamous	5.5 g	5.5 kg	1.0	18×10^6
Silvery gibbon (*Hylobates moloch*)	monogamous	6.1 g	5.4 kg	1.1	5×10^6
Orangutan (*Pongo pygmaeus*)	monogamous	35 g	75 kg		
Chimpanzee (*Pan troglodytes*)	polygamous	119 g	44 kg	2.7	273×10^6
Gorilla (*Gorilla gorilla*)	monogamous	30 g	200 kg	0.15	42×10^6
Humans (*Homo sapiens sapiens*)	monogamous	41 g	64 kg	0.6	153×10^6

Man is placed among the monogamous species in terms of relative testicular size; total motile sperm number is less than among the promiscuous primates; and humans are the only primates to use sex for marital bonding during times of physiological infertility.

circumstances, and the denial of his own reproductive choices, that Onan as the surviving brother decided instead to spill his semen onto the ground (Genesis 3: 9-10). This gives us the best biblical precedent for the importance a man attaches to his genetic product and to his reproductive destiny.

Concern with genetic destiny and lineage, added to the generally sound sociobiological principle of husbands providing for wife and children, has throughout ancient, mediaeval and modern times resulted in elaborate social and cultural constraints on female freedom – all in order to promote female fidelity. Human males' modern preoccupation with genetic destiny among offspring is thus well enough known for it now to attract much critical feminist comment.

Leaving aside its exaggerated forms, a man's concern with his genetic destiny is a social force that is biologically fundamental enough to require serious respect. To some this conclusion is selfevident. To others, who may think that human culture can or should rise above its biological foundations, an argument from sociobiological principles will not itself be convincing (e.g. Rose, Kamin & Lewontin, 1984). But an examination of the modern practice of sperm donation, which follows, will bring us to the same conclusion.

Sperm donation

When a man's fertility fails because of a low sperm count, the personal consequences are complicated and sad (Van Thiel *et al.*, 1992). Impotence, usually temporary, loss of self-esteem and withdrawal are common among husbands; anger, guilt and a wish to make reparations are common among wives (Czyba & Chevret, 1980; Berger, 1980; Teper & Symonds, 1983; Berger *et al.*, 1992). Increasingly, reproductive technology is resorted to whenever possible before couples turn to a donor sperm bank (Oldereid, Rui & Purvis, 1992; Lippi, Mortimer & Jansen, 1993). This technology, involving as it can the use of *in vitro* fertilization with sperm micromanipulation procedures, is generally at or beyond the limit of what is medically practicable and financially affordable.

Secrecy

Of the several people involved in donor insemination (DI), it is the infertile husband for whom maintaining secrecy is the most important (David *et al.*, 1992). This is more so in some cultures than in others. For example, enlisting the help of a brother as sperm donor is an option generally rejected in favour of maintaining secrecy in the United States (Sauer *et al.*, 1992), where modern family structures are nuclear and insular. Among Indian Hindus, however, where more open and extended family networks persist, fraternal semen donation is an option favoured on genetic and cultural grounds. In Western societies, therefore, anonymous donor sperm banks have replaced acceptance, adoption, prudent adultery and divorce as the ways in which a woman might adjust to her partner's sterility.

The ostensible reason for sperm donors to be anonymous has been a perceived need to protect the social father, the recipient woman and the child from the embarassment of acknowledging the child's genetic father. Many Western countries have now enacted laws whereby the social father, after a birth resulting from donor insemination, is recorded as the legal and only father on the birth certificate (to the irritation of genealogists, Blizzard, 1976). Several authors, however, have drawn attention to the duty DI practitioners also have to sperm donors (Dunstan, 1975; Jansen, 1987), many of whom in surveys have expressed willingness to be approached by their DI offspring, although their recruitment as donors has taken place with the expectation and the promise of anonymity (Rowland, 1983; Daniels, 1987; Mahlstedt & Probasco, 1991).

Donors' reasons

The motives sperm donors have in donating their semen varies with the prevalent methods used to recruit the donors. If donors are paid well (the United States is the one country where sperm donation is overtly commercial, see below), most donors will be discovered to have become sperm 'donors' for the money (Sauer *et al.*, 1992). Outside the United States, sperm donation has mainly been an altruistic activity, with reimbursement of costs common, but with the idea that it is lucrative held only by relatively impoverished donors, such as students. Nevertheless a small financial reimbursement seems to have a facilitatory effect in donating sperm, justifying or neutralizing (Nijs, Steeno & Steepe, 1980) an act that may seem otherwise to be a bit too self-consciously altruistic. Table 2 shows that the attitude of donors towards remaining anonymous to their unknown offspring may not be as different as might be expected between donors ostensibly donating for money and those ostensibly donating for other reasons.

The non-financial motives recorded among sperm donors include personal knowledge of and sympathy for infertile couples (Huerre, 1980; Daniels, 1987) and, especially among unmarried donors, a general desire to father a child or to pass on genes (Nijs *et al.*, 1980; Kovacs, Clayton & McGowan, 1983); occasional donors are simply curious about their own fertility. Sperm donors as a group, unless screened, will include homosexual men (Heurre, 1980; Rowland, 1983; Stewart *et al.*, 1985). In France, where DI is coordinated nationally through the Federation Française des Centres d'Etudes et de Conservation du Sperme Humain (CECOS) (Jalbert *et al.*, 1989), only men who are fathers are eligible to be sperm donors, a restriction that excludes well-motivated single men who want to be donors because they have no other hope of securing genetic descendants.

A curious phenomenon is alluded to by the results of one Australian study. Rowland (1983) found that the majority of donors who already had children were separated from their wives at the time they became sperm donors. From other sources we know that most marital separations in Australia are initiated by the wife, who more often than not receives custody of the children. The French experience, too, with married donors, mentions semen donation as 'balm for a wounded ego' (Huerre, 1980). There may, therefore, be an element of compensation, spite or revenge for some sperm donors. In Rowland's study, a third of donors still living with a female partner had not and did not intend telling her. Otherwise, however, secrecy is not much of an issue for most sperm donors. Daniels (1987) found in reviewing six New Zealand DI programmes that 89% of donors had told other people of their involvement in sperm donation (Daniels, 1987).

Irrespective of the main motive for donating sperm, studies in all countries where sperm donation is accepted show great interest among donors in furnishing

Table 2. *Predominant or ostensible method of recruiting sperm donors and donors'*
acceptance of disclosure of identifying information to the recipients and the offspring

Year	Author	Country	Main motive	Acceptance of disclosure[a]
1983	Kovacs *et al.*	Australia	altruism	32%
1983	Nicholas & Tyler	Australia	altruism	56%
1983	Rowland	Australia	altruism	60%
1985	Handelsman *et al.*	Australia	altruism	33%
1987	Daniels	New Zealand	altruism	24% + 30%[b]
1989	Sauer *et al.*	USA	financial	low
1991	Mahlstedt & Probasco	USA	financial	60%

Kovacs, Clayton & McGowan, 1983; Sauer *et al.*, 1992; Mahlstedt & Probasco, 1991;
Handelsman *et al.*, 1984; Rowland, 1983; Nicholas & Tyler, 1983; Daniels, 1987.
[a]Generally defined as willingness to be sought out by offspring.
[b]Unsure.

useful information on personal and professional characteristics beyond the
physical features that form the usual basis for matching donor with intended
social father (Handelsman *et al.*, 1984; Mahlstedt & Probasco, 1991). There is
also a complementary interest among sperm recipients to know more than just
the medical and physical features of the sperm donor. In our own DI programme
at Royal Prince Alfred Hospital in Sydney we invite donors to write a paragraph
or two to their anonymous offspring – a device that is more and more popular
among donors and recipients alike.

The high level of curiosity donors show in the outcome of their donations is
today still not often rewarded by their receiving much information in return
about outcomes. In 1975 Schoysman argued that 'there is no reason whatsover
that he (the donor) should know the result' and that donors with their own
children who tragically had died would be 'troubled by the fact that somewhere
there is another child alive' (Schoysman, 1975). Times obviously have changed,
but donors are still mostly told nothing, unless a congenital abnormality or an
inherited disease appears among the offspring, information about which might
be medically important to the donor. Nowadays there is more and more support
for retaining identifying information, even if, for the present, it is not used.

Discussions of donors meeting their 'child' have, curiously, expressed the
offspring in the singular (Rowland, 1983), in parallel, presumably, with the
experience of adoption. But five or six children is by no means unusual for a
sperm donor, additional to his own natural ones. Whether they all wish to make

contact or not is beside the point: merely knowing that there are so many children about may itself be worrying. The student who sells his sperm by repeated donations through medical school may come to regret the folly of his genetic excess. Developing new respect for sperm donors should have one immediate consequence, namely to limit the number of pregnancies from each donor – or at least to ask donors how many anonymous offspring they would be happy with. This principle is not new, but the reason for the limit till now has generally been to reduce the chance of inadvertent consanguinity should DI offspring and the donor's natural children happen to marry.

Genetic paternity

One lesson learned from the practice of adoption has been that the discovery by an adolescent of his or her true genetic origins is too serious a hazard to allow even a small chance of inadvertent disclosure. Such a discovery means that the qualities most expected by a child of its parents, namely frankness and truthfulness, will have been assumed mistakenly – a dreadful revelation. If the risk of disclosure is small, the hazard, the penalty, is great. But today's DI children will be adults at a time when genetic testing for heritable vulnerability to disease may well be common. The risk of inadvertent discovery can only increase. Meanwhile the anecdotal experience that social workers are gaining from meetings between genetic parents and their adopted offspring is shifting prevailing opinion away from the notion that behaviour and personality are mainly determined culturally towards, instead, a recognition of the importance of genetic influences. This is a change from the emphasis traditionally placed on nurture over nature in most university courses in the social sciences. Such a move towards appreciating genetic determinants of behaviour, more and more evident elsewhere (Plomin, 1990), will increase DI recipients' desire to know more of sperm donors; but it should also sharpen our duty to inform the providers of sperm of the outcome of their donations.

In time, a more sensitive and sensible approach to genetic parenting will probably prevail. Meanwhile the first social experiment with mandatory removal of anonymity in sperm donation has not been encouraging. Since 1985, legislation in Sweden has demanded disclosure of identifying information concerning donors of sperm to recipients. Despite predictions that donors would be frightened off by being known, it seems instead that the motives among sperm donors have shifted. The decline in DI in Sweden seems to be attributable more to the couple's wish for secrecy than to the donor's, with travel to Denmark or Norway for the sake of anonymity advised by many practitioners (Dr Mats Ahlgren, Stockholm, personal communication). Teper and Symonds wrote in 1983 that the absence of longitudinal studies precluded an examination of how couples cope with secrecy during their careers as DI parents. Today, we are no wiser (Schover, Collins & Richards, 1992).

The anonymous use of sperm has been made possible by the simplicity of obtaining semen. Programmes of anonymous oocyte donation have, in contrast, been slow to develop, relying as they mostly have on spare eggs from women undergoing oocyte collection for IVF and related infertility procedures. As embryo freezing programmes have developed, fewer and fewer eggs incidentally obtained are available for donation. Oocyte donation, therefore, is more and more likely to come from a donor who undergoes ovarian stimulation and follicle aspiration just for the donation, and who is usually known to (indeed is often very close to) the egg recipient. This development, together with the risks of semen-mediated diseases and the general trend away from genetic secrecy, has caused patients and health care workers, including doctors, to question why sperm donors should be anonymous, especially for patients from societies where extended family structures are common and brothers as semen donors are morally preferable to strangers. Many in Western society too are realizing that loosening the nuclear family to allow a greater role for close relations and friends is a sociological approach worth exploring.

Commerical spermatozoa

There are commercial sperm banks in several countries, but only in the United States, with its strong national philosophy of pragmatism, is the sale of sperm for reproductive ends an industry. Practitioners can order semen through the mail for their infertile patients matched to order by physical and other attributes. In 1993, prepared semen cost about US $150 to $250 per 0.5 ml straw. In America, the presumption remains strong that buying sperm from a donor excludes DI professionals from further duties to the donor. Anonymity seems sacrosanct.

By 1980, a commercial sperm bank had been established where Nobel Prize winners could be immortalized, if they wished, through commercial sale of their semen (Broad, 1980). At least two sperm banks in California in 1992 specialized in the sale of sperm from gifted men. At the Repository for Germinal Choice, described as a project of the Foundation for the Advancement of Man, approved applicants are given thorough descriptions of each available donor, from which they can make their selection. The price of the sperm depends on the donor's popularity.

Such is the state of sperm producers' determination of their genetic destiny ('spermatozoa out'). It is much further developed in society than is its female complement, control over the genetic destiny of oocytes among the women who provide them ('oocytes given'). Before we look at the more subtle matters of female reproductive choice in Volume 2 ('oocytes kept'), we turn to the ethics of what sperm can do in women ('spermatozoa in').

Spermatozoa in: the sociobiology of impregnation

Natural fertilization in mammals takes place internally. Impregnation, or the entry of sperm into the female body, may be straightforward, but it is a powerful biological, social and emotional event. The outcome can be welcome or it can be catastrophic. Impregnation has many ethical and moral complexities.

Semen in women

The intrusion

The frequent exposure of a woman's reproductive tract and abdomen to the components of semen constitutes an immunological, and sometimes infective, challenge. The human body is no zoological fortress, as the medical fields of virology, bacteriology, and parasitology make clear (Forrest, 1991).

Spermatozoa in a woman's body, too, have a deserved reputation for intrepidity (Verkuyl, 1988). Through their display in the sperm head of polycationic binding sites, spermatozoa can act as vectors for foreign DNA (Lavitrano *et al.*, 1992), perhaps infective, to enter through the cervix in circumstances where an absence of sperm in the ejaculate might be less of a challenge. For more than one reason, vasectomy as a choice for contraceptive sterilization can be a special kindness (Cooper, 1991). HIV, however, is apparently concentrated in seminal plasma (Forrest, 1991) and its transmission therefore does not require sperm to be present. At vaginal intercourse, given an equal chance of man or woman being already infected, male to female transmission of HIV is twice as likely to happen as female to male transmission (European Study Group on Heterosexual Transmission of HIV, 1992). The use of barrier contraception provides a sensible balance in a society titillated daily by the erotic (Madonnna, 1992).

There are three early fates for spermatozoa ejaculated into the vagina or placed there by artificial insemination: (1) loss to the exterior, which happens normally to much of the semen after sexual intercourse; (2) phagocytosis, associated with a rapid leukocytic response to sperm entry into the female tract (the response is specific for spermatozoa: it does not follow injection of sperm-free semen) (Pandya & Cohen, 1985); or (3) colonization of oestrogenized, receptive cervical mucus in a way that keeps sperm viable for days, as a reservoir, when intercourse has taken place at the time of ovulation (Zinaman *et al.*, 1989). Non-ovulatory mucus will effectively keep most spermatozoa out. What determines the balance between phagocytosis or maintenance of a spermatozoon in the cervix, either of which can happen when mucus is receptive, is not known (Barratt, Bolton & Cooke, 1990). Nonetheless it is a fact that natural human fertility is low enough for most women take several ovulatory cycles to conceive; on these occasions at least, sperm penetration into the body is an ordinary event. How benign the repeated exposure of the female body is to sperm will depend on the circumstances of the challenge.

Spermatozoa are phagocytosed by macrophages and by epithelial cells lining the reproductive tract. The result can be destruction or informational presentation to the reticuloendothelial or immune system. Sperm heads are known to persist morphologically in macrophages for seven days or more (Ball, Scott & Mitchinson, 1984). In mice, tritiated-thymidine-labelled DNA in sperm heads finds its way into the ovaries, lymph nodes, spleen, uterus and the heart! Despite this deep penetration by sperm-borne material, the development of antibodies to spermatozoa in women is uncommon (except, perhaps, with anal intercourse, when the ejaculate is received into the rectum) (Chacho, Hage & Shulman, 1991). Sperm agglutinating antibodies are increasingly likely to develop the longer the exposure to sperm takes place in the absence of pregnancy (Ingerslev & Ingerslev, 1980).

Are there biological benefits to non-conceptional exposure of the female body to spermatozoa via the vagina? It does seem probable that there is a biological purpose for exposing the female immune system to her mate's antigens before pregnancy. Especially short periods of exposure to sperm prior to conception make pre-eclampsia in pregnancy more common and more serious (Duenhoelter, Jiminez & Baumann, 1975). Craft found a higher incidence than expected of pre-eclampsia in women who by receiving donated embryos had no prior exposure at all to the developing fetus's paternal antigens (Serhal & Craft, 1989). Exposure to sperm during a conception cycle may also improve the chance that an embryo will survive. Chaykin and Watson (1983) found that transferred two-cell mouse embryos were more likely to implant in virgin recipients if dead spermatozoa were inserted into the vagina than if there was no exposure of the recipient's genital tract to spermatozoa. Human data, though, are less convincing. Bellings *et al.* (1986) concluded from results in a clinical *in vitro* fertilization programme that pregnancy rates were higher if sexual intercourse preceded follicle aspiration, but other investigators have found no such benefit from insemination (Fishel *et al.*, 1989). It remains possible that sperm need to reach the tubes or the peritoneal cavity to exert a beneficial effect.

On the harmful side of impregnation, incorporation of either sperm-head DNA itself or vector-bound foreign DNA into endocervical epithelium of the cervical transformation zone still competes with viral genome theories to explain the association there is between squamous cell neoplasia of the cervix and multiple sexual partners or early age of first sexual intercourse (Reid *et al.*, 1978). Epidemiological studies of cervical carcinoma have led to an hypothesis that there may be 'high risk males' for this condition. As well as spermatozoa, semen contains B-cell and T-cell lymphocytes (Wolff & Anderson, 1988), which are known to colonize host immune systems in some circumstances. There is little information, though, on the fate of ejaculated lymphocytes in the mammalian female reproductive system. Feminists might justly deplore how little research has been done on the fate in the female body of male antigens and the male genome after impregnation.

Because of the falling average age at menarche in modern societies and the rising average age at marriage, and because of efficient and easy methods of contraception, commentators, parents and the young themselves all justify the practice of premarital sex. This sociological justification contradicts more traditional social values, but these values are now maintained against the odds. Such sexual liberation for women (and hence for men) has been behind the increasing number of sexual partners many young women are exposed to. But this is a social phenomenon that has risks other than unwanted pregnancy. With the prominence now given to the risk a woman has of acquiring, venereally, such untreatable viral diseases as genital herpes, papillomavirus and, especially, HIV, there has been an understandable and biologically sensible public promotion of the use of condoms (e.g. Making Sense of Sex Hotline, 1992). There has also been some re-establishment of the virtues of sexual abstinence and retaining virginity.

The biological and social demand for sex and the realization of its risks inevitably creates a tension we need to accommodate. The spoken or unspoken compromise of the twenty-first century may define a virgin as a woman or a man who has not had condom-free intercourse, and that this biologically important first event will be saved for a permanent relationship, which will in due course preface pregnancy.

Sperm selection

The female reproductive tract has a limited capacity to segregate normal from abnormal sperm. Because the incidence of fetal trisomies is higher with maternal balanced translocations (10%) than with paternal balanced translocations (2% to 3%) (Simpson & Martin, 1976), it is thought that some degree of sperm selection on the basis of abnormality takes place physiologically. Whether this selection occurs on the journey from cervix to oocyte or whether it takes place after the male chromosomes are displayed in the egg cytoplasm prior to syngamy is not known. Studies do show that barriers located from the vagina (Hanson & Overstreet, 1981; Barros *et al.*, 1984) to the oocyte's zona pellucida (Menkveld *et al.*, 1991) can influence the proportion of normal sperm that get past them. In nature, though, sperm motility counts for more than normal-sperm-shape in sperm reaching the oocyte.

The most obvious process of sperm selection for impregnation based on sperm appearance takes place in IVF laboratories. Preliminary studies on the chromosomes of embryos produced by microinjection of individually selected, normal-looking spermatozoa into the perivitelline space have shown a slightly lower likelihood of karyotypic abnormality than is likely either naturally or with conventional IVF (Kola *et al.*, 1990).

Sex preselection and gene choice

The technology for separating X-bearing sperm from Y-bearing sperm and so influencing the gender of the offspring seems to be reasonably reliable now in rabbits (Johnson, Flook & Hawk, 1989). Effective technology for separating human sperm may not be far off (Zarutskie *et al.*, 1989). Will the use of such technology be dangerous? Can or should parents have this perogative?

For most people in the foreseeable future it will remain more fun to become pregnant by having sex and taking one's chances with the baby's gender than it will be to choose to experience an IVF programme to get a gender-designated embryo. It is popularly predicted that sex preselection for social reasons would favour the conception of boys. A gross trend towards boys-first families, however, would confer such an advantage on being a first-born girl (Leading Article, 1990) that it is curious why there is not more enthusiasm among feminists for sex-preselection research. Even if, one day, the exercise of reproductive choice means that one might decide whether one gestates the smart but not-so-pretty embryo or the good-looking but dim one, it will be just a few prospective parents who will want to go to the trouble and expense such an *in vitro* rigmarole would involve instead of spending their money on a better education for whoever is born. For now the point to note is that it is the parents themselves who need to live with the consequences of such intervention, not outsiders.

Artificial insemination

Husband's semen

Artificial insemination with husband's semen (AIH) is the simplest and the oldest of the reproductive technologies (Beck, 1984). When impregnation through sexual intercourse fails to secure pregnancy it may be due, for example, to retrograde ejaculation, sexual impotence, severe hypospadias or disease of the female lower genital tract. In these circumstances, AIH can be practised with effect. AIH is also the means by which semen banked by men who are to receive cytotoxic drugs that can be expected to cause azoospermia is used to try and secure pregnancy. Failure to offer semen cryobanking to such a man in 1981, was, in 1991, the subject of an unsuccessful action for damages in Britain, but now that sperm-banking is more generally available, a future action based on such an omission today might well succeed (Brahams, 1992).

Notwithstanding the Roman Catholic Church's condemnation of masturbation, semen for AIH is almost always obtained this way. Surveys consistently show that there is moral acceptance of both masturbation and AIH among virtually all groups in society, to the point where prohibition of AIH is regarded as practically absurd by the more critical of the Catholic Church's intelligensia (McCormick, 1989). Obsolete values like these should now have just historical importance.

AIH is thus mostly untroubled ethically, but there are three exceptions: when it is accompanied by ovarian stimulation with the intention of inducing multiple follicular development and ovulation (e.g. Remohi *et al.*, 1989); when the semen comes from a prisoner, separated from his wife or previous partner by the command of society; and when the semen is to be used posthumously, after the death of the sperm provider (Cusine, 1977).

The use of multiple ovulation-induction in association with intrauterine AIH has become a popular form of assisting conception, especially when there is oligospermia. The arithmetic to justify it is simple: if few spermatozoa are reaching the fallopian tubes, then the presence of two oocytes at the site of fertilization will double the chance of pregnancy; four oocytes will approximately quadruple it, and so on. The hazard that is thereby introduced is the one of high multiple pregnancy, possibly then managed by selective feticide, which has its own ethical dangers (Jansen, 1990).

If most sperm in the world are produced to be lost, it is especially true for all of a prisoner's gametes. It is said that gaols can stink of semen (Banville, 1990). While prisons are for punishment, so reproductive destiny will be locked up with the prisoner. The occasional requests we receive at our DI programme in Sydney for help in obtaining, storing and using semen from a prisoner have quickly become submerged in confused motives, administrative resistance and the general helplessness that afflicts inmates and their dependants. The Virginia Supreme Court has recently denied the appeals of two prisoners under sentences of death who wanted to freeze their sperm in an attempt to preserve 'their bloodline' (Crockin, 1992); at least one man's girlfriend agreed to be named as the legal recipient of the sperm. The men's invocations were apparently described by Virginia's Governor as 'brazen' and 'appalling', while the court characterized them as 'frivolous'; rejecting all arguments, the court ruled that it was not unconstitutionally cruel or unusual punishment to execute the men without first freezing their sperm for possible future use.

The Warnock Report in the UK sought to stop semen being used by a woman after the death of her husband (Warnock, 1984), and under the UK Human Fertilisation and Embryology Act, 1990, the male whose sperm is used successfully after his death is not to be treated as the father of the child. The grounds given for this infringement of the reproductive and social autonomy of women who have once chosen a mate were the expected psychological complications for the child and the mother. Warnock did not explain why and how these problems (if they truly are problems) might come to be the primary concern of people other than the woman herself.

Proper consideration of gamete provenance based on genetic potential put such inflexible laws in a different light. A similar case in France was decided in favour of the recipient woman after strong expression of public opinion forced the release of semen posthumously from the National Sperm Bank. The woman's perspective in such circumstances has been considered elsewhere (Jansen, 1987) and it is enough here to say that she should have a large part in making the final decision on the matter (and obviously an unhampered right to decline).

From the husband's perspective, we observe that men often store semen when they learn they have a disease that threatens life. On the face of it the reason is that they are to receive cancer-killing drugs, which are likely , as a side effect, to destroy the sperm-forming tissues in the testes. But consciously or subconsciously they also want to preserve their genetic potential in case they die from their disease. Many dying patients take comfort from having children, because it means that it is not strictly the end of the road biologically. On the other hand, among the reasons for the anguish adolescents have in facing death is that their procreative instincts have not been fulfilled. This does not give society an obligation to use reproductive technology to grant all their wishes (or those of their distressed parents) (Rothman, 1990), but, if the reason a husband leaves stored semen behind after death is to secure descendants, then an explicit or testamentary wish for passage of inheritance rights during the reproductive life of his partner should be able to be considered, if she wants it that way. In New South Wales, the Law Reform Commission has sympathetically and sensibly recommended that the deceased husband be recognized as the father, provided that the woman is his widow and is unmarried at the time of insemination and the birth, but that the child have a right to the father's inheritance only if specifically provided for in his will (New South Wales Law Reform Commission, 1986).

Similarly the death through non-inheritable cause of a gamete donor should not necessarily mean withdrawal of his semen from a donor programme.

Donor insemination

For the recipient couple, donor insemination (DI) is a substantial moral challenge to their emotional stability and to their marriage. The infertile woman generally accepts the idea of DI faster than her husband does, although in my medical practice I occasionally hear descriptions of disquiet by a woman about the thought of a stranger's sperm coursing through her body. The normal, social matter of choosing a genetic mate in effect is annulled and instead, with anonymous sperm banks, reproductive choice passes to someone else.

For the infertile husband, however, the start of DI for his wife demands an acknowledgement of biological loss and a genetic dead-end. The lasting, personal importance of such a loss will depend on the man's ideas of social and genetic fatherhood, the supportive or otherwise attitude of his wife and friends, and, probably least but nonetheless important, the compassionate approaches taken by the nurses, social workers and doctors.

All published studies on the outcomes for children born of DI show that they develop as well as, or better than, their naturally conceived peers. They are healthy, wanted and loved (King & Pattison, 1991; Teper & Symonds, 1983). Their parents are less likely than average to separate and to divorce (Leeton & Backwell, 1982; Bendvold *et al.*, 1989; Amuzu, Laxonva & Shapiro, 1990).

Virgin births and lesbian motherhood

Like celibate priests, devoted homosexuals and committed virgins have been pushed to the side in transmission of the human gene pool. Now, with artificial insemination and with someone else's help in providing sperm, the last two of these three groups can bear genetic fruit without either purposeful transgression or divine intervention.

Childlessness for a coitally active heterosexual couple of reproductive age is a disability that calls for professional medical help. A doctor can, and should, be able to restrict his or her professional duties to treating such medical infertility without venturing into areas of considerable social controversy or moral uneasiness. But artificial insemination itself needs no medical help: masturbation and injection of semen into the vagina allows conception to take place with neither intercourse nor an invoice for professional medical fees. Homosexuals, virgins and others can in this way conceive and have children without sex.

Homosexuals face resistance in the community if they want to become parents. I considered briefly, above, the likelihood that male homosexuals will enter the group of men who are sperm donors in society unless special measures are taken to exclude them. Because of the risk of transmitting HIV by donor insemination (Stewart *et al.*, 1985), many jurisdictions now require the same declaration of a safe 'life-style' from prospective sperm donors as they do from blood donors. None the less the simplicity of self-insemination means that some women who seek pregnancy and children without heterosexual intercourse will turn to homosexual men as sources of semen. Given the inevitability of this biosocial phenomen, the compassionate physician concerned about the risk of infection with donations of fresh semen may offer sperm banking to quarantine such dedicated semen while the donor is tested serially for HIV antibodies.

Do medical professionals, or does society, have other duties to a virgin's (Jennings, 1991; Silman, 1993) and lesbian woman's (Brewaeys *et al.*, 1989) procreative wants? The stable-mother-father model for the psychological nurture of children that is held up as the disqualifying criterion for virgins and lesbians is nowadays a fractured one. Whether it is the resilience of children or the resourcefulness of single parents, there are today such a lot of examples of successful departures from the traditional two-parent ideal that the argument that nothing be done to facilitate breaks from this standard is unrealistic and unsympathetic. Ultimately, however, applying public resources to such an extension of reproductive medical responsibility will be a matter for society to decide and for individual doctors to accommodate or to reject. Meanwhile the question remains open whether the loneliness of a child brought up by a virgin with firm ideas of the repulsiveness of sex can be overcome by its peers and education. Such fears may or may not turn out to be well founded.

It should now be plain that the doctor has a primary duty to the wishes of the sperm donor, anonymous or not. No person has a right to be impregnated if there is no person who has a duty to provide the semen and no person who has the duty to perform the insemination. Many modern studies of donors' attitudes to insemination of single women and lesbians show, however, that a sizeable minority of donors feel no inhibitions with regard to the use of their semen for these people (Table 3). It would be safe to say that publicly sponsored donor insemination of such women is not imminent in most western countries, but access can be available in some places. Anonymous donor insemination for lesbian couples has, for example, been available in Belgium since the early 1980s (Brewaeys *et al.*, 1989). In America, where sperm can simply be bought, there is no legal or constitutional barrier for unmarried women who wish to become pregnant by artificial insemination (McGuire & Alexander, 1985). In practice, lesbian mothers have often used sperm donated by their lover's brother, keeping (they say) the genes in the family (Field, 1989). Consideration of the social and biological facts is warranted.

Table 3. *Sperm donors' attitudes to the use of their semen for unmarried women*

				Acceptance of		
Year	Author	Country	$n =$	widows	single	lesbians
1983	Nicholas & Tyler	Australia	50	41%	30%	30%
1983	Rowland	Australia	67	80%	75%	70%
1984	Handelsman *et al.*	Australia	75	44%	44%	44%
1987	Daniels	New Zealand	37	41%	30%	30%

Enough children have been brought up by lesbian social mothers for early conclusions to be drawn from this odd but interesting social experiment, in which children are reared by homosexual women. In an anecdotal report, a lesbian feminist magazine editor expressed amused chagrin that of 30 boys and girls aged 4 to 19 she had heard of brought up by lesbian households only one, a girl, had had a homosexual relationship, and had since 'moved in with a man' (Forster, 1978). In controlled studies reviewed by King and Pattison (1991), children from female homosexual households did not differ from children from heterosexual single-parent households in gender identity, sex role behaviour, sexual orientation, emotions, behaviour and personal relationships.

Data for children brought up in male homosexual households are harder to come by, given the great difficulty homosexual men face obtaining custody of or even access to their children after marriage fails. Such information that we have does not reveal abnormal trends in psychosexual and emotional development of children raised in such families (King & Pattison, 1991).

How strong is the heritability of homosexuality? The biologist must conclude that genetic determinants of homosexuality are likely substantially to outweigh social ones (Kallmann, 1952; Bailey & Pillard, 1991; Maddox, 1991; Hamer *et al.*, 1993). Not the least of the indirect evidence for this is the strongly heterosexual environment in which homosexuals are usually reared and the generally heterosexual orientation of children who come from homosexual households. Recent genetic pedigree and linkage analysis locates a gene or genes predisposing to male homosexuality on the X-chromosome, in a region designated Xq28 (Hamer *et al.*, 1993).

The data are intriguing not so much because they contradict predictions that homosexual social households will foster homosexuality among children raised in them. Rather, for the first time in hominid evolution, children will be born who genetically may be endowed with whatever hereditary basis there is for homosexuality, including circumstances in which both parents are so homosexual in orientation that ordinarily they would have eschewed heterosexual sex, and hence reproduction, completely. (For later speculation is the evolutionary advantage to human society of maternal uncles devoted not to reproduction but, on modern sociological evidence, to caring and to cultural roles perhaps beyond those of more ordinary men.)

What will the genetic and social outcome be for the children of homosexual men? How will society and culture gain? All we can presently say is that it is an experiment that is taking place.

Uninvited insemination: the bioethics of rape

> Morally, those of us who have a high opinion of sex cannot accept the idea of passive consent sanctioning all kinds of carnal communication; rather than rely on the negative criterion that absence of resistance justifies sexual congress, we must insist that evidence of positive desire alone dignifies sexual intercourse and makes it joyful. From a proud and passionate woman's point of view, anything less is rape. (Greer, 1973).

Feminist writing can be polemical, ultimately isolating, but Germaine Greer surpasses lesser writers by bringing her arguments powerfully to the point where a unifying ethic of male–female relations is possible. In Greer's essay, published in *Playboy*, she describes violent rape satirically as 'a crime against legitimacy of issue and the correct transmission of patrimony'. It could have been said in a gender-neutral way, but she describes adequately the genetic plunder and personal devastation that is rape. She goes on to show why women 'have been known to vomit and vomit, to wash themselves compulsively, to burn their clothes, even to attempt suicide, after a rape', and what it is for a woman's life to be ruined by 'a child whom she could never leave and never love'.

Grand rape

The bioethics of uninvited impregnation is inherently shocking. Violent rape, with personal and social havoc on a large scale, is one aspect of the genocide that has been part of conquest in war. Historically, and appallingly in modern times too, such conquest has meant the slaughter of men and babies, while women 'were impregnated with the spawn of the conqueror' (Greer, 1987). Socio-biologically, similar behaviour has evolved in a large number of mammalian species with roughly comparable social groupings (e.g. rodents, ungulates, carnivores, monkeys and apes). Among these disparate species, an invasion by new males typically leads to expulsion of their male predecessors and, for females, abortion, infanticide and copulation with a new partner (Berger, 1983). In this way the invading males' genetic representation and destiny is imposed for reproductive success at the expense of that of the males they replace. Our awareness of consequences and our cultural development now mean that such behaviour is abhorrent and intolerable, whether we are directly affected or not. Whatever its sociobiological roots, human forethought, compassion and conscience must now preclude uninvited impregnation, whether the males stay with their new females (which is what usually happens in nature and which was for humans the probable case prehistorically) or leave them. The malicious impregnation that comes with violence, and with knowing what semen is capable of, is a peculiarly human horror. Two examples will do.

In 1972, invading Punjabi soldiers did not stay to live with the consequences of their genocide in East Pakistan (Greer, 1987). Bengali women were raped in Dacca and their children and their husbands were murdered. Many of these women, having been left naked, hanged themselves when they were given saris by rescuers. The Planned Parenthood Federation set up abortion clinics in newly constituted Bangladesh. Destitute women in isolated areas of Bengal walked away from or smothered new-born Punjabis.

A more individual example took place while this essay was being written. The grand-daughter of the first Muslim prime minister of the Punjab was gang-raped in Karachi on November 27, 1991, by assailants who scorned her political associates and, by claiming protection from 'higher-up friends', implied that the rape was at the behest of the province's authorities. There was no doubt about this in the mind of her father, a former president of the Muslim league, who was interviewed, sobbing (Anonymous, 1991).

Seduction

On an everyday level, women writers effectively point out too that a lasting sexual empathy between men and women is made more difficult because of the uninvited impregnation of petty rape, which as Greer (1973) puts it, is sex legally consented to but either forced or practised deceitfully – the 'phoney tenderness', the 'false promises of an enduring relationship', the 'sexual rip-offs ... (which) wear down the contours of emotional contacts and gradually brutalize all those who are party to them'. Spermatozoa entering a woman's body in such circumstances convey arrogance and disdain, whether momentarily welcome or not.

The bioethical terror of malicious impregnation and the slow grief of unwelcome impregnation are important to consider in this chapter because of their thorough immorality. They contravene every sphere of ethics: their deontological contravention of empathy, of our personal duties to each other; their teleologically inescapable and starkly sad consequences for the victims; and their utilitarian social repugnance and havoc.

Unwelcome ejaculatory violence thus lies behind at least some feminist criticism of masculineness – and behind how a feminist might write about sperm bioethics. The bioethics of femineity, the oocyte, and reproductive choice I consider further in Volume 2. Meanwhile, to a biologist, the invasive property of spermatozoa should have special biosocial importance. The 10^{17} or so sperm cells turned out each day in a crowded world need to be accommodated more thoughtfully.

References

Amuzu B, Laxova R, Shapiro SS. Pregnancy outcome, health of children, and family adjustment after donor insemination. *Obstet Gynecol* 1990; **75**: 899–905.

Anonymous. Pakistan: peccaverunt. The rule of Sind's law. *The Economist* 1991; December 14: 31.

Bailey JM, Pillard RC. A genetic study of male sexual orientation. *Arch Gen Psychiat* 1991; **48**: 1089–96.

Ball RY, Scott N, Mitchinson MJ. Further observations on spermiophagy by murine peritoneal macrophages *in vitro*. *J Reprod Fertil* 1984; **71**: 221–6.

Banville, J. *The Book of Evidence*. London: Minerva, 1990; 220 p.

Barratt CLR, Bolton AE, Cooke ID. Functional significance of white blood cells in the male and female reproductive tract. *Hum Reprod* 1990; **5**: 639–48.

Barros C, Vigil P, Herrera E, Arguello B, Walker R. Selection of morphologically abnormal sperm by human cervical mucus. *Arch Androl* 1994; 12 Suppl.: 95–107.

Beck WB Jr. Two hundred years of artificial insemination. *Fertil Steril* 1984; **41**: 193–5.

Bellings BS, Copeland CM, Thomas TD, Mazzuccheli RE, O'Neil G, Cohen MK. The influence of patient insemination on the implantation rate in an *in vitro* fertilization and embryo transfer program. *Fertil Steril* 1986; **46**: 252–6.

Bendvold E, Sjoberg D, Skjaeraasen J, Kravdal O, Moe N. Marital break-up among couples raising families by artificial insemination by donor. *Fertil Steril* 1989; **51**: 980–3.

Berger DM. Impotence following the discovery of azoospermia. *Fertil Steril* 1980; **34**: 154–6.

Berger DM, Eisen A, Shuber J, Doody KF. Psychological patterns in donor insemination couples. *Can J Psychiat 1986 Dec* 1992; **31**: 818–23.

Berger J. Induced abortion and social factors in wild horses. *Nature* 1983; **303**: 59–61.

Blizzard J. Balls to the heralds rampant. *World Med 1976;* October 6: 17–19.

Brahams D. Chlorambucil infertility and sperm banking. *Lancet* 1992; **339**: 420.

Brewaeys A, Olbrechts H, Devroey P, Van Steirteghem AC. Counselling and selection of homosexual couples in fertility treatment. *Hum Reprod* 1989; **4**: 850–3.

Broad WJ. A bank for nobel sperm. *Science* 1980; **207**: 1326–7.

Chacho KJ, Hage CW, Shulman S. The relationship between female sexual practices and the development of antisperm antibodies. *Fertil Steril* 1991; **56**: 461–4.

Chaykin S, Watson JG. Reproduction in mice: spermatozoa as factors in the development and implantation of embryos. *Gamete Res* 1983; **7**: 63–73.

Clutton-Brock TH. *The Evolution of Parental Care*. Princeton, NJ: Princeton University Press, 1991: 352 pp.

Cooper J. *Super Men and Super Women*. London: Mandarin, 1991: 72.

Crockin SL. Death row inmates denied claims to freeze sperm. *Fertil News* 1992; 16.

Cusine DJ. Artificial insemination with the husband's semen after the husband's death. *J Med Ethics* 1977; **3**: 163–5.

Czyba JC, Chevret M. Psychological reactions of couples to artificial insemination with donor sperm. *Int J Fertil* 1980; **24**: 240–5.

Daniels KR. Semen donors in New Zealand: their characteristics and attitudes. *Clin Reprod Fertil* 1987; **5**: 177–90.

Darlington CD. *The Evolution of Man and Society*. London: George Allen and Unwin, 1969: 360.

David D, Soulse M, Mayaux MJ *et al.*: Donor artificial insemination. Psychological survey of 830 couples. *J Gynecol Obstet Biol Reprod (Paris) 1988* 1992; **17**: 67–74.

Duenhoelter JH, Jimenez JM, Baumann G. Pregnancy performance in patients under fifteen years of age. *Obstet Gynecol* 1975; **46**: 49.

Dunstan GR. Ethical aspects of donor insemination. *J Med Ethics* 1975; **1**: 42–4.

European Study Group on Heterosexual Transmission of HIV. Comparison of female to male and male to female transmission of HIV in 563 stable couples. *Br Med J* 1992; **304**: 809–13.

Fiedler H. HIV seropositivity in paid blood donors. *Lancet* 1992; **339**: 551.

Field NE. Evolving conceputualizations of property: a proposal to de-commercialize the value of fetal tissue. *Yale Law J* 1989; **99**: 169–86.

Fishel S, Webster J, Jackson P, Faratian B. Evaluation of high vaginal insemination at oocyte recovery in patients undergoing *in vitro* fertilization. *Fertil Steril* 1989; **51**: 135–8.

Fleagle JG. *Primate Adaptation and Evolution*. San Diego, CA: Academic Press, 1988: 203–29.

Foley RA, Lee PC. Finite social space, evolutionary pathways, and reconstructing hominid behavior. *Science* 1989; **243**: 901–6.

Forrest BD. Women, HIV, and mucosal immunity. *Lancet* 1991; **337**: 835–6.

Forster J. Lesbian couples: should help extend to AID? *J Med Ethics* 1978; **4**: 91–5.

Greer G. Seduction is a four-letter word. *Playboy* 1973; January: 80–228.

Greer G. Raped women in refuge camps. In: *The Madwoman's Underclothes. Essays and Occasional Writings 1968–85*. London: Pan Books, 1987: 108–10.

Hamer DH, Hu S, Magnuson VL, Hu N, Pattatucci AML. A linkage between DNA markers on the X chromosome and male sexual orientation. *Science* 1993; **261**: 321–7.

Handelsman DJ, Dunn SJ, Conway AJ, Boylan LM, Jansen RPS. Psychological and attitudinal profiles in donors for artificial insemination. *Fertil Steril* 1984; **43**: 95–101.

Hanson FW, Overstreet JW. The interaction of human spermatozoa with cervical mucus *in vivo. Am J Obstet Gynecol* 1981; **140**: 173–8.

Harvey PH, May RM. Out for the sperm count. *Nature* 1989; **337**: 508–9.

Huerre P. Psychological aspects of semen donation. In: David G, Price WS, eds. *Human Artificial Insemination and Semen Preservation*. New York: Plenum Press, 1980: 461–5.

Ingersvel HK, Ingerslev M. Clinical findings in infertile women with cirulating antibodies against spermatozoa *Fertil Steril* 1980; **33**: 514–20.

Jalbert P, Leonard C, Selva J, David G. Genetic aspects of artificial insemination with donor semen: the French CECOS Federation Guidelines. *Am J Med Genet* 1989; **33**: 269–75.

Jansen R. Bioethics of the oocyte. In: Grudzinskas JG, Yovich, JL, Simpson JL, Chard T. eds. *Cambridge Reviews in Human Reproduction*. Cambridge: Cambridge University Press, 1995.

Jansen RPS. Sperm and ova as property. *J Med Ethics* 1985; **11**: 123–6.

Jansen R. Ethics in infertility treatment. In: Pepperell R, Woods C, Hudson B, eds. *The Infertile Couple*. Edinburgh: Churchill Livingstone, 1987: 346–87.

Jansen RPS. Unfinished feticide. *J Med Ethics* 1990; **16**: 61–5.

Jennings S. Virgin birth syndrome. *Lancet* 1991; **337**; 559–60.

Johnson LA, Flook JP, Hawk HW. Sex preselection in rabbits: live births from X and Y sperm separated by DNA and cell sorting. *Biol Reprod* 1989; **41**: 199–203.

Kallmann FJ. Comparative twin study on the genetic aspects of male homosexuality. *J Nerv Mental Dis* 1952; **115**: 283–98.

King MB, Pattison P. Homosexuality and parenthood. *Br Med J* 1991; 303: 295–7.

Kola I, Lacham O, Jansen RPS, Turner M, Trounson A. Chromosomal analysis of human oocytes fertilized by microinjection of spermatozoa into the perivitelline space. *Hum Reprod* 1990; **5**: 575–7.

Kovacs GT, Clayton CE, McGowan P. The attitudes of semen donors. *Clin Reprod Fertil* 1983; **2**: 73–5.

Lavitrano M, French D, Zani M, Frati L, Spadafora C. The interaction between exogenous DNA and sperm cells. *Mol Reprod Dev* 1992; **31**: 161–9.

Leading Article. Boy or girl? *The Economist* 1990; July **28**: 16.

Leeton J, Backwell J. A preliminary psychosocial follow-up of parents and their children conceived by artificial insemination by donor (AID). *Clinical Reproduction and Fertility* 1982; **1**: 307–10.

Lippi J, Mortimer D, Jansen RPS. Sub-zonal insemination for extreme male-factor infertility *Hum Reprod* 1993; **8**: 908–15.

Lovejoy CO. The origin of man. *Science* 1981; **211**: 341–50.

Madonna. *Sex*. London: Martin Secker & Warburg, 1992.

Maddox J. Is homosexuality hard-wired? *Nature* 1991; **353**: 13.

Mahlstedt PP, Probasco KA. Sperm donors: their attitudes toward providing medical and psychosocial information for recipient couples and donor offspring. *Fertil Steril* 1991; **56**: 747–53.

Making Sense of Sex Hotline. *Fact and Fantasy File Diary 1992*. Canberra: Commonwealth Department of Health, Housing and Community Services, 1992.

McCormick RA. *The Critical Calling. Reflection on Moral Dilemmas since Vatican II*. Washington DC: Georgetown University Press, 1989: 329–52.

McGuire M, Alexander NJ. Artificial insemination of single women. *Fertil Steril* 1985; **43**: 182–4.

Menkveld R, Franken DR, Kruger TF, Oehinger S, Hodgen GD. Sperm selection capacity of the human zona pellucida. *Mol Reprod Dev* 1991; **30**: 346–52.

Moller AP. Ejaculate quality, testes size and sperm competition in primates. *J Hum Evol* 1988; **17**: 479–88.

Morris D. *The Illustrated Naked Ape*. London: Jonathan Cape, 1986: 14–73.

Mortimer D, Leslie EE, Kelly RW, Templeton AA. Morphological selection of human spermatozoa *in vivo* and *in vitro*. *J Reprod Fertil* 1982; **64**: 391–9.

New South Wales Law Reform Commission. *Artificial Conception Report 1. Human Artificial Insemination*. Sydney: NSWLRC, 1986: 79–83.

Nicholas MK, Tyler JPP. Characteristics, attitudes and personalities of AI donors. *Clin Reprod Fertil* 1983; **2**: 47–54.

Nijs P, Steeno O, Steppe A. Evaluation of AID donors: medical and psychological aspects.

A preliminary report. In: David G, Price WS, eds. *Human Artificial Insemination and Semen Preservation.* New York: Plenum Press, 1980: 453–9.

Oldereid NB, Rui H, Purvis K. Male partners in infertile couples. Personal attitudes and contact with the Norwegian health service. *Scand J Soc Med 1990 Sep* 1992; **18**: 207–11.

Pandya IL, Cohen J. The leukocytic reaction of the human cervix to spermatozoa. *Fertil Steril* 1985; **43**: 417–21.

Parker ST. Early hominid mating system [letter]. *Science* 1989; **244**: 195.

Plomin R. The role of inheritance in behavior. *Science* 1990; **248**: 183–8.

Reid BL, French P, Singer A, Hagan BE, Coppleson M. Sperm basic proteins in cervical carcinogenesis: correlation with socio-economic class. *Lancet* 1978, **ii**: 60.

Remohi J, Gastaldi C, Patrizio P *et al.* Intrauterine insemination and controlled ovarian hyperstimulation in cycles before GIFT. *Hum Reprod* 1989; **4**: 918–20.

Rose S, Kamin LJ, Lewontin RC. *Not in Our Genes: Biology, Ideology and Human Nature.* Harmondsworth, Middlesex: Penguin, 1984: 322 pp.

Rothman CM. Live sperm, dead bodies. Commentary. *Hastings Center Rep* 1990; **20**(1): 33–4.

Rowland R. Attitudes and opinions of donors on an artificial insemination by donor (AID) program. *Clin Reprod Fertil* 1983; **2**: 249–59.

Rowland R, Ruffin C. Community attitudes to artificial insemination by husband or donor, *in vitro* fertilization, and adoption. *Clin Reprod Fertil* 1983; **2**: 195–206.

Sauer MV, Gorrill MJ, Zeffer KB, Bustillo M. Attitudinal survey of sperm donors to an artificial insemination clinic. *J Reprod Med 1989 May* 1992; **34**: 362–4.

Sauer MV, Todi IA, Scrooc M, Bustillo M, Buster JE. Survey of attitudes regarding the use of siblings for gamete donation. *Fertil Steril 1988 Apr* 1992; **49**: 721–2.

Schover LR, Collins RL, Richards S. Psychological aspects of donor insemination: evaluation and follow-up of recipient couples. *Fertil Steril* 1992; **57**: 583–90.

Schoysman R. Problems of selecting donors for artificial insemination. *J Med Ethics* 1975; **1**: 34–5.

Serhal PF, Craft IL. Oocyte donation in 61 patients. *Lancet* 1989; **1**, 1185–7.

Short RV. Sexual selection and its component parts, somatic and genital selection, as illustrated by man and the great apes. *Adv Stud Behav* 1979; **9**: 131–58.

Silman R. *Virgin Birth.* WFT Press London, 1993.

Simpson JL, Martin AO. Prenatal diagnosis of cytogenetic disorders. *Clin Obstet Gynecol* 1976; **19**: 841–53.

Stewart GJ, Tyler JPP, Cunningham AL *et al.* Transmission of human T-cell lymphotropic virus type 111 by artificial insemination by donor. *Lancet* 1985; **2**: 581.

Teper S, Symonds EM. Artificial insemination by donor: problems and perspectives. In: Carter CO, ed. *Developments in Human Reproduction and their Eugenic, Ethical Implications.* London: Academic Press, 1983: 19–52.

Van Thiel M, Mantadakis E. Vekemans M, Gillot de Vries F. A psychological study, using interviews and projective tests, of patients seeking anonymous donor artificial insemination. *J. Gynecol Obstet Biol Reprod (Paris) 1990* 1992; **19**: 823–8.

Verkuyl DAA. Oral conception. Impregnation via the proximal gastrointestinal tract in a patient with an aplastic distal vagina. Case report. *Br J Obstet Gynaecol* 1988; **95**: 933–4.

Warnock M (Chairman). *Report of the Committee of Inquiry into Human Fertilisation and Embryology.* London: HMSO, 1984; 18–55.

Wolff H, Anderson DJ. Immunohistologic characterization and quantitation of leukocyte subpopulations in human semen. *Fertil Steril* 1988; **49**: 497–509.

Wolff H, Schill W-B. Antisperm antibodies in infertile and homosexual men: relationship to serologic and clinical findings. *Fertil Steril* 1985; **44**: 673–7.

Zarutskie PW, Muller CH, Magone M, Soules MR. The clinical relevance of sex selection techniques. *Fertil Steril* 1989; **52**: 891–905.

Zinaman M, Drobnis EZ, Morales P *et al.* The physiology of sperm recovered from the human cervix: acrosomal status and response to inducers of the acrosome reaction. *Biol Reprod* 1989; **41**: 790–7.

Index

Printed in the United Kingdom
by Lightning Source UK Ltd.
134359UK00002B/119-120/A

9 780521 479967